Veterinary Forensics:

Animal Cruelty Investigations

Melinda D. Merck, DVM
Editor

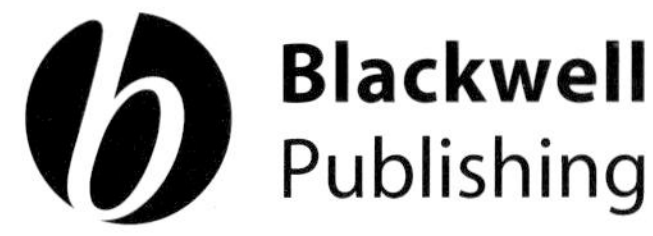

Melinda D. Merck, D.V.M., received her veterinary medicine degree from Michigan State University in 1988. In addition to practicing small animal medicine, she began working on animal cruelty cases with local shelters and animal control in 1989. She opened her private practice, The Cat Clinic of Roswell in Roswell, Ga., in June 1990. She sold her practice after receiving a full-time appointment to ASPCA as a Forensic Veterinarian with the organization's Anticruelty Initiatives in 2007. She is the Vice President of Veterinary and Forensic Affairs for the Georgia Legal Professionals for Animals. Dr. Merck testifies as a forensic veterinary expert for animal cruelty cases around the country. She is a veterinary forensics consultant for the Fulton County District Attorney's Office in Atlanta, Ga., and conducts veterinary forensic examinations for Gwinnett County Animal Control. She provides training for veterinary and law enforcement professionals nationwide on the use of veterinary medical knowledge in the investigation and prosecution of animal cruelty cases.

Blackwell Publishing Professional
2121 State Avenue, Ames, Iowa 50014, USA

Orders: 1-800-862-6657
Office: 1-515-292-0140
Fax: 1-515-292-3348
Web site: www.blackwellprofessional.com

Blackwell Publishing Ltd
9600 Garsington Road, Oxford OX4 2DQ, UK
Tel.: +44 (0)1865 776868

Blackwell Publishing Asia
550 Swanston Street, Carlton, Victoria 3053, Australia
Tel.: +61 (0)3 8359 1011

First edition, 2007

Library of Congress Cataloging-in-Publication Data
Veterinary forensics : animal cruelty investigations / Melinda Merck, editor. – 1st ed.
p. ; cm.
Includes bibliographical references and index.

ISBN-13: 978-0-8138-1501-5 (alk. paper)
ISBN-10: 0-8138-1501-0 (alk. paper)

1. Veterinary forensic medicine. 2. Animal welfare. I. Merck, Melinda.
[DNLM: 1. Animal Welfare. 2. Forensic Medicine. 3. Veterinary Medicine. SF 769.47 V586 2007]

SF769.47.V48 2007
636.089′4—dc22

2006036916

The last digit is the print number: 9 8 7 6 5 4 3

Veterinary Forensics:

Animal Cruelty Investigations

Dedication

This book is dedicated to all the animals who have suffered abuse. May this book empower us to go further and seek justice for the innocent victims.

Table of Contents

	List of Contributors	xi
	Foreword	xiii
	Preface	xv
	Acknowledgments	xvii
	Introduction	xix
Chapter 1	The Legal System and the Veterinarian's Role	3
	Introduction	3
	The Laws	4
	The Legal System	5
	Preparing for Trial	9
	Expert Witness Testimony	11
Chapter 2	Crime Scene Investigation	19
	Introduction	19
	CSI: The Veterinarian's Role	20
	Environment: Weather Data	21
	Photography and Videography	21
	Evidence Recognition and Collection	22
	Blood Evidence	23
	Grave Detection and Excavation	26
Chapter 3	CSI: The Animal as Evidence	31
	Introduction	31
	Determining Non-accidental Injury	31
	Behavioral Considerations of Animals	34
	Evidence Collection	35
	Chain of Custody	36
	Photography and Videography	36
	Examination of the Live Animal	37
	Forensic Necropsy	46
	Special Considerations	52

Chapter 4 Special Considerations in Animal Cruelty Cases 59
Trace Evidence 59
Forensic Botany 63
Forensic Palynology 64
DNA: Deoxyribonucleic Acid 65
Other Unique Identifiers of Animals 68
Münchausen Syndrome by Proxy 69
Stress 71
Suffering 72
Pain 75

Chapter 5 Patterns of Non-accidental Injury: Non-penetrating Injuries 79
Overview of Blunt Force Trauma 79
Abrasions 80
Bruising/Contusions 81
Fractures 84
Hit-by-Car/Motor Vehicle Accident Injuries 85
Fall Injuries 85
Swinging/Dragging Injuries 86
Head Trauma 86
Neck and Spinal Injuries 95
Chest Injuries 97
Abdominal Injuries 98
Ligature Injuries 99

Chapter 6 Patterns of Non-accidental Injury: Penetrating Injuries 101
Introduction 101
Lacerations 101
Avulsion Injuries 102
Stab Wounds 103
Incised-Stab Wounds 107
Incised Wounds 108
Chop Wounds 109
Therapeutic or Diagnostic Wounds 110
Mutilation 110
Ritualistic Crimes 110

Chapter 7 Patterns of Non-accidental Injury: Burns 115
Interpreting Burn Patterns 115
Collection of Evidence 115
Burn Classification 117
Systemic Effects of Burns 118
General Histopathological Findings in Burns 119
Thermal Burns 119
Chemical Burns 122
Electrical Burns 123
Fires: Thermal Injury and Smoke Inhalation 125

Chapter 8	Patterns of Non-accidental Injury: Gunshot Wounds	131
	Introduction	131
	Overview of Firearms	131
	Examination of Gunshot Victims	134
	Wound Ballistics	135
	Determining Entrance and Exit Wounds	136
	Determining Gunshot Range	141
	Retrieving Gunshot Residue	150
	Retrieving Projectile and Wadding	150
	Retrieving the Cartridge Cases	151
	Determining Trajectory	151
	Recording the Injuries	152
Chapter 9	Patterns of Non-accidental Injury: Asphyxia and Drowning	155
	Overview of Asphyxia	155
	Suffocation	156
	Strangulation	158
	Drowning	163
Chapter 10	Patterns of Non-accidental Injury: Poisoning	169
	Overview of Intentional Poisonings	169
	Evidence and History	171
	Diagnostics	172
	Agents Used in Animal Poisonings	175
	Summary	199
Chapter 11	Patterns of Non-accidental Injury: Neglect	201
	Introduction	201
	Environment Examination	201
	Starvation	202
	Animal Hoarders	210
	Heat Stroke	215
	Hypothermia	218
	Embedded Collars	220
	Demodicosis	221
	Untreated Injuries	221
Chapter 12	Sexual Assault	225
	Overview	225
	Crime Scene Investigation	226
	General Findings	226
	Examination of the Victim	227
	Suspicious Exam Findings	230
	Zoonotic Disease	231
	Evaluation of Assailant's Sperm and Semen	232

Color Plate Section

Chapter 13	Animal Fighting	235
	Overview of Dog Fighting	235
	The Pit Bull Breed	235
	Fighting Classifications	236
	The Dog Fight Pit	236
	Training and Fighting Paraphernalia	236
	Examination of the Animal	237
	Overview of Cockfighting	239
	The Fighting Gamecock	239
Chapter 14	Time of Death	241
	Overview	241
	Determining the Postmortem Interval	242
	Examination of the Body	242
	Determining the PMI: Forensic Entomology	249
	Determining the PMI: Examination of the Crime Scene	258
	Final Analysis: The Report of Exam Findings	259
Appendix 1	Evidence Log	267
Appendix 2	Cruelty Case Samples Packaging Record	268
Appendix 3	Cruelty Case Samples Receipt Record	269
Appendix 4	Live SOAP Form	270
Appendix 5	Weight Change	272
Appendix 6	Body Condition Assessment	273
Appendix 7	Skin Condition: Cat	274
Appendix 8	Skin Condition: Dog	275
Appendix 9	Condition of Haircoat and Nails: Cat	276
Appendix 10	Condition of Haircoat and Nails: Dog	277
Appendix 11	Physical Care Scale: Haircoat and Nails	278
Appendix 12	Necropsy History	279
Appendix 13	Necropsy Worksheet	280
Appendix 14	External Wounds: Cat	283
Appendix 15	External Wounds: Dog	284
Appendix 16	Fixed Tissue Histology Checklist	285
Appendix 17	Preliminary Veterinarian Statement	286
Appendix 18	Final Veterinarian Statement	287
Appendix 19	Medical Record Certification	288
Appendix 20	Exam/Necropsy Report	289
Appendix 21	Tufts Animal Care and Condition Scale	291
Appendix 22	Forensic Entomology Data Form	293
Appendix 23	Entomology Specimen Disposition/ID Log	294
Appendix 24	Entomological Sample Log Sheet	295
Appendix 25	Forensic Specialists and Laboratories	296
Appendix 26	Animal Cruelty Forensic Kits	308
Appendix 27	Webliography	312
	Index	315

List of Contributors

Sharon M. Gwaltney-Brant, DVM, PhD, DABVT, DABT
Medical Director
ASPCA Animal Poison Control Center
1717 S. Philo Road, Suite 36
Urbana, IL 61802
(217) 337-9744
gwalt@apcc.aspca.org
Wrote Chapter 10: Patterns of Non-Accidental Injury: Poisoning

Laura A. Janssen, J.D.
Senior Assistant District Attorney
Fulton County District Attorney's Office
136 Pryor Street, 3rd Floor
Atlanta, Georgia 30303
(404) 730-4980
Laura.Janssen@fultoncountyga.gov
Wrote Chapter 1: The Legal System and the Veterinarian's Role

Doris M. Miller, DVM, PhD, Diplomate ACVP
Director, Athens Veterinary Diagnostic Laboratory
College of Veterinary Medicine
The University of Georgia
Athens, Georgia 30602
Phone: (706)542-5568
Fax: (706)542-5977
miller@vet.uga.edu

Contributed pathology throughout the book

Foreword

Late one afternoon a couple of years ago, one of my Assistant District Attorneys informed me that she would be spending the entire night in our Grand Jury Room working on an animal cruelty case with her expert witness. Ordinarily, I would be curious about any expert's willingness to work an 8- to 10-hour day at her own office, and then head to the Fulton County District Attorney's Office in downtown Atlanta to pull an all-nighter; but this was no ordinary expert witness. It was Dr. Melinda Merck.

About halfway through my first term in office, in 2000, the Georgia General Assembly upgraded the crime of animal cruelty to a felony. I had studied the sinister and ominous nature of this crime for two decades. As the District Attorney of a large metropolitan community, I vowed to make up for time lost when animal cruelty was not taken seriously. I share that vision with the author of this book.

As I read Dr. Merck's first draft of this book on veterinary forensics, I could see her own lifelong mission to fight animal cruelty materialize. This textbook has the distinction of being literally the first of its kind and is written by a laudable pioneer in this field. I have seen firsthand the ease with which Dr. Merck navigates through animal crime scenes that have left other investigators confounded. That said, even the most indefatigable leaders can be only one place at a time. This book allows Dr. Merck to be a guiding influence to an expanded audience of veterinarians since her brilliant grasp of this subject and singularity of focus lends itself to classrooms in veterinary schools across the country.

Having prosecuted several felony animal cruelty cases over the years, I can attest to the vital importance of having a veterinary expert trained in forensics in every case. Based on the unusual forms of evidence used in these types of cases, I created an "Animal Cruelty Unit" within my own office and assigned a dedicated prosecutor to be on call 24 hours a day, 7 days a week, to go out to the crime scenes to oversee investigations. Unsurprisingly, Dr. Merck adopted those same hours and took my animal cruelty prosecutor under her tutelage to ensure that our office was equipped with the resources needed for trial.

The object of every legal investigation is the discovery of the truth. Suffice it to say, this author has become an invaluable member of our prosecution team. I sincerely hope that this book will create a large, national pool of expert forensic veterinarians. Then, it is only a matter of time before my colleagues across the country witness the same galvanizing effect such experts have on animal cruelty prosecutions as I have seen with Dr. Melinda Merck.

Paul L. Howard, Jr.
Fulton County District Attorney
Atlanta, Georgia

Preface

The day will come when men such as I will look upon the murder of animals the way we look upon the murder of man.

—Leonardo da Vinci, 1452–1519

This book is about the veterinary forensic findings in animal cruelty cases. Veterinary forensics refers to the application of veterinary medical knowledge to matters of law. Very little has been written on the subject of veterinary forensics. With more states passing mandatory reporting requirements for veterinarians and the rise of prosecution of animal cruelty, veterinarians need more medical resources to properly assist in these cases. Most information for this book comes from the editor's and contributors' personal experiences with animal abuse cases. Additional information for this book has been gleaned from human forensic pathology and crime scene investigation textbooks. A large portion of human pathology findings can be applied to animals, although many areas of research are still needed on animals. This book primarily focuses on dogs and cats, except for cockfighting in Chapter 13. The principles and techniques in this book can be applied easily to other species as well.

The book begins with a brief look at the legal system in the United States and the veterinarian's role in cruelty cases. Becoming involved in the legal system is very intimidating and the thought of testifying can be terrifying. This chapter explains the process from the beginning of an investigation to its conclusion in court.

Animal cruelty is a crime often without a witness or with a witness that cannot testify. It is imperative that veterinarians understand crime scene investigation. The case is often won or lost at the beginning of the case. Chapter 2 covers CSI and the role of the veterinarian at the scene or examining evidence collected from the scene. The animal's body is an extension of the crime scene and is considered evidence. Chapter 3 goes into detail on the examination of the animal, chain of custody procedures, and how to perform a proper necropsy. Chapter 4 covers the special considerations of all animal abuse cases, such as DNA and trace evidence. Certain elements of animal cruelty crimes are often required to be proved, such as pain and suffering. This is also addressed in Chapter 4.

Chapters 5 through 12 deal with patterns of non-accidental injury found in abused animals. Each chapter discusses the gross and microscopic findings, clinical pathology, and evidence collection. Chapter 13 covers dog and cockfighting, the injuries commonly seen, and the associated paraphernalia associated with each blood sport. The final chapter deals with determination of time of death and the report of the veterinarian's exam findings. Time of death is a compilation of several findings to arrive at the best estimate. The most conclusive analysis for time of death is forensic entomology, which is covered extensively in this chapter.

Finally, several photographs within the book highlight pertinent forensic findings in animals. Extensive appendices are provided with forms for examination, report writing, entomology collection, body condition scoring, forensic kits, and forensic specialists and labs; as well as a webliography.

I believe this book will provide veterinarians with the background and resources needed to work with animal abuses cases. I hope this book stimulates them to conduct the research needed to further support the prosecution of these heinous acts against animals.

Melinda Merck

Acknowledgments

I want to thank all the wonderfully gifted contributors to this book. Their individual work in animal cruelty has provided a standard for others to follow. Their knowledge and input was vital to the creation of this textbook. I am grateful to Mel Bishop and Dr. Jason Byrd for their contributions to the entomology section. I thank my friend and colleague, Cheryl Good, DVM, and my father, Jerry Merck, for their hours of editing. Their insight, counsel, and support made this book possible. I am eternally grateful for the continued support and patience of my friends, family, and clients while I devoted time to forensic investigations of animal cruelty and the research necessary for this book.

Thanks to all the people at the American Society for the Prevention of Cruelty to Animals, most especially Randall Lockwood, PhD. His knowledge and compassion is without equal and his counsel invaluable.

Lastly, I want to thank all of the people at the Fulton County District Attorney's Office; Gwinnett County Animal Control, Police Department, Solicitor's Office, and District Attorney's Office; and the Georgia Legal Professionals for Animals. It is their perseverance in the pursuit of justice for animal cruelty that has created a demand for veterinary forensics and the need for this book.

Thank you all.

Melinda Merck

Introduction

Our lives begin to end the day we become silent about things that matter.

—Martin Luther King, Jr.

Forensic science is the application of science to matters of law. Forensic science is actually a combination of diverse disciplines such as chemistry, physics, geology, and biology that includes medicine and pathology. Forensic science can impeach an alibi or statement. Jurors expect forensic science in the case and expect it to be interesting. This is called the *CSI effect*. They will question the lack of forensic tests based on what they "know" from television. This places a huge burden on the prosecution and investigators. It also stresses the need to address the absence of evidence such as fingerprints, DNA, and gunshot residue as well as the presence of evidence. Jurors will interpret evidence based on their "knowledge."

A medicolegal investigator is someone who investigates the body and evidence on the body. The fields of medicolegal investigator, crime scene technicians, law enforcement, and criminalists may overlap when looking at evidence. The veterinarian functions as medical examiner, medicolegal investigator, and crime scene investigator in animal cruelty cases. So much of the case depends on the veterinarian's actions and findings that it is critical to involve the veterinarian at the beginning of the case. Veterinarians are natural investigators. Logical, deductive reasoning is the very essence of veterinary medicine. In veterinary forensics, the list of rule-outs expands to include the horrific. The conclusions formed are derived from the variety of information gathered from the forensic investigation. Each finding is a piece of a puzzle; together they tell the story.

The animal's body holds the hidden story. The victim that can never speak may provide the most eloquent testimony with their DNA and body of evidence. The veterinarian's job is to glean all the pieces of information from the body and put them together to determine the most probable scenario. All pieces of information must be accounted for and explained. The veterinarian gives each individual finding its appropriate importance and places it in the proper context. Consulting with human forensic experts can aid in the evaluation of the examination findings. It is crucial not to ignore a piece of the puzzle that appears not to fit, for it is likely the key to the case.

The crime of animal cruelty is underreported and often goes without investigation. The American Veterinary Medical Association, Canadian Veterinary Medical Association, and American Animal Hospital Association have supported the reporting of animal cruelty and have indicated they believe it is the veterinarian's responsibility to do so. Several states have passed laws making it mandatory for veterinarians to report animal cruelty. A study of Massachusetts veterinarians found that 93.6 percent believed they had an ethical responsibility to report suspicions of animal abuse, but only 44.5 percent believed this responsibility should be mandated (Donley et al. 1999). It is disturbing that veterinarians cited client contrition as a reason not to report abuse, viewing those who expressed remorse more favorably than those who did not. Since veterinarians lack training in psychology and criminology, they are not in a position to make assessments regarding their clients' abilities or desires to improve the care of the animal (Morgan 2005). Ethicist Bernard Rollin stated that "veterinarians are the rational, natural advocates for animals in society and, furthermore, that society expects them to fill this role . . . they must act to ferret out those individuals likely to move from animal abuse to human abuse, particularly child abuse" (Rollin 1998).

People may question the importance of investigation or prosecuting animal cruelty. They may even make comments that it is "just an animal." Whenever anyone says "it is just an animal" he or she becomes a co-conspirator with the perpetrator. Whenever someone objectifies the victim he or she becomes part of the problem. Violence against animals IS violence, period. If we accept a certain level of deviance and do not intervene, then it can escalate to another level, and we send a message that violence is acceptable.

People are upset by acts of animal cruelty because it makes them feel more unsafe than do drugs or prostitution. People are afraid of people who abuse animals. Arson parallels animal cruelty in several ways: It is an easy crime to commit; it is about increased power and control; it is disturbing to the community; it shocks and offends; and it is easy to get away with. Another reason animal abuse causes such a public outcry is the helplessness of the victim. It is an act of such obvious depravity that the public demands action by the legal system. This is a crime that often goes on behind closed doors where there are rarely witnesses. An animal that is being abused can never go to someone and report what is being done, as can a child. An animal can never testify. It is these two elements that truly define the helplessness of the victim.

Animal cruelty may be committed by anyone, including the veterinarian's clients. It is not limited by age, gender, or any socioeconomic boundaries. There is a proven link between animal cruelty and other acts of violence such as child abuse and domestic violence. There is a historical link of serial killers with a criminal past that involves animal abuse. This has been seen in the most notorious serial killers, such as Jeffrey Dahmer, Ted Bundy, and Henry Lee Lucas. Even John Wilkes Booth killed all the cats on his farm.

There is a link between childhood animal cruelty and adult violence, family violence, or abuse. In 1987, the *Diagnostics and Statistical Manual of Mental Disorders* (DSM III) included animal cruelty as a symptom of conduct disorder in children. Later animal cruelty was deemed a reliable diagnostic criterion for this conduct disorder (Haden and Scarpa 2005). Several studies have been conducted on children and adolescents. They show that an average of 20 percent have committed animal abuse—one in five children and adolescents—with a male-to-female preponderance of 3:1 (Haden and Scarpa 2005). In 1999, a clinical study by E.S. Luk et al found that children who had committed animal cruelty had a higher number of and more severe conduct disorder symptoms, poorer family functioning, and greater perceptions of themselves, especially in academic and sports abilities. It has been suggested that this elevated sense of self associated with perpetration of animal cruelty may be the link between childhood cruelty to animals and adult psychopathology (Haden and Scarpa 2005).

Animal cruelty is the act of abusing a helpless victim who has no recourse and no voice. It is our role, as veterinarians, to be their voice and seek justice for their suffering. Animal cruelty occurs in conjunction with or as a prelude to the perpetrator's first act of assault against a human, or even homicide. The act of animal abuse is a window to the future—and veterinarians are in a position to change that future.

References

Donely, L., G.J. Patronek, and C. Luke. 1999. Animal Abuse in Massachusetts: A Summary of Case Reports at the MSPCS and Attitudes of Massachusetts Veterinarians. *Journal of Applied Animal Welfare Science* 2:59–73.

Haden, S.C., and A. Scarpa. 2005. Childhood Animal Cruelty: A Review of Research, Assessment and Therapeutic Issues. *The Forensic Examiner*. 14:23–32.

Morgan, C. 2005. *"But They Said They Were Sorry": Veterinarians' Reasons for Not Reporting Animal Abuse*. Presented at the 30th World Congress of World Small Animal Veterinary Association, May 11–14, 2005. Mexico City, Mexico.

Rollin, B. 1998. Veterinary Medical Ethics. In *Cruelty to Animals and Interpersonal Violence: Readings in Research and Application*, ed. Randall Lockwood and Frank R. Ascione. West Lafayette, IN: Purdue University Press.

Veterinary Forensics:
Animal Cruelty Investigations

Chapter 1

The Legal System and the Veterinarian's Role

Laura A. Janssen

Introduction

The veterinarian's role in successful animal cruelty prosecution cannot be overstated. The veterinarian is as essential to animal cruelty cases as the medical examiner is to homicide cases. As in all criminal cases, the ultimate goal of animal cruelty investigation is to gather evidence showing that the crime was committed and determine the perpetrator. At that point, the perpetrator is charged and prosecuted in court. The offender can only be sentenced after a guilty verdict or guilty plea. The severity of the sentence largely depends on the facts and strength of the case. Sentencing can have a huge impact on the recidivist (repeat offender) rate in animal cruelty cases. Prosecutors agree that the ideal way to achieve these important goals is to involve the veterinarian in every stage of the legal process, from the commencement of the investigation through sentencing.

Prosecutors experienced in animal cruelty cases often view the veterinarian as an expert with whom they consult in preparing for the case, not merely an expert witness who is only involved during the guilt-or-innocence phase of the trial. That is not to say that the veterinarian's role is constant from one stage to the next. In fact, the veterinarian trained in forensics contributes to the success of animal cruelty prosecutions through assisting and teaching law enforcement at the crime scene, seeking evidence that may be irrelevant or non-existent in other types of cases, suggesting more particularized questions for witnesses, establishing an accurate timeline, formulating a theory behind the crime, proving malice and intent through necropsy findings and evidence collected at the scene, assisting the prosecutor with charging decisions, helping the prosecutor prepare demonstrative aids for use by the veterinarian at trial, arming the prosecution with the tools to overcome defenses to the crime, and testifying as an expert witness. Such dependence by the prosecution on its expert is unique to animal cruelty cases.

In addition to a veterinarian's immense contribution to prosecutors in individual cases, the veterinarian's ability to increase public awareness is a true sign of the times. Although animal cruelty itself dates back many centuries, its classification as a crime has gained momentum only in the past decade. The treatment of animal cruelty cases by the judiciary is often reminiscent of courts' early dealings with domestic violence cases. Widespread use of experts who testified about the cycle of violence gave judges the insight they needed to hand down more appropriate sentences for domestic violence offenders. Similarly, veterinarians testifying as expert witnesses should use court appearances as opportunities to educate the courts about animal cruelty whenever possible. Bond hearings, bench/non-jury trials and sentencing hearings are often suitable for such testimony. By contrast, the defendant's propensity to commit future acts of violence may be considered inadmissible character evidence during a jury trial.

Although the main thrust of this chapter is the veterinarian's involvement with law enforcement and prosecutors in seeking justice against the crime of animal cruelty, it is not unusual for veterinarians to be called as defense witnesses. One reason it is so important to build a solid case of animal cruelty from the beginning is to prevent a defense expert from taking the stand and citing all the essential evidence that could have been collected and tested, but was not. This shows the jury that the investigation was incomplete, leaving them with insufficient information to arrive at a guilty verdict. A veterinarian who uses all techniques available in forensics and pathology and helps build the case based on sound legal reasoning cannot be touched by a defense expert.

The Laws

It is essential for veterinarians to know what prosecutors refer to as the elements of the crime of animal cruelty in their jurisdiction. In order to secure a guilty verdict, the State must prove each element of the crime or crimes charged beyond a reasonable doubt. Elements of the crime of animal cruelty vary among the states. One basic element contained in all animal cruelty statutes is the definition of the word *animal*. How each state defines animal varies. As odd as it seems, proof that the victim is an animal under the law may be an issue raised by the defense. The only witness qualified to prove this element in court is the veterinarian.

More often than not, the most contentious issues in court are the cause of death and proof of intent. It is important for the veterinarian to know all local, state, and federal laws regarding animal crimes before arriving at the crime scene or performing an exam or necropsy. The laws may be found on the Internet and humane organizations' websites that keep a current list of animal laws. All states have laws regarding animal cruelty and most have separate laws for animal fighting. These laws, which may be classed as misdemeanors or felonies, define cruelty and the punishment for crimes. Separate laws may govern the seizure of the animals.

A working knowledge of the applicable laws establishes the direction and extent of the veterinarian's investigation. As evidence is discovered, the informed veterinarian can determine if his or her findings meet the laws. Knowledge of the governing laws also is an excellent way to establish the veterinarian's credibility with law enforcement officers on the scene. When it is obvious to law enforcement that the veterinarian shares their goals, the veterinarian will more readily become a part of the investigatory team.

Some state laws contain language regarding immunity for veterinarians who report animal cruelty to law enforcement. Depending on the jurisdiction, these laws may apply to veterinarians and/or the veterinary staff. Fortunately, Good Samaritan immunity exists in all states. This type of immunity is triggered when a person reports a suspected crime in good faith. By definition, good faith is a state of mind with an honest purpose, free from any intent to defraud, in which a person's acts reflect faithfulness to his or her duty or obligation. When good faith is established, the reporter is immune from both civil and criminal liability. Of course, this type of immunity applies to all citizens, not just veterinarians.

Recently, several states have passed mandatory reporting requirements for veterinarians regarding their duty to report animal cruelty and/or animal fighting. Veterinarians practicing in states in which no mandatory reporting laws exist are still bound by the professional code of ethics. The American Veterinary Medical Association, American Animal Hospital Association, and most state veterinary boards support (and some even require) the reporting of animal abuse by veterinarians.

Taken one step further, veterinarians even may be found culpable in cases in which they repeatedly see animals that have been abused by the same owner and fail to report their findings or suspicions. From the prosecutor's viewpoint, a veterinarian has the expertise to easily recognize abused animals, such as dogs with dog fighting injuries, then receives money for services rendered, and then knowingly fails to report the crime. The issue is not the treatment of the animal or the receiving of money; the failure to report the crime is the determining factor. The veterinarian then may be charged as a party to the crime of animal cruelty.

When reporting animal cruelty, there are issues regarding the confidentiality of the patient records. A report of animal cruelty may be made without turning over the patient records. Each state has laws under the veterinary practice act that deal with the client/patient records. Some states have specific language in their laws that allows the release of records when an animal is the victim of a crime. Depending on the statutes, a subpoena for the production of evidence or an Open Records Request may be required for the veterinarian to be able to legally turn over the records.

The Legal System

General Overview

The initial report of a crime triggers an on-scene investigation. In some instances, a 911 call may not indicate animal cruelty. For example, the call may indicate domestic violence. Once law enforcement officers arrive on the scene, they may discover a beaten puppy in the home along with an injured woman. At this point a veterinarian should be called to the scene. Of course, delay is inherent based on the fact that the emergency call did not indicate an animal was involved.

The presence of an injured or deceased animal at a crime scene should obviate the need for a veterinarian to be present. However, in reality, a veterinarian's presence at a crime scene is more the exception than the rule. Once again, this is due to the lack of public awareness that animal cruelty itself is a serious crime rather than a secondary or residual crime. Failure to call a veterinarian to the scene also may result from a lack of knowledge among law enforcement officers and prosecutors as to the enormous insight and skill veterinarians can bring to a criminal investigation.

Once their true value becomes known, veterinarians are indispensable to such agencies. Until then, veterinarians committed to working on animal cruelty cases must be persistent in contacting the elected official in their jurisdiction who is responsible for prosecuting animal cruelty and other crimes. The title of this official varies among states. District attorneys, attorneys general, and solicitors general are some common examples. By virtue of representing the state, prosecution offices are government agencies with a limited budget for experts. If financially feasible, veterinarians may choose to initially volunteer to assist prosecutors as consultants and/or expert witnesses in order to avoid the risk of being turned away unwittingly based on cost. Ideally, once a prosecutor sees first-hand that veterinarians are the cornerstone of the animal cruelty case, the office will make allowances in its budget for expert funds in all animal cruelty cases.

Although prosecution follows investigation in the chronology of the legal process, veterinarians interested in working on animal cruelty cases should team up with the prosecutor first. The prosecutor's success in court rises and falls on a good investigation. If the prosecution sees that specialized veterinary investigation dramatically strengthens the State's case, the prosecuting official can then mandate that law enforcement include the prosecutor's appointed veterinarian at every animal cruelty crime scene. If a veterinarian is fortunate enough to be part of the investigation team, the veterinarian's schedule, fees, and other concerns should be discussed with the prosecutor upfront.

Once contacted, veterinarians need to treat the call as an emergency and rush to the scene. Veterinarians may not realize that their early arrival on the scene may literally save the case. The idea of preserving the body of a deceased animal and arranging for a necropsy is foreign to most law enforcement officers because they have not been trained or told to do so. In hoarding cases, for example, officers' protocol may be to call the sanitation department, or that jurisdiction's equivalent to the sanitation department, to clean up the scene as they do with animals lying in or on the side of the roadway after being struck by a car. Even when crime scene technicians take photos of the deceased animals, they are unaware that photos alone are insufficient to prove the animal's cause of death in court. The case cannot survive this fatal flaw. That is why the presence of a veterinarian on the scene to stop officers from disposing of the body is tantamount.

Similarly, it is often unheard of that investigators must seize an injured animal from the hands of an alleged perpetrator like any other piece of evidence. In fact, when the animal is alive but injured, officers often leave the pet at the abusive home, relying on assurances by friends or relatives of the perpetrator that they will take the animal to a veterinarian. The case diminishes when the animal is not treated at all, or the animal is treated, but the officer does not know that he or she must follow up on the veterinary findings to establish the cause of the injuries. The prosecution then has no idea where the animal was taken for treatment and cannot subpoena veterinary records. There is no going back to do this. By this time, the animal may have mysteriously disappeared or may be present but free from signs of injury or evidence. The case must then be dismissed. However, if a veterinarian were present from the start, this issue would not have arisen.

Finally, in the worst-case scenario, the perpetrator is released from jail on bond or bail and returns to the home only to re-injure, hide, or even kill the animal. In a domestic violence case, the victim may now be too frightened to report another crime. Again, an informed veterinarian on the scene could convey to the officers the risk of re-offending and, unlike the officers, could take and transport the animal to the veterinarian's clinic for the treatment and tests needed for evidence at trial. Although many jurisdictions require the seizure of animal victims, veterinarians may be more familiar with such rules than investigators by virtue of their profession. As with all legal procedures discussed in this chapter, methods of animal seizure vary among jurisdictions.

It should be noted that in cases in which animal abuse is associated with domestic violence, a growing number of jurisdictions now include animals in Temporary Protective Orders. In some states, such a condition is within the discretion of the court, and in other states, such as Massachusetts, the state law mandates such a condition. Temporary Protective Orders are often referred to by the acronym TPO, and are used in virtually all pending domestic violence and other victim-based cases. They are, at their core, court-issued orders designed to protect victims from their alleged aggressors while awaiting trial or other disposition of the case. Aggressors are commonly ordered to have no contact or no violent contact with victims, thereby protecting them from further injury or intimidation.

The addition of a "no contact with animals" clause or some form of this clause is a substantial step toward protection of animal victims in domestic cases. More advanced jurisdictions issue animal protective orders even when domestic violence is absent, thereby recognizing animal cruelty as an autonomous crime and one that is often repeated. Still other jurisdictions may impose a "no contact with animals" condition on violent perpetrators who have no animals, but should be precluded from obtaining them because of their violent tendencies. It should be noted that a prosecutor's request alone may not be sufficient for the court to issue any type of animal protection order, in which case the testimony of a veterinarian may be key in protecting the animals from future harm.

Issues of Live Animals as Evidence

The seizure of live and/or injured animals from a seemingly cruel environment gives rise to another important role in the legal process that only a veterinarian can adequately fill. Animals seized from a crime scene are characterized as the State's evidence if animal cruelty is alleged. As with all evidence, live animal evidence must be preserved and kept within the possession of the State. At first glimpse, this concept strikes most veterinarians as inhumane and unnecessary, conjuring up images of countless caged animals living in solitude or a crowded shelter with no hope of being adopted for months or even years while the case drags on. Fortunately, animal cruelty prosecutors consider such an ill-fated existence to be in direct contravention of evidence laws. Their duty to adhere to evidence laws need not contradict veterinarians' duty to improve and maintain the animal's health and welfare.

Prosecutors' legal concerns with animal evidence in a pending case should be twofold: (1) once an animal cruelty victim's health is restored, make sure the animal is not exposed to unhealthy conditions that could compromise its health and/or compromise the veterinarian's ability to accurately pinpoint the cause of the animal's condition at the time of the crime; and (2) keep track of the animal's whereabouts so the prosecutor can comply in good faith if the defendant, through his or her attorney, opts to have an expert perform independent tests on the animal or otherwise examine or observe it.

Compliance with the prosecutor's first concern protects the veterinarian's findings while protecting the evidence. For example, take a case involving ten deceased animals and three live animals. The ten deceased animals appear to have starved to death. Before the prosecutor can charge someone with cruelty to animals, the veterinarian must prove that there was no other possible cause of death, such as a contagious disease. Once the veterinarian has eliminated other possible causes of death, and the case has been charged, the three live animals, deemed to be evidence, must be handled carefully. If these three animals are placed in an unhealthy environment, they may contract a debilitating illness. If their bodies succumb to such illness, this may cast doubt on the veterinarian's original findings regarding the cause of death for the other ten animals. The defense can easily argue that these three animals, like the other ten, were sickly and weak to begin with and there was nothing the defendant could have done to reverse the inevitable.

Prosecutors' second legal concern with live animal evidence is questioned by many veterinarians. The idea of putting animal victims through the same battery of tests by the defense seems gratuitous. Veterinarians and prosecutors cannot take away the defendant's right to independent testing of the evidence, but they can remain present during the defense expert's examination, closely monitor the animal during testing, and, when such testing may jeopardize the animal's health, testify that the inherent danger to the animal overrides any possible benefit that could come from the testing.

There is no universal rule among the states concerning legal transfer of ownership of animals who survived animal cruelty. When the rules are ambiguous or nonexistent, veterinarians are the best ones to advise prosecutors on recommended foster homes and adoption programs. Ideally, a perpetrator will forfeit his or her right to reclaim live animals that have been seized. If such forfeiture is not provided for in the law, prosecutors should ask for forfeiture of the animals as part of the sentence.

Discovery

Once law enforcement officers and investigators establish probable cause that the crime of animal cruelty as defined in their jurisdiction has taken place, the prosecuting agency formally accuses or indicts the perpetrator on an official charging document. This document should place the defendant on notice of the criminal law or laws violated and describe the illegal acts. The veterinarian can be instrumental during the drafting of the charges because, by design, the necropsy, examination, and/or tests performed by the veterinarian describe what happened.

After the case is charged, the perpetrator, or defendant, is prosecuted. The State, or prosecuting agency, is required to serve the defendant or his or her attorney, with the evidence it plans to use. What is discoverable and the procedure for service varies among jurisdictions and also may depend on whether the crime charged is a felony or misdemeanor. As a general rule, the State opts to receive reciprocal discovery, or the defendant's evidence.

The rules of discovery must be strictly adhered to and are ongoing until the final disposition of the case. Failure of either party to comply with the rules of discovery in good faith may result in dismissal of the case. At no time is this more crucial than when the State possesses evidence that may be favorable to the defense. Such evidence is characterized as exculpatory, or favorable, to the defense, and is governed by the U.S. Supreme Court case *Brady vs. Maryland.* For this reason, such evidence is commonly referred to as *Brady* material.

Veterinarians, as witnesses for the State, must be cognizant of the rules of discovery and *Brady*. All of the veterinarian's notes, photographs, radiographs, medical records, and communications regarding the case (including e-mails) may be subject to discovery rules. Because discovery is all-encompassing, the veterinarian should exercise appropriate caution when writing notes and communications to parties involved in the case. When asked by the State or defense to turn over all veterinary records, the veterinarians should ask what this entails rather than omit something based on what he or she personally believes is irrelevant.

Because discovery is ongoing in a criminal case, any change in the integrity of the evidence should be reported immediately to the prosecutor. Failure to report all changes, whether they help or hurt the State's case, is unethical and unacceptable. Ideally, the veterinarian who treated the animal(s) initially after the crime will do all follow-up exams in order to maintain consistency. These exams should include weight, status of recovery from injury or disease, and the length of time for recovery. Veterinarians may want to remind the prosecutor that medical records from veterinarians who saw the animal before the crime may assist their expert testimony by comparing the health of the animal before and after the criminal act.

Preparing for Trial

In the grand scheme of things, only a small percentage of animal cruelty cases actually go to trial. This is reflective of the percentage of all criminal cases that result in a trial. A criminal defendant can plead guilty, thereby waiving his or her Constitutional right to a trial and dispose of the case minutes before the trial begins. The veterinarian, like the prosecutor, always should be prepared for trial, because the outcome of any case is often unpredictable, untimely, and unexpected. If the case does go to trial, it means that the defendant has entered a not-guilty plea and the State has the burden of proving its case beyond a reasonable doubt.

Because the burden of proof falls on the State, and the defendant has no obligation to prove innocence, it is crucial for the State to understand how both the veterinarian and veterinary evidence factor into the case. Veterinary evidence will not be treated or presented as the crux of the case unless it is properly communicated to the prosecutor and the prosecutor sees it for what it is worth. Likewise, the veterinarian will not fully see how his or her investigation can make or break a case without spending time with the prosecutor both before and during trial.

Depending on the size of the jurisdiction, communicating one-on-one with the prosecutor for any length of time may require persistence and creativity on the part of the veterinarian. It is not unusual for prosecutors in a busy jurisdiction to have hundreds of cases in addition to their animal cruelty cases. Their caseload may not allow them to spend as much time as they would like to spend on each individual case. On the other hand, inviting prosecutors to visit the veterinarian's clinic, where they would be surrounded by animals, may be just the incentive they need to leave their courthouse for an afternoon to see the veterinarian's work firsthand.

The veterinarian must state what all the veterinary findings mean to the prosecutor in plain language. This will require patience on the veterinarian's part because this field is foreign to the majority of prosecutors. It is not a topic that even experienced prosecutors have dealt with until very recently, given its slow evolution into the legal arena. The veterinarian should bring all demonstrative materials, such as radiographs, diagrams, and photographs with him or her, not only to describe what the findings mean visually, but also to give the prosecutor an opportunity to decide which visuals should be enlarged or otherwise displayed in court. This is an important part of the preparation, because visualization has been shown in jury surveys to be the best method for a jury to retain information.

It is common for photographs depicting deceased and/or mutilated animals to draw vigorous objections from the defense. Defense attorneys argue that such grim images are more prejudicial than probative and thus will likely enflame the jury and therefore are inadmissible and cannot be shown to the jury. Experienced prosecutors anticipate such objections during trial preparation, especially when they plan to show the enlarged version of such photos. The key to overcome these objections and make sure the jury views all of the evidence is to demonstrate that the expert veterinarian needs the gruesome exhibit to assist him or her in driving a point home. If showing such a photo will assist the expert to explain a certain theory or finding to the jury, the photograph may be viewed by the court as having a purpose other than running the jury through the gamut of emotions. The expert also needs to convey to the court the usefulness of enlarging such an image for the jury to easily observe something in the picture that is otherwise undetectable to anyone but the expert.

Of course, the veterinarian can and should bring all notes and other medical documents to both the meeting and court. It is never necessary for the veterinarian to memorize all records ahead of time. He or she may reference such documents in court in order to refresh recollection so long as the documents have been provided to the defense counsel by the State. If the prosecutor writes some or all of his or her expected questions for the veterinarian during pre-trial preparation, it is not advisable for the veterinarian to respond to the prosecutor with written responses. This would be considered discoverable and would have to be served to the defense attorney.

Given the enormous amount of work and time veterinarians put into animal cruelty cases, it is best to leave the legal decisions and strategies to the prosecutors, whose duty it is to direct the courtroom production. Veterinarians possess unique insight into the world of animals that cannot be matched by experts in the legal profession. Prosecutors depend on them heavily, viewing them as endless sources of knowledge on the topic. Legal theories are not empirical and reliable like science and can change in an instant. Each twist and turn in the legal landscape of the case often leads the prosecutor back to the expert to discuss a new scientific angle. The veterinarian who focuses on what he or she does best will contribute the most to the case.

A prime example is one in which the veterinarian is a member of the investigative team and accompanies law enforcement personnel on an assignment. The team finds evidence of animal cruelty and the perpetrator makes a written confession to the police. The veterinarian's knowledge of the confession causes a myopic view of the case. The evidence may seem overwhelming without any veterinary tests, so the veterinarian takes a more cursory approach when performing the necropsy, taking photos, documenting findings, and may even decide not to perform certain routine tests because the case seems solid without them.

The results of such a decision may prove devastating. Confessions and/or searches are suppressed or ruled inadmissible every day in court. This occurs even when the law to admit this evidence seems directly on point. When an admission or confession is ruled inadmissible, for example, the State's case will disappear unless other evidence exists to prove the allegations. As for legal strategy, it is common for one or both lawyers to change their strategies several times before and during trial, given the countless number of unexpected events that can and do occur as a trial unfolds. Veterinarian experts should not be distracted by any chaos, drama, or conflict in the courtroom, because such theatrics cannot shake the reliability of their scientific findings.

Expert Witness Testimony

General Overview

Prosecutors across the country struggle daily with the impact the popular television show "C.S.I." has on jurors. Trying to extract such unrealistic expectations from jurors' minds is like un-ringing a bell. Prosecutors repeatedly tell juries during closing arguments that the tests done on "C.S.I." are not possible in real life. They may even ask scientific experts to testify on the ridiculousness and impossibility of performing such tests. However, jurors consistently return not-guilty verdicts if the State's case lacks the "C.S.I." effect.

Veterinary tests are foreign, yet fascinating to jurors and judges alike. Prosecutors are discovering that the tests performed by veterinarians in animal cruelty cases resemble a real-life version of "C.S.I." Nevertheless, the tests cannot speak for themselves. Without a well-executed presentation in court, the jurors will not appreciate the unique revelations that veterinary science has to offer.

There are two types of witnesses: factual and expert. A factual witness can only testify to what he or she saw, heard, felt, tasted, smelled, or did in association with an event. In a criminal case, examples of factual witnesses include eyewitnesses, law enforcement officers, and victims. An expert witness can testify to facts and offer opinions on evidence as well as hypothetical questions posed in court. Unlike a factual witness, a scientific expert witness will be asked repeatedly if his or her opinion is based on a "reasonable degree of scientific certainty." Veterinarians are accustomed to viewing a colleague as an expert through board certification in a particular field. In the legal setting, an expert is someone capable of rendering an opinion on the evidence that falls within his or her area of expertise. Veterinarians, by the nature of their training and practice, are qualified in numerous fields, unlike their human medical counterparts. Depending on the years of experience, focus of practice, and particulars of the case, most veterinarians can be qualified as expert witnesses.

The Federal Rules of Evidence contain the general guidelines for expert testimony followed by most courts in the country. The following passages contain pertinent parts of Rules 702 and 703, which explain the unique nature of expert testimony and the type of facts experts may use to form their opinions.

Rule 702
If scientific, technical or other specialized knowledge will assist the trier of fact to understand the evidence or to determine a fact in issue, a witness qualified as an expert by knowledge, skill, experience, training, or education may testify thereto in the form of an opinion or otherwise.

Rule 703
[T]he facts or data in the particular case upon which an expert bases an opinion or inference may be those perceived by or made known to the expert at or before the hearing.

Courts subject expert veterinarian witnesses to the same scrutiny as all other expert witnesses when deciding whether to allow their testimony. The United States Supreme Court and the Court of Appeals of the District of Columbia created formulas for measuring the admissibility of expert testimony in two seminal cases: *Daubert v. Merrell Dow Pharmaceuticals, Inc.*, 509 U.S. 579 (1993) and *United States v. Frye,* 293 F. 1013 (D.C. Cir 1923). Because the standards in each case differ, states either follow *Daubert* or *Frye,* or portions of both in their determination of expertise. Veterinarians should become familiar with their own jurisdiction's criteria. The following is a brief summary of each case.

Courts using *Daubert* hold that general acceptance of the underlying principle of the scientific evidence is not required. Instead, they consider:

1. whether the theory or technique can be and has been tested;
2. whether the theory or technique has been subjected to peer review and publication;
3. the known or potential rate of error;
4. the existence and maintenance of standards controlling its operation; and
5. the degree to which the theory or technique has been generally accepted by the relevant scientific community.

Courts using *Frye* do require general acceptance of the principle underlying the scientific evidence in order for it to be admissible, stating:

> Just when a scientific principle or discovery crosses the line between the experimental and demonstrable stages is difficult to define. Somewhere in this twilight zone the evidential force of the principle must be recognized, and while courts will go a long way in admitting expert testimony deduced from a well-recognized scientific principle or discovery, the thing from which the deduction is made must be sufficiently established to have gained general acceptance in the particular field in which it belongs.

Scientific publications, judicial precedent, practical applications, or testimony from scientists as the beliefs of their fellow scientists are suggested methods to prove this acceptance.

Veterinarians asked to testify at trial can expect to be served with a *subpoena*, which requires them to literally "lay all business aside" in order to come to court at the date and time listed on it. Depending on the jurisdiction, the date may span weeks or even months, because that is the length of the trial calendar/docket, not because that is the length of the case. Unless the animal cruelty case that is the subject of the subpoena is specially set on a certain date, it shares a position on that calendar with many other criminal cases set for jury trials. It is not unusual for larger jurisdictions to have hundreds of cases on their trial docket and perhaps several animal cruelty cases.

Veterinarians' time is limited among their practice and their animal cruelty investigations and court appearances. For that reason, those testifying as experts should call the prosecutor handling their case immediately upon receiving their *subpoena* and ask to be placed on call. In reality, the State, defense attorney, or both, will ask the judge to invoke the rule of witness sequestration, which means that all witnesses will be sequestered, or not allowed in the courtroom, until they are called to the witness stand. Because most witnesses are available by cell phone or pager, it is highly unusual for the prosecution to ask their witness to wait outside the courtroom for the duration of the trial until it is their turn to testify. In addition to requesting the State to place the veterinarian on call, the veterinarian also should inform the State as to how much time is needed from the time of the phone call until the time the expert can realistically arrive at the courthouse.

Depending on the jurisdiction, the trial may be before a jury or judge. Whoever hears the case is known as the trier of fact. Some jurisdictions do not allow the defendant to have a trial by judge only, also referred to a bench trial, without the consent of the State. If the parties proceed to a jury trial, the attorneys begin by striking a jury in a process known as *voir dire*. The attorneys then make opening statements. What follows is called the guilt-innocence phase, in which the prosecutor presents different forms of evidence, including testimony, to meet the burden of proof of guilty beyond a reasonable doubt. The expert veterinarian testifies during the guilt-innocence phase.

Experts' testimony takes place during the State's case, the defense's case, or both. Finally, the attorneys give their closing arguments and the jury is read jury charges by the judge. These are instructions regarding the applicable law and burden of proof. A specific charge concerning expert testimony is included in these instruction. It may say, for example, "Testimony has been given by certain witnesses who, in law, are termed experts. The law permits persons expert in certain areas to give their opinion derived from their knowledge of that area. The weight which is given to the testimony of expert witnesses is a question to be determined by the jury. The testimony of an expert, like that of any other witness, is to be received by you and given only such weight as you think it is properly entitled to receive. You are not required to accept the opinion testimony of any witness, expert or otherwise." Suffice it to say, a juror's decision to accept or reject expert testimony depends entirely on the content of the testimony and the manner in which it is presented.

A Note about Juries

Expert veterinarians must never assume they are preaching to the choir when testifying in a jury trial. Although *voir dire* is widely known as a process for selecting a jury, it is more accurately viewed by attorneys as striking a jury. The actual jurors who are sworn in to hear the case are the jurors who are remaining after both the State and defense have exhausted their number of permitted strikes to eliminate jurors who they believe cannot be fair and impartial to one or both sides.

Special consideration is given in many states to the jurors who state in *voir dire* that they, for some reason, whether philosophical, emotional, or otherwise, cannot bear to sit through a case involving animal cruelty. As in child molestation, murder, and rape cases, the number of people who express this concern can be high. If a potential juror goes so far as to say that he or she cannot possibly be fair, this may trigger a strike for cause, which is a strike by the court that does not count against either party's number of strikes. This strategy allows the defense to use further strikes to eliminate the remaining jurors who are empathetic to animals' pain and suffering.

The end result might actually be a panel of jurors who have never owned pets, do not like animals, and/or do not take the crime of animal cruelty seriously. This is one more reason it is so important for veterinarian experts to assume in all cases that the prosecutor, jury, and judge know no more than the most basic facts about animals.

As a rule, jurors respond more positively to witnesses who are organized and prepared, speak with authority, and testify without hesitation (Call 1999). In general, if an expert witness speaks too slowly, it will cause him or her to lose the jury's attention. The average person speaks about 120 words per minute and the average listener comprehends twice that many words in a minute (Adler and Rodman 1998). By the same token, although repetition of crucial facts is a good strategy, the rule of moderation still controls. Studies show that repeating the same information more than five times may actually make the jurors discount it (Wenner 1998).

The order in which prosecutors call their witnesses is as much a strategy decision as closing arguments. Often, some witnesses will be more persuasive, credible, and/or memorable than others. Trained prosecutors adhere to the rule of primacy—information presented toward the beginning is remembered more easily; and the rule of recency—information presented last is easier to retain (Sannito and

McGovern 1985). This often results in the expert veterinarian being called to testify last when the prosecutor is depending on the expert to deliver the final blow by testifying to a reasonable degree of scientific certainty that the elements of the crime were met. The veterinarian's testimony assures jurors that despite any doubts they may have had from factual witnesses up to this point, the science speaks for itself through the expert witness. It is reminiscent of a final scene of "C.S.I."

Qualifying the Expert

What sets one veterinarian expert witness apart from another can be a combination of factors, including experience, training, specialty areas, and academic achievement. Aside from handing the prosecutor their *curriculum vitae,* or C.V., as part of case preparation, veterinarians should explain their credentials in terms of the minimum requirements to be a licensed veterinarian and what features of their C.V. are above and beyond minimum standards, and also point out which entries account for their specialty areas. This is important for the prosecutor to understand before trial in the event that the expert is objected to by the defense.

When the expert veterinarian finally takes the witness stand and is sworn in by either the court's deputy or the prosecutor, depending on the jurisdiction, the first order of business is to qualify him or her as an expert. Prosecutors do this by laying a foundation, just as they do with any other piece of evidence they seek to admit. Other non-expert witnesses are sworn in but they do not have to be qualified. Veterinarians, by the nature of their training, typically are experts in all aspects of medicine, including infectious disease, surgery, radiology, and emergency medicine. This is not the case for their human medical counterparts, who have subspecialties of expertise (board certification) in all of these areas. The prosecutor must go through the steps to clarify all the areas of expertise in which the veterinarian is considered an expert. The following is a set of standard questions usually asked in some form or another in the qualification process.

- Would you please state your name and address?
- What is your occupation/profession?
- Are you a duly licensed veterinarian and surgeon?
- In what state(s)?
- How long have you been licensed to practice your profession?
- Are you presently engaged in the practice of your profession?
- Where did you receive your training in veterinary medicine?
- What duties were you asked to perform by the ________ County District Attorney's Office?
- Does that work include the performance of necropsies?
- During your training and experience, how many necropsies have you performed?
- Are you on the staff, or are you affiliated in any way, with any universities or academic institutions?
- Do you specialize in any particular type of animal?
- Exactly what does veterinary medicine mean?
- What is a necropsy?

- Are you a member of any specialized medical or scientific group or association?
- You have mentioned veterinary forensics. Will you explain what that term means?
- Are you trained in this area?
- Is training and experience over and above your license to practice veterinary medicine?
- Is certification on a national basis?
- Are you the author of any textbooks or any specific papers in the field of veterinary forensics?
- Of the _____ (number of) necropsies you have performed or observed, approximately how many times were you able to determine the cause of death?

After this line of questioning, the prosecutor asks the judge to declare the veterinarian an expert in the field of veterinary medicine and veterinary forensics in dogs and cats, for example. The defense attorney then takes one of three actions: objects, states that he or she has no objection, or takes the opportunity to *voir dire* the witness. This means that the defense attorney questions the veterinarian expert about his or her qualifications. This is the point at which the veterinarian is asked more pointed questions about a specific area of veterinary medicine. The defense attorney likely inquires about how many times the veterinarian has testified in court, whether such testimony was for the State or the defense, and how much money the veterinarian is being paid by the State to testify in court. Of course, the veterinarian must answer all of these questions to the best of his or her knowledge.

It is not difficult for the State to overcome an objection to the veterinarian as an expert in the treatment of animals. The challenge lies in the veterinarian's qualifications for necropsies and cause of death and crime scene investigation and pathology. The best way for a veterinarian to be declared an expert in the area of veterinary medicine, which enables him or her to prove the elements of the crime, is to explain the area of expertise in plain language that a jury of non-scientists can understand. If jurors do not understand a term, they will likely ignore it altogether, or assign it their own meaning.

Although the essence of veterinarian experts' testimony is scientific and their demeanor on the witness stand should reflect professionalism, this does not exempt them from humanizing scientific facts whenever possible. Studies done on actual jurors showed that they recall testimony that triggered their emotions more than they recall straight facts. For that reason alone, all experts should learn to humanize veterinary findings as part of their presentation skills. The ideal example is the description of pain and suffering an animal endured at the hands of the defendant. It is one thing to say that an animal suffered. It is quite another to testify as an expert, in the context of describing the degree of excruciating pain, to the amount, frequency, and over what period of time narcotic pain medicine was administered to control the pain. When a feeling such as pain is conveyed by an actual veterinarian, that pain comes alive and becomes empirical, leaving no room for argument or doubt as to that element of the crime.

Once the veterinarian is qualified as an expert, the State moves on to direct examination. At trial, the expert veterinarian has the advantage of speaking directly to the jury, whereas the prosecutor and defense attorney may only address the jury during opening statements and closing arguments. Of course, all parties can address the judge directly at all phases of trial. Prosecutors analogize the courtroom to a theater production when explaining the roles of the different parties. The prosecutor is not the star of the show. The expert witness is the star of the show and the prosecutor is the director. Ideally, all eyes should stay on the veterinarian during expert testimony.

Veterinarians should not talk down to the jurors, but perhaps address them as they do their clients. Interruptions can and will occur. When an objection is voiced to the prosecutor's question, the veterinarian should stop talking and wait for direction. The attorney argues to the judge and at some point, the prosecutor instructs the expert to answer the same question or asks a new question. The key is to listen.

When the prosecutor finishes direct examination, the defense attorney cross examines the expert. Again, the key is to listen and answer accordingly. The most damaging thing a veterinarian expert can do during cross examination is to use sarcasm, show exasperation, or become angry or condescending. No matter how well direct examination went, the veterinarian expert will lose all credibility with the jury by acting less than professional.

Veterinarians who are committed to their role in animal cruelty prosecution convey their belief in their science through their passion and hard work. When communicated to non-scientists at the crime scene, in the prosecutor's office, and in the courtroom in such a way that allows them to share this passion, the "C.S.I." effect becomes real and contagious to everyone in the audience.

References

Adler, R.A., and G. Rodman. 1998. *Understanding Human Communication*. New York: Holt, Rinehart, and Winston.

Call, J.A. 1999. Making the Research Work for You. *Trial Magazine* 32(4):20–27.

Fed. R. Evid. 702, 703.

Sannito, T., and P.J. McGovern. 1985. *Courtroom Psychology for Trial Lawyers*. New York: John Wiley and Sons.

Wenner, D.A. 1998. Preparing for Trial: An Uncommon Approach; the Trial Lawyer Can Use Focus Groups to Flag Potential Juror Reactions and Prepare Effective Arguments for Trial. *Trial Magazine* 34(1):34–35.

Chapter 2
Crime Scene Investigation

Introduction

Crime scene investigation is the first and most critical step in any investigation. There are three important steps at a crime scene: recognition of evidence, proper collection of evidence, and adequate preservation of evidence. In animal cruelty investigations, what could be considered evidence is not always obvious. Furthermore, the evidence collected may hold more value than the investigator or prosecutor realizes. With animal abuse cases, the first responder's actions are critical for successful collection and analysis of the evidence and directly affect the success of prosecution. In homicides, the medical examiner's involvement begins at the scene, and so should it be for animal cruelty cases. The veterinarian must be familiar with proper crime scene investigation because most investigators are inexperienced in animal cruelty cases. Involving the veterinarian at the very beginning of the investigation helps ensure that all the evidence is properly identified and analyzed.

The crime scene speaks a silent language. It holds information about the victim, the suspect, and the crime that took place. To understand everything a crime scene has to say requires time and meticulous attention to detail. One of the most powerful processes is to take all the findings and create a reconstruction of the crime scene before the story is known from the suspect or witnesses. Whatever the suspect (or witness) says is going to be tested against the crime scene findings.

The goal of any criminal investigation is to solve the forensic triad: Link the victim to a suspect and connect them to a crime scene. Crime scene investigation is based on Locard's Exchange Principle: Every contact leaves a trace. Another important principle is: The absence of evidence is not evidence of absence. Forensic evidence also may be used to validate or disprove an alibi or witness statements, reconstruct the crime scene, or develop important investigative leads. Ultimately, recreation of the event tells the story of the animal's suffering.

There are actually two crime scenes present: the macro crime scene, which is the location and surrounding area of the crime, the victim, and the suspect's body; and the micro crime scene, which is the body itself. Forensic science begins at the crime scene. There must be a thorough forensic exam of the crime scene and those findings must be shared with the veterinarian. The veterinarian must rely on evidence (or lack thereof) gathered at the scene to help determine proximate cause of death/injury, mechanism of death, and manner of death/injury.

Physical evidence may be classified as chemical, biological, or pattern evidence. In may be further classified as transient, conditional, pattern, transfer, or associative. *Transient* refers to evidence that is easily lost or changed over time, such as body temperature and decomposition. *Conditional* refers to evidence resulting from an action or event that can be transient as well, such as rigor, weather conditions, entomology, and stomach contents. *Pattern* refer to evidence with imprints, markings, or other patterns such as bite marks, blood spatter, wound patterns, and weapon patterns. *Transfer evidence* is the physical exchange of material between objects after contact, such as fibers, hair, or plant matter. *Associative evidence* is anything that can link a suspect or victim to the scene or each other (Ladd and Lee 2005).

All evidence must be preserved for later testing and use at trial. In addition to testing performed for the prosecution side, the defense has the right to perform independent tests and analysis. Every reasonable effort should be made to preserve evidence and make it available for the defense team, even though this may not take place for a lengthy time period.

CSI: The Veterinarian's Role

The veterinarian's role at a crime scene is to assist investigators and examine any animals at the scene. The veterinarian should assist in the collection of evidence, examine the evidence, and assess the evidence and the crime scene. It is important to meet with the lead investigator, discuss the situation, and develop a plan for investigating the scene. Several things usually need to be addressed simultaneously, and the veterinarian can be of invaluable assistance. The situation often requires working under time pressures resulting from weather or other environmental conditions that could alter or destroy potential physical evidence. There may be sick or critical animals that must be triaged for transport to veterinary hospitals. It is important to record all initial observations of the scene and the animals. The status of each animal at the scene must be recorded because it may change for better or worse after arrival at a veterinary facility.

There may be decomposing animals that must be examined to preserve any evidence. There are certain on-scene tasks that must be performed in order to determine the time of death. An investigator should interview the owner and any witnesses to determine when the animal was last seen alive. A rectal temperature should be taken of all deceased animals. A minimum of two readings should be taken over a 1-hour period to determine the rate of cooling (see Chapter 14). Any entomological evidence related to the body should be gathered at the scene (see Chapter 14). It should be noted if the animal was in direct sunlight, shade, under any cover, or exposed. A determination of the state of rigor and lividity should be made and recorded (see Chapter 14). Paper bags should be placed on the feet of all deceased animals at the scene. Plastic bags should not be used, especially if the body is placed in a cooler prior to examination because of water condensation, which can destroy potential evidence. The body should be wrapped in a clean white sheet and then placed in a clean body bag or plastic bag prior to transport.

Environment: Weather Data

The most important information to initially document at the scene is the weather. The environmental temperature, either with indoor or outdoor settings, must be recorded, noting the time it was taken. A temperature should be taken of the general area, where any deceased animals were found, and at the level of the body. This information is critical to time-of-death estimates. It also can be a factor in neglect charges. Often, the first responders open doors or windows, which changes the enclosed structure's temperature; however, temperature information can be determined. Was the air conditioning or furnace on; if so, at what setting? Confirmation should be made that the power is on and that the heating and air conditioning works. If it has been turned off, or the power has been disconnected, it is important to get the outside temperature. The times of any temperature readings must be noted.

Photography and Videography

Photography is the most important function at a crime scene. Animal cruelty crime scenes, especially hoarding cases, can be chaotic and the evidence is often overwhelming. Photographic preservation of evidence helps minimize the possibility of overlooking something important. In some cases, a crime scene unit may be called in to take general photographs and video. The veterinarian may need to take additional photographs, especially close-ups, of evidence as well as the individual animals and any injuries. It is important to take pictures of the general area, the animals, the housing, all areas the animal could have access to, any insects on the animals, any fluids, weapons, and anything else pertinent to the case.

The type of camera used is important. Polaroid cameras should not be used because the photograph can fade over time and the case can take months to years to be resolved. Digital cameras are ideal because the quality of the photograph is immediately evident. There are digital SLR cameras with interchangeable lenses that are great for clear close-up shots. For 35-mm cameras, the negatives must be kept to authenticate the photographs in court. For digital cameras, the pictures may be copied and preserved on a CD for authentication and the digital card may be re-used.

Photographs should be first of the general area and then more detailed. It is standard to start with photographs of the home or facility, including a picture of the address. A photo log should be kept for each picture taken. When taking pictures of the animals, there should be a card next to the animal identifying the case number, animal ID number, and date.

Ideally, a video should be taken of the scene and the animals. It is important to show the condition of the animal, such as weakness, limping, injuries, or vocalizing. When taking video, it is important to inform the others at the scene so they can minimize other noise.

Evidence Recognition and Collection

Crime scenes are complex and chaotic, requiring systematic evaluation. The recognition of evidence involves the ability to identify probative evidence that is among irrelevant or unrelated evidence at the scene. It is especially important to recognize evidence that warrants further testing. At the beginning of the case it is difficult to know what evidence may become important to the case. Often the seemingly most insignificant piece of evidence breaks the case wide open.

When evaluating the scene for evidence, the investigator is looking for evidence of what happened, what can support or refute the suspect's statement, and evidence of how the animal was or was not cared for. A diagram of the scene should be done describing and assigning a name to the different areas. Any evidence collected must be labeled with the location it was found. All evidence collection should be done with the proper equipment and follow the proper chain of custody procedures (see Chapter 3). Evidence should be gathered that points to the length of time for the conditions of the animals and their injuries. Any evidence that shows ownership or how the suspect obtained the animals should be collected. The refrigerator and freezer should be searched for medications.

The housing of the animal, the availability and condition of the food and water, and the appropriateness of the food should be recorded (Fig. 2.1). The level of the water should be measured from the surface to the top of the container to determine if the animal could reach it. The area should be searched for any extra food the owner had to feed the animals and the expiration date on the package. It is important to ask the owner what food they normally fed the animal for comparison of vomit or stomach contents, especially in suspected poisoning cases. If the animal was tied up, the length of the tie should be measured and collected with the knot intact. If a chain was used, it should be collected and weighed. Any dog house should be evaluated

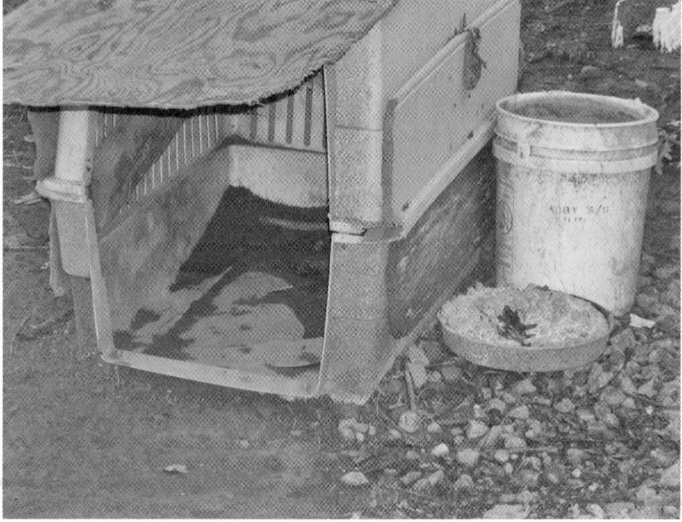

Figure 2.1 Inadequate housing with torn floor, open sides and front; moldy food. For color detail, please see color plate section.

for size and condition. The bedding and underneath the dog house should be searched for hidden evidence.

The scene should be examined for bodily fluids, such as vomit, urine, or feces. The lack of feces can be indicative of starvation and the lack of urine can be indicative of dehydration. The condition of the feces should be noted, such as diarrhea or formed, and fresh or moldy. Animals often lose bladder and bowel control under extreme fear or distress. Samples of any urine, vomit, or feces should be collected. When animals are starving they may exhibit pica and ingest inanimate objects. The feces should be inspected at the scene and for the following 24 hours for evidence of any foreign material.

The investigator should look for blood and note the location and quantity by taking measurements of the blood stain (see Blood Evidence). Samples should be taken of any blood found. If blood has soaked into an absorbent surface, the item may be weighed and compared with a clean similar item as a control. The difference in weight provides the estimated blood volume loss (1 kg = 1 L).

Blood Evidence

Overview

Although in-depth interpretation of blood spatter and blood stains require extensive training, an investigator should be able to look at blood patterns and make some basic deductions. Veterinarians have the best understanding of animal behavior and therefore should be most qualified to re-create the events of the crime. It is imperative that veterinarians be able to understand basic blood spatter analysis to analyze crime scenes, crime scene photos, and assist law enforcement. Interpretation of blood spatter can reveal the position of the victim, attacker(s), presence of a witness, type of weapon used, number of blows, movement of the victim and/or the attacker, height of the attacker, and sequence of events. This evidence can determine the events, what did not occur, and the presence of other individuals at the time of the event.

When analyzing a crime scene, the absence of blood spatter is just as important as the presence of blood spatter. It should be recorded where blood is present and where it is not, such as where something blocked the spatter, creating a void. One needs to look for voids where the victim, attacker, or an object blocked the blood from striking a surface. This also can help determine if a crime scene was staged.

It is important to gather all the evidence at the scene for a blood spatter expert to analyze. A diagram should be made of all blood spatter and photographs taken using a photographic scale. Measurements should be taken from the floor, walls, and/or ceiling. Additional measurements should be taken from the nearest object to the blood drop. The width and length of the blood drop should be measured. The shape and characteristics of the drops should be documented.

Blood Stain Analysis

An investigator can interpret certain basic patterns at the scene, such as drag marks, smears, or blood trails. There are some generalities of blood stain interpretation. When a drop of blood falls to a smooth floor, it remains basically spherical

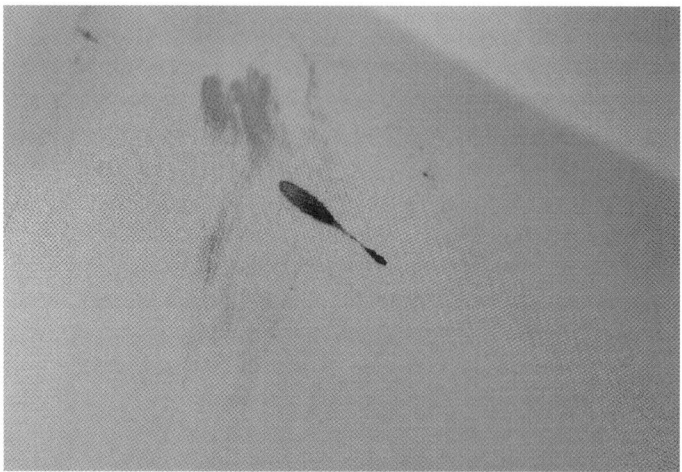

Figure 2.2 Wave cast-off blood spatter. For color detail, please see color plate section.

depending on the velocity. If it lands on a rough surface, it may appear star shaped. Drops that fall from great heights also are star shaped. If the blood strikes the wall at a right angle, it is round. Blood drops that land at other angles are elongated, with the narrower part indicating the direction of travel. The blood drop may have a wave cast-off as it lands, giving the appearance of an exclamation point (Fig. 2.2). The direction of the smaller drop of blood indicates the direction of travel.

Passive bloodstain patterns are drops formed by the force of gravity alone. Transfer or contact stains are formed when something comes into contact with the blood and transfers it onto another surface. Projected blood stains are created when an exposed blood source is subjected to a force greater than the force of gravity. These may be externally or internally produced, such as with an arterial spurt. A flow pattern may be seen whenever there is a change in the shape and direction of a blood stain caused by the influence of gravity or movement of the object. A drip pattern is the result of blood dripping into blood. A perimeter stain consists of only its outer periphery, the central area having been removed by wiping or flaking off after the blood has partially or completely dried. A swipe pattern is caused by the transfer of blood from a moving source onto an unstained surface. The direction of travel may be determined by the feathered edge. A wipe pattern is created when an object moves through an existing stain, removing and/or altering the bloodstain's appearance.

It is important to keep in mind that an injured animal may be mobile and may shake his head or body, causing spatter. Sneezed blood may be diluted or have air vacuoles, creating *ghost drops* or *bubble drops*. Ghost drops, or ghost-centered drops, are hollow-centered blood drops. They are formed when blood mixes with air, creating an air bubble; this eventually pops, leaving a hollow center. Ghost drops are indicative of coughing or vomiting blood and can be a mixture of sizes. Insects can cause blood artifacts moving through the blood and creating a false blood trail.

Blood Spatter Analysis

Blood spatter can be categorized based on the size of the blood drops, which is directly related to the force that caused the spatter. The velocities of blood spatter refer to the force that caused the blood to move and is measured in feet per second (fps). It should be noted that there is a gap of 25–100 fps in the following categories. The analysis of these blood drops requires interpretation of events such as weapon acceleration (Akin 2005).

High-Velocity Blood Spatter

High-velocity blood spatter (HVBS) are drops of blood propelled by an explosive force greater than 100 feet per second. The blood spatter droplets are less than 1 mm in size, and the spatter pattern is usually called a mist. HVBS does not travel far because of the small mass and resistance of air. Tissue fragments may be propelled further because of their larger mass. These are seen usually with gunshots, explosives, machinery, expired air, coughing, and sneezing (Akin 2005).

Medium-Velocity Blood Spatter

Medium-velocity blood spatter (MVBS) are drops of blood propelled by an external force of greater than 5 feet per second and less than 25 feet per second. The drops are usually 1–3 mm in size. Usually they are caused by blunt- or sharp-force trauma, such as stabbing, weapons, punches, arterial spurts, and some cast-off from weapons (Akin 2005). Arterial spurts create a large amount of blood that can be confusing to interpret. The victim may still be under attack while bleeding, creating overlying patterns. There may be swipes caused by transfer from the attacker or the victim falling against the arterial spurt pattern. Or there may be swipes where blood is transferred and smeared from the attacker or victim's body or clothes (Akin 2005). The arterial spurt pattern is created by the contraction of the left ventricle of the heart. It creates an arcing pattern because it begins with low pressure that then increases followed by low pressure again (Akin 2005).

Weapon cast-off blood spatter, also known as *cast-off,* is caused by blood flung off a weapon when the weapon is swung upward or backward. These blood stains may be elliptical or oval. They are more spherical when the blood hits at a 90-degree angle to the attacker. When the body is struck with a weapon, there is no cast-off blood spatter from the weapon with the first strike. The first strike initiates the bleeding. The second and any subsequent strikes to the now-bloody area produce cast-off blood spatter. This cast-off can be very small and easily missed at a crime scene. Cast-off also can be classified as low velocity blood spatter if the drops measure 8 mm or larger (Akin 2005).

Low-Velocity Blood Spatter

Low-velocity blood spatter (LVBS) is caused by a force less than 5 fps, equivalent to the force of normal gravity. These drops usually measure 3 mm or higher. They are most often caused by blood dripping from someone who is still, walking, or running (Akin 2005). Blood dripping from a body or object usually falls at a 90-degree angle, forming a sphere when it hits a flat perpendicular surface. The sphere is usually smooth if the surface is smooth. Spikes or crenations may be caused if the surface has texture, or several drops repeatedly land in the same spot or fall from a distance. When blood falls from someone who is walking or running, the blood stain is more elliptical or angular with a point at one end. These stains also may have a wave cast-off, a smaller drop. The point of the angular drop and the wave cast-off indicate the direction of travel (Akin 2005). Larger pools of blood may be seen if the animal or person who is bleeding paused in one area.

Blood Spatter Analysis of Dog Fighting Pit

A dog fighting pit is often covered in blood spatter on the walls and flooring. If the flooring is made of absorbent material it is possible to estimate the amount of blood loss. Because there is blood from several dogs on the surfaces, it is important to look for any discrete blood drops to decrease the chance of getting a mixed DNA profile. The walls and floor inside the pit should be analyzed as well as any blood found on the outside. For blood stains on carpet, a 2- to 3-inch-square area should be cut out. All distinct blood stains should be swabbed (see Chapter 4). After the sample is taken, it is best to do a second swab and perform a presumptive test for blood on-site with phenolphthalein. The strongest positive should be the priority swabs to test for DNA.

The height should be measured from the floor of all blood spatter found. The blood drops should be photographed, measured, and categorized as low-, medium-, or high-velocity spatter. Any large blood stains should be documented and sampled. The floor and walls should be examined with a UV light to detect urine and appropriate samples taken. Certain measurements should be taken of any dogs that were associated with the fighting pit. Measurements should be taken from the end of the muzzle to the caudal pelvis and from the end of the muzzle to end of the tail. The height should be measured from the floor the top of the head, the shoulders, and the hips. These measurements may be needed to compare to the blood spatter.

Grave Detection and Excavation

The veterinarian may be called to assist the detection and excavation of a grave suspected to hold the body of an animal. A forensic anthropologist or archeologist should be called to the scene to assist in these cases.

Stratigraphy

Stratigraphy refers to the study of the soil layers in a grave. These are different than the surrounding natural and undisturbed area. One cannot dig a grave and then fill it back in without causing disruption to the normal soil layers. The top layer may be mixed with deeper layers. The fill may contain artificial layers such as lyme. These layers can help determine how the evidence became interred. When excavating a grave, care should be taken to document these layers through photography and sampling.

Tool Mark Evidence

Tool mark evidence may be present at a grave either subterranean or on the surface ground. These marks are important forensically in that they indicate the tool or tools used to dig the grave. They may provide insight to the planning if the tool used was one of opportunity and readily available at the grave site. If more than one tool was used it may indicate there was an accomplice. Subterranean tool marks have been found many years later and under different environmental conditions (Hochrein 2002). The type of soil affects the retention of tool marks; gravels or dry sandy soils are the least conducive. Handle tool marks may be at or near the surface edges of the grave. As the grave is dug deeper with a long tool, such as a shovel, the edges of the grave may be used as a fulcrum for the handle. This can indicate the position of the person digging the grave. The back fill dirt may hold tool marks such as in clumps of sod or clods of soil.

The surface of the grave often contains hand, shoe, or knee impressions. These impressions are unavoidable in digging a grave regardless of the instrument used. When using small digging tools, the digger must kneel or sit around the edges. Fabric impressions on the soil may be found where the person was kneeling. When using a shovel, the digger must put his foot on the top of the blade, often leaving heel impressions. These may be misinterpreted as two different instruments used instead of the heel of the foot in conjunction with a shovel blade tool mark. Often the digger stomps or tamps the surface to pack the fill, leaving shoe or foot impressions (Hochrein 2002).

Bioturbation

Bioturbation refers to the environmental factors that turbate or naturally churn, displace, or modify the position and nature of the remains (Hochrein 2002). These can include plant (floral turbation) and animal (fauna turbation). The animal factors include rodent burrows, which are often at the upper edge of the grave pit. The species of animal and the behavior of burrowing related to season may be used to determine timelines related to the burial. These burrow routes also may be examined for scavenged evidence. The roots inside a grave also may provide evidence of the instrument used to dig the grave. Large, broad-bladed tools, such as shovels, tend to tear and slice the roots at the edges of the walls. Thinner-profile tools, such as pitchforks and crowbars, tend to preserve root networks within the grave usually located beneath the body.

Burial Features

Burial features are affected by water as well. The pooling, evaporation, drying, and fine sediments in an open and filled pit create patterns of cracking (Hochrein 2002). Surface cracks may occur at the edges of the grave, helping to identify the boundaries for excavation. The cracks may disappear with rainfall but consistently reappear along the same margins. In contrast, sedimentation over shallow or flat surfaces causes patterns of cracking in irregular, spider web–like fashion (Hochrein 2002). The width of the cracks should be measured. In dry conditions, the crack widens at a rate of approximately 1 mm per day. Heavy rainfalls cause rapid closure of these cracks. By using the soil type and historical weather information, it may be possible to determine the post-deposition time interval to the last rainfall (Hochrein 2002).

Compression and depression of the burial site change the surface contours in and around the pit. These changes may be seen through aerial or pedestrian observations. Primary depressions occur as the fresh fill dirt settles. Secondary depressions are caused by the body bloating because of putrefaction and then collapsing of the abdomen as the gases and fluid are released. The body must be placed in such a way that the bloating and subsequent collapse causes the change within the burial pit and enough time has elapsed for the putrefaction process to have occurred (Hochrein 2002). If a body has been placed in a container, the secondary depressions also may be created as the container deteriorates. Holes dug by scavengers may be misinterpreted as secondary depressions. As time goes on, the evidence of both primary and secondary surface depressions becomes more subtle and harder to detect. Eventually, all evidence may be obliterated by bioturbation, sedimentation, and other changes to the landscape.

Excavation of the Grave

Excavation techniques of a grave must take into account the forensic nature of the case. It must be systematic, consider the environment and context of the burial, and take precautions to look for all evidence and document accordingly. The grave should be examined initially for defects and trace evidence. A grid should be established using a three-dimensional system around the immediate grave site boundaries to use as recording points for evidence collection. This should take into account the surrounding topography and elevation, which should be documented to address groundwater flow, surface erosions, and biota (Hochrein 2002).

The surface should be examined for evidence of surface sedimentation and cracking, bioturbation, compression and depression, and tool marks. Botanical and entomological samples should be taken. Progressive defoliation of the surface of the grave site should be done taking plant samples. Plants surrounding the area beyond the grave site boundaries should be taken for comparison. The removal of vegetation reveals the surface of the grave, allowing for closer examination. Photographs of all samples should be taken prior to their collection and their location should be documented in relation to the grid system.

A small rectangular window should be excavated at the center of the site down to the level of the remains. This allows a quick assessment of the depth and stratification of the soil. All excavated fill must be sifted through screens for evidence related to weapons, projectiles, ligatures, textile materials or other trace related to the suspect, the cause of death, and what was used to transport the body. The excavation should proceed from the center outward, keeping one to two sides of the box intact to maintain a profile section above and across the remains. Any evidence or stratigraphic change should be photographed and mapped. To map the area, a transparent plastic sheet may be placed across the section and the evidence and strata traced onto the sheet (Hochrein 2002). Heavy equipment should be avoided if at all possible. The tools used to excavate should not be something the suspect may have used, to avoid contamination of the scene with false or confusing tool marks. A wet-dry vacuum should be used to evacuate the excavated fill from the burial site and the contents screened for evidence. Care should be taken to avoid ground water or purge contamination.

Examination of the Body

An important consideration is whether or not the victim was alive when buried. Depending on the amount of decomposition and if the body was wrapped, it may be impossible to determine if the soil was inhaled. Evidence of internal compaction has been seen in cases of humans buried alive. The soil was compacted where the victim pressed on the sides with bound legs; their shoulders, knees, or any other area of the body could have moved side to side or bottom to top. Scratching and biting of any external wrapping and the compacted areas may be expected findings with animals. The animals may have frayed or broken nails on their feet.

Any roots in the grave and around the body should be noted. The position of the roots and the penetration in and around bones should be documented. These roots should be collected for analysis of the rate of growth. This can provide a time line for the date of interment of the body.

References

Akin, L.L. 2005. Blood Spatter Interpretation at Crime Scenes. *The Forensic Examiner* 14(2):6–10.

Hochrein, M.J. 2002. An Autopsy of the Grave: Recognizing, Collecting, and Preserving Forensic Geotaphonomic Evidence. In *Advances in Forensic Taphonomy*, ed. W.D. Haglund, and M.H. Sorg, pp. 45–70. Boca Raton, FL: CRC Press.

Ladd, C., and H.C. Lee. 2005. The Use of Biological and Botanical Evidence in Criminal Investigations. In *Forensic Botany: Principles and Applications to Criminal Casework*, ed. H.M. Coyle, pp. 97–115. Boca Raton, FL: CRC Press.

Chapter 3
CSI: The Animal as Evidence

Introduction

The animal itself is considered part of the crime scene and as such must be treated as evidence. The animal's body contains the story of what happened, and it is the veterinarian's job to find it. It is important to have all the available crime scene and investigation information prior to examining a suspected victim of animal cruelty. The veterinarian must collect and analyze all the evidence from the animal in context with the history, crime scene, and investigation findings. Each piece of information obtained from the animal must be accounted for and explained. It is crucial to never disregard a seemingly insignificant piece of evidence, because that evidence could be the key to the investigation.

Determining Non-accidental Injury

Overview

Determining accidental vs. non-accidental injury (i.e. abuse) begins with an index of suspicion when the exam findings are not supportive of the initial history. All aspects of the case must be considered to determine if the injury could have been accidental or was non-accidental. The question is: Does the explanation by the owner, the environmental conditions, and the medical history explain the extent of the injuries? A conclusive determination may not be possible until the history and/or the environment are further investigated and compared with the examination findings.

Certain types of injury and conditions raise suspicion of abuse in and of themselves. The pathognomonic features for child abuse include fingertip bruising, cigarette burns, and lash marks. Features that are highly suggestive of abuse are retinal hemorrhages, unexplained subdural hematomas, and torn lingual frenula. The most pathognomonic feature of abuse in animals is repetitive injuries. This may present as multiple injuries in different stages of healing, indicating that they occurred at different times; or the animal may have a medical history of repeat injuries. The Munro and Thrusfield study revealed repetitive injury in 16 dogs out of 243 reported cases of non-accidental injury; in 13 cats out of 182 cases (Munro and Thrusfield 2001b). Another consideration is households in which the patient or other animals have suffered from similar injuries or unexplained death or disappearance. The patient may have a pattern of unexplained symptoms or injuries. The owner may have several animals listed that the veterinarian has only seen once, or they may adopt frequently from their local shelter because their pets never live long or always "run away."

Extensive data published on child abuse parallel findings in animal abuse; these data may be used for identification and classification of injuries resulting from animal abuse (Munro and Thrusfield 2001a). Child abuse can be categorized as physical abuse (non-accidental injury), psychological abuse, sexual abuse, and neglect. A study of non-accidental injury in animals was conducted by Munro and Thrusfield of 1,000 veterinarians in the United Kingdom. The study found that certain things either raised suspicion or caused recognition of non-accidental injury. These features included something indicative in the history, the behavior of the animal and/or owner, the type of injury, implication of a particular person, or involvement of the police or animal control in the case. These are very similar to diagnostic pointers to non-accidental injury in children (Munro and Thrusfield 2001a).

It is interesting to note that Munro and Thrusfield found age, gender, and breed factors in the reported cases of non-accidental injury. They found that there were a higher number of dogs (63 percent) and cats (71 percent) less than 2 years of age compared with the general population. This may result from the fact that younger animals are harder to manage, possibly more aggravating to the owner, and more likely to incite aggressive acts by the owner (Munro and Thrusfield 2001b). It may be that older animals are not victims as often because there has been time for the human–animal bond to strengthen. The study found that male dogs were abused in a higher proportion to female dogs. This may be because violent offenders tend to prefer male dogs or that male dogs may be more aggressive and less manageable than female dogs (Munro and Thrusfield 2001b). No statistical gender difference was found in the cases involving cats. The study also considered breed differences and compared those with the general population in the United Kingdom. They found that the Staffordshire bull terrier, Staffordshire bull terrier cross, and mixed breed dogs were at increased risk of abuse. The study suggests that possible explanations for the breed risk may result from the nature of the person who seeks to own the Staffordshire bull terrier, and that more cross- or mixed-breed dogs are owned by people of lower socioeconomic status. They also found that the Labrador retriever showed a lower risk of abuse (Munro and Thrusfield 2001b).

Abused Animals in the Practice Setting

It is very difficult for veterinarians to realize and accept the fact that animals who are victims of abuse will be brought into their practice. The Munro and Thrusfield study demonstrates that this is actually quite common. The person who brings in the animal may or may not be aware that the animal has been abused. That person, or a child, also may be a victim of abuse in the home. Often, the person bringing the animal in has a close relationship with the abuser. It is very important for veterinarians to realize that their discussions with the owner may elicit important information, including possible confessions. The study by Munro and Thrusfield reported that in several cases a family member was implicated by the owner. In 25 cases, the owner admitted to committing the abuse. It is of particular interest that in five cases, the admission came after the veterinarian had merely discussed the possibility of abuse as the cause of the injuries (Munro and Thrusfield 2001a).

Taking the History in a Potential Abuse Case

Things may not always be what they appear to be when examining a victim of animal cruelty. The suspicion of non-accidental injury should be raised when there is significant discrepancy between the history provided and the clinical findings. Suspicion also should be raised when explanations are vague, inconsistent, or contradictory.

It is important to get a more thorough history in animal abuse cases than routinely performed in veterinary medicine. In abuse cases, certain questions need to be answered to investigate, charge, and prosecute these crimes. Questions should be asked to determine who had access to the animal (including other animals), what the animal had access to, when the event occurred, where the event occurred, how it happened, and why it happened. Details are needed about the environment, including does the animal have access to the outside, is it allowed outside unattended, and when outside is the animal confined, how is it confined, is a gate present on the fence, and if so is it locked. If the animal lives strictly indoors, then the layout of the home is needed, including the presence and location of stairs. Specific information is needed regarding where the animal was found, what was present around the animal (e.g. blood or other bodily fluids), and its initial symptoms. In addition, a history should be obtained regarding what food the animal eats (including brand, dry or can), how often the animal is fed, if it is known when the animal last ate or drank, and when the animal last had access to food or water.

It is important for the veterinarian to use common sense combined with experience to analyze all the information to determine if there is an increased likelihood that the injury is non-accidental. Often, the owner claims the animal fell off something within the home or outside. The veterinarian must consider the height of the object and the species involved and compare that with the extent of the animal's injuries to determine if that scenario is plausible. It is important to ask specific questions of any witnesses to the incident to gather as much information as possible.

Another common explanation given by owners is that the animal was hit by a motor vehicle. The injuries found on an abused animal are often caused by blunt force trauma and may resemble those found in hit-by-car (HBC) victims. The injuries seen in HBC animals depend on the speed of the vehicle, where the animal was hit, if the animal was knocked to the side of the vehicle, or if it tumbled under the car and possibly run over by one or more tires. The injuries sustained by HBC victims range from very mild to severe. They may involve the limbs, pelvis, abdomen, thorax, head, or any combination of areas depending on the size of the animal and how it was hit. However, there are consistent findings in HBC victims regardless of other injuries to the body. These include frayed nails, torn foot pads, skin abrasions (often medial on one side of the body and lateral on the other), and dirt, debris, or gravel on the fur or in the mouth. When an animal is struck with the force of a moving vehicle, it tumbles under the car or is thrown to the side. This causes forceful contact with the ground and possible dragging of the body. The animal instinctively puts his feet and nails out to brace against these forces. The physical impact projects the animal's body into motion, which in turn results in external injuries.

The behavior of the owner may raise suspicion as to the cause of the animal's injury. The owner may be apathetic, uneasy, angry with routine history questions, embarrassed, or his or her responses may be generally inappropriate to the situation, especially as he or she is apprised of the gravity of the situation. If the behavior of the owner is of concern, it may be prudent to have someone else in the room for safety. It should be noted that animal abusers come from all socioeconomic classes. There may be parallels to those found in child abuse, which is more common in the lower socioeconomic class where there is more social deprivation and family dysfunction (Munro and Thrusfield 2001a).

Hearsay

Veterinarians often make the incorrect assumption that what a client tells them is admissible in court. This is considered hearsay and is not admissible even with a witness to the statement or a signed statement. An exception to hearsay is when a person makes a statement against self-interest. For example, if a person makes a statement implicating him- or herself in the crime it is not considered hearsay. Otherwise, whatever a client tells the veterinarian or staff must be repeated to an officer of the law for the statement to be admissible in court.

Behavioral Considerations of Animals

The behavior of animals in response to a threat or injury can determine what evidence is found on examination and at the crime scene. The behavior may be influenced by the species of animal, breed, age, gender, size, and whether the animal is sexually intact. When an animal is wounded, it often licks at the area, potentially removing crucial evidence. When in pain, the animal may roll, hide, and/or vocalize. This knowledge can be vital when evaluating a crime scene to determine the sequence of events and where to look for evidence.

It is important to consider what the animal's behavior might have been in response to the assault to determine what evidence may be found on a suspect. The animal's defense reactions to an assault are highly variable. The animal may scratch or bite the assailant. If the animal tried to run or struggled to get away, the wounds may be located toward the rear of the body. The animal may curl up to protect the head and underbelly, exposing the sides and top of the body to assault. There may be additional injuries caused by the assailant grabbing the animal and/or the restraints used. Defense wounds on an animal may not be present or may be difficult to interpret.

Several forms of asphyxia require that the assailant be in close proximity to the victim. It is probable that the victim inflicted some kind of injury to the assailant during the struggle. It is also highly likely that there was a transfer of evidence from the assailant to the victim and from the victim to the assailant. Consideration should be given in all cases of abuse to these scenarios and appropriate measures taken to identify and collect this evidence.

The animal's behavior may raise suspicion of abuse, such as fear toward the owner, dullness, depression, or anxiousness. The fear and anxiety reactions of the animal may be so severe as to cause the animal to vocalize, urinate, or defecate when the owner is present. It is important to note if this behavior goes away when the person leaves and especially if it returns when he or she reappears. It should be documented if it recurs with a person of the same sex, similar body type, and if it is linked with specific items, such as baseball caps or eyeglasses. These behavior manifestations may not be admissible in court but they are certainly clues to the possible abuser that should be conveyed to the investigator. It should be noted that animals may have seemingly normal "happy" responses to their abuser, including wagging the tail and licking the hand.

Evidence Collection

Evidence collection from the animal follows the same protocols as in crime scene investigation (see Chapter 2). All evidence should be photographed *in situ* prior to collection and packaging. Precautions should be taken to minimize contamination of evidence by wearing cap, mask, gloves, and a clean gown. It is imperative to realize that anything can be important as evidence. The significance of a piece of evidence may change later based on crime scene findings, additional investigation, witness statements, or the suspect's statement. A suspect or defendant is free to change his or her statement and the veterinarian needs to anticipate all possible defenses in the forensic evaluation of the animal. There is only one chance to gather all the evidence from the animal.

It is important to have the proper tools to detect and collect evidence from the animal (see Appendix 26). The body should be inspected with a UV light source to detect fluids and trace evidence. A flashlight may be used and held at an angle to detect trace evidence, such as foreign hairs and fibers (see Chapter 4). A magnifying glass is helpful when examining the body for small pieces of evidence. Plastic tweezers are needed to retrieve fine pieces of evidence without causing damage. Evidence tape is needed to seal all evidence, whether it is contained in bags, boxes, or envelopes. Evidence labels and tags are used on the outside of the containers and on body bags. All evidence bags and envelopes should be paper instead of plastic. Moisture can build up in plastic bags, which can cause damage to the evidence inside. If the evidence is wet, it may be placed in a plastic bag first for transport up to a maximum of 2 hours. Then the item should be removed, allowed to dry, and placed in a paper or otherwise breathable evidence bag.

When taking swabs of evidence, only sterile swabs should be used. It is helpful to have a Styrofoam block to hold the swabs while they dry. A wooden block with drilled holes also can work. It may be useful to have the blocks divided into sections such as *blood, skin, vaginal, rectal,* and *oral,* denoting the source of the swab. If the area of interest is dried fluid, a wet–dry technique may be used. First swab the area with a sterile swab that is moistened with saline, which rehydrates the dried cells. Then roll a dry sterile swab on the moistened area, which absorbs the rehydrated fluid. When taking samples, a control swab should be collected adjacent to the area of interest and labeled a control swab. All swabs should be individually placed in a swab box or paper envelope after drying.

Chain of Custody

Any evidence related to a crime must follow a chain of custody. This refers to a process of documentation in which the evidence is accounted for at all times. *Evidence* is anything collected from the crime scene: all samples, all photographs taken, the photo card or negatives, and the animal itself. In all cases of suspected cruelty it should be the police or animal control that transports the body to the veterinarian to maintain the chain of custody.

All evidence must be labeled with the date, time, and description of the item; and the person who collected it should initial or sign across the seal. An evidence log must be maintained showing the same information and the location in which the item is stored (see Appendix 1). All evidence should be kept in a locked cabinet with restricted access. If the evidence must be kept in a refrigerator or freezer without a lock, it should be located in an area with limited access. If the evidence is transferred to another person, location, or laboratory, it must be noted in the evidence log with the time, date, and a signature from the sender and/or recipient. This applies to the body of the animal as well.

Human labs already have a system in place to record chain of custody when dealing with criminal cases. But most veterinary facilities do not. When sending a sample, a Cruelty Case Samples Packaging Record (see Appendix 2) must be filled out. This form is used to record in detail the description of the samples submitted, how they are packaged, by whom, the date and time, the carrier, and the case number. On any testing request form it must be noted and highlighted that the samples are part of a criminal investigation. Along with the test request, a Cruelty Case Samples Receipt Record (see Appendix 3) must be submitted for the receiving lab to fill out. This form serves as the legal document that testifies that the chain of custody has been maintained and the evidence has not been compromised. It should be partially filled out by the sender with the identifying case information only. The form should be completed by the receiving lab describing the samples that were received and faxed back immediately to the sender on the day the sample is received. Both forms should match in their descriptions of the samples to show that their integrity was maintained. These steps are crucial for the test results to stand up to scrutiny and be admissible in court.

Photography and Videography

With all suspected victims of animal cruelty there should be photographic documentation of the exam. It is preferable to use digital cameras over 35 mm because the quality of the photograph is known immediately. It is better not to use Polaroid cameras because the photographs fade with time. This can present a significant problem because some cases can take several months or even years to come to court. Regardless of the type of camera used, it is important for the photographs to be authenticated in court. With 35 mm pictures, the negatives must be kept as evidence. With digital cameras, the memory cards or sticks may be copied onto a CD. The CD may be used to authenticate the photographs in court and the memory cards or sticks may be re-used. The computer adds the date and time that the CD was created, so this data transfer should done in a timely manner.

When taking photos, the series should start with general shots of the animal, including the case and animal ID number. A photo log should be kept of each photograph taken. Distant photos should be taken showing the entire body of the animal: right and left side, front, and dorsal views. Photographs should be taken of any obvious lesions, abnormal physical findings, and any evidence found on the body. It is best to include a special photographic scale in most pictures to show dimensions and proximity to physical landmarks.

Clear close-up views should be taken of any pertinent findings. These photographs may need to be enlarged to 8 × 10 for court so the resolution of the photographs should be one that will not lose the detail with this enlargement. The digital SLR cameras are similar to 35-mm cameras in that they have interchangeable lenses. A macro lens may be used for clear close-ups of tiny lesions measuring 1–2 mm. Because of the sensitivity of fine detail lenses to movement, it is recommended to use a mini-tripod for stability when taking photos.

Whenever possible, video should be taken of the exam and the animal. The video should begin with a picture of the case and animal ID number. It is preferable to have the time and date showing on the recording. Videography is most valuable when an animal shows obvious difficulty performing certain functions, such as neurological problems or limping. It is also helpful to show certain behaviors, such as vocalizing because of pain or severe brain injury. In starvation cases, it is useful to video the animal's response when first given water and food. It is best to videotape anything that can be better appreciated through live recording rather than take still photos. The video may be converted to a tape or DVD, which can be used as evidence.

Examination of the Live Animal

When examining the animal, the veterinarian looks for evidence that either supports or refutes the suspect's statement, investigation findings, or circumstances surrounding the incident. It is important to fully document all the injuries and identify all the problems. Once the problems are well defined, they are half solved. Ideally, no examination should be conducted without all the information from the investigators and/or the owner, including photographs and the officer's report. The initial observations from the exam may be accurate but they may be misinterpreted without the proper information to put things in context, which can lead to incorrect conclusions.

Documentation

When examining an animal, there must be full documentation of all the findings. The exam should include written and photographic documentation. Diagrams and videos should be used whenever possible. It is helpful to have a recording device when examining the animal to dictate examination findings. All notes, recordings, photographs, and reports are considered evidence and will be reviewed by the investigator, prosecutor, defense attorney, and judge. There are several forms from the American Society for the Prevention of Cruelty to Animals (ASPCA) that may be helpful to document the exam findings (see Appendices 4–11, 17–20). The Examination Report form also can be a guideline for the examination. The veterinarian may be asked for a preliminary report or statement. This should only contain confirmed findings and pending tests. It is difficult to retract written statements later without a valid reason.

It is important to do a complete physical exam, including blood work, fecal, and radiographs on a victim of animal cruelty. Every effort should be made to collect evidence prior to treatment to prevent contamination of the evidence. After treating the animal, it is vital to document the process of the animal's recovery, including weight gain, and repeat appropriate tests. As the animal recovers, the medical records and/or reports should include the timelines for treatments and assessment of the reasons for the animal's recovery.

External Exam

A full physical exam should be conducted, noting all normal and abnormal findings. It is not acceptable to just record abnormal findings because it can imply that a full exam was not performed. The case number, animal identification number, a description of the animal, including breed, coloring, hair coat length (in mixed breeds), gender, sex status, and estimation of the age should be noted. A general assessment of the animal's overall condition is made, including hair coat, skin, nails, and body condition (see Body Condition Scoring). The animal's mental status, strength, activity level, and interaction with people and animals should be assessed as well.

The exam should include the weight, temperature, pulse, respiration, mucous membrane color, capillary refill time, and assessment of hydration status. The temperature may be taken rectally if there is no evidence of sexual assault. Otherwise, the temperature should be taken after sample collection from the rectum (see Chapter 12). All animals should be scanned for the presence of a microchip.

The fur should be inspected using a UV light source for trace evidence, saliva, blood (the animal's, another animal, or human), or other bodily fluids. Any evidence should be collected prior to proceeding with the exam (see Chapter 4). The body should be inspected for any bruises, obvious wounds, or lesions. The fur may need to be shaved to show the extent of injury. These should be documented by their location, distribution, and size. An estimate of the age of wounds should be given. A granulation bed forms in approximately 1 week. Granulation tissue grows at a rate of approximately 1 mm/day and slows over time to 1 cm/month (Reisman 2004).

The head should be examined for evidence of trauma including a fundic, oral, and otoscopic exam (see Chapter 5). The head should be palpated for fractures and swellings. The mouth should be inspected for injury and foreign material. Injuries to the tongue may be caused by head trauma, burns, strangulation of tissue because of foreign bodies, or the chewing/ingestion of plants, sharp objects, or chemicals.

The animal should be evaluated for any signs of pain, especially related to a specific area. The presence and degree of pain play an important role in animal abuse cases. Pain is indicative of the amount of suffering and severity of injury. It is also something that a judge, attorney, and jurors can understand. Every animal is different in how it presents pain depending on the species, breed, and personality. The veterinarian must be able to recognize even the subtlest sign of pain, such as pupil dilation or licking. It is important to describe the degree of pain, document any medications given, and any response. The body should be palpated for swellings, area of tenderness, and other signs of injury. The tail is often injured in animal cruelty situations, although it may often go unnoticed because fearful animals usually tuck in their tails. The most common injuries are vertebral separation and fractures. Separation near the base of the tail may present as subcutaneous hemorrhage in the perineal region (Fig. 3.1).

The examination of the feet is a crucial part of the physical exam. The feet may hold valuable trace evidence embedded in the fur or nails. Frayed nails are indicative that the animal was dragged on a hard surface or the animal struggled and clawed against a hard surface. These nails may be slightly frayed or worn down to the base of the nail. The foot pads may show evidence of injury such as abrasions, lacerations, or punctures, or the feet may appear completely unremarkable, which, when placed in context with the rest of the exam findings, may be the key to what happened to the animal. For most accidental causes of severe trauma, such as a motor vehicle accident, there is usually injury to the feet. It is crucial to keep in mind that the absence of findings speaks the loudest about what did or did not happen.

Measurements of the body should be taken and recorded, especially if any blood stains or blood spatter are found at the crime scene. These measurements may be needed to properly analyze and interpret any blood spatter found at the scene. The

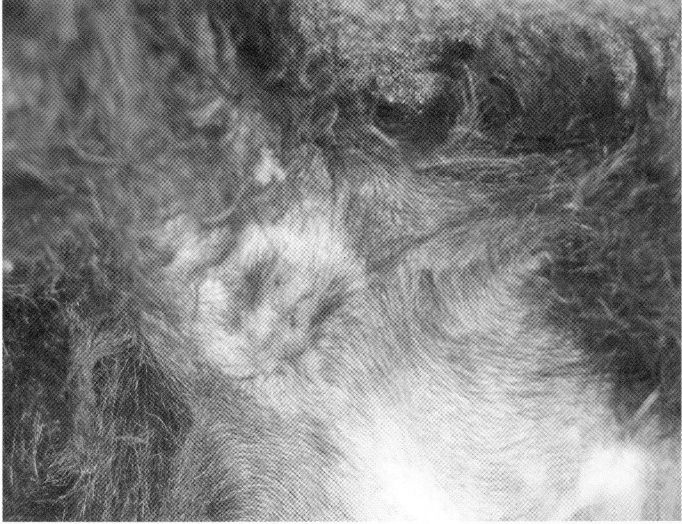

Fig. 3.1 Dissecting subcutaneous hemorrhage around anus resulting from proximal tail fracture and dislocation. For color detail, please see color plate section.

measurements will be compared to those taken at the scene to determine if the animal may have caused the blood stain or if it was from the perpetrator. Measurements should be taken of the length of the body from the head, starting from the muzzle to the rear, and ending at the caudal pelvis. Measurements should be taken of the height of the animal from the feet to the top of the cranium, feet to the point of the shoulder area, and feet to the top of the pelvis. Whenever there is a wound on the body that could have created blood spatter at the crime scene, measurements should be taken from the wound to the muzzle, tail, and floor. Additional measurements should be taken of any area of interest based on circumstances surrounding the death or injury, crime scene findings, or the initial exam.

Body Condition Scoring

Body condition scoring (BCS) refers to a system of scoring the animal's body fat and muscle mass. In animal cruelty cases it is primarily used in cases of starvation. It also may be used with large animal seizures such as hoarding or puppy mill cases. In these cases the animals may range in condition from emaciated to overweight. There are several BCS systems that may be used. The simplest is best for the attorneys and jury to understand. When dealing with a wide range of body conditions, it is best to use the 1–5 system: 1 = emaciated; 2 = thin; 3 = normal; 4 = overweight; 5 = obese.

Tufts University has developed a system called the Tufts Animal Care and Condition (TACC) scales (see Appendix 21). This system is more descriptive, containing five categories: 1 = ideal; 2 = underweight/lean; 3 = thin; 4 = very underweight; 5 = emaciated. It should be noted on the report which BCS system is being used and provide a reference scale. The TACC also has a scoring system for weather safety, environmental health, and physical care scale that is useful in neglect cases. The TACC system provides more detailed descriptions of the conditions, is easy to use, and provides uniformity for all veterinarians and investigators.

Radiographs

Most victims of animal cruelty have been subject to repetitive abuse. Blunt force trauma is the most common type of abuse in homes in which there is domestic or family violence. It is crucial to take radiographs of all suspected victims of cruelty, regardless of the physical exam findings.

Radiographs can detect occult injuries as well as past fractures. They should be taken of live and deceased animals with views starting at the head and ending at the tail.

Fractures seen on radiographs without bony callus may be acute or non-acute fractures. Palpation may reveal non–bony callus indicative of an older fracture. Some fractures cannot be palpated and the callus may be detected only on necropsy exam (Fig. 3.2). The time for healing of a fracture is variable depending largely on the degree of displacement, stability of the fracture, and age of the animal. With rib fractures, the surrounding rib cage serves as a stabilizer to allow these fractures to heal, even though there is a good bit of movement with respiration. A minimally displaced rib fracture can be expected to heal in 8–16 weeks.

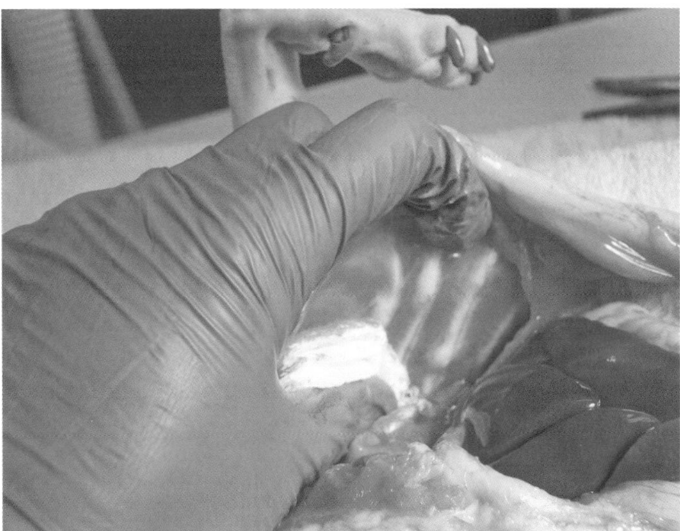

Fig. 3.2 Older, healing rib fracture. For color detail, please see color plate section.

Radiographs also can be useful in poisoning cases in which it is suspected that tainted food is source of the poison. Most fish-flavored commercial cat food contains bits of bone. If the radiographs reveal bits of bone in the stomach or intestine and the cat is not normally fed this type of food, it is indicative that the cat ate a foreign food source that may have been the source of poison. The same scenario applies to dogs or cats if bone-containing chicken or beef was used to poison the animal.

Samples

With any cruelty case, a sample of the animal's DNA and fur of each color should be collected and held. Further into the investigation testing of these samples may become critical for the case. A fecal sample should be obtained from the animal for parasite testing, DNA, or other tests (see Chapter 4). In starvation cases, it is important to inspect the feces in the first 24 hours for evidence of what the animal had recently ingested, such as foreign material resulting from pica. For suspected poisoning cases, the veterinarian should collect any vomitus, blood, and urine for possible testing (see Chapter 10). Blood and urine should be taken in all cruelty cases prior to any treatment and held in refrigeration until a decision is made regarding any testing.

Clinical Pathology

All suspected victims of animal abuse should have a minimum data base of blood work performed. This can help to detect underlying problems and contributing causes, and confirm physical exam findings. It is important to rule out infectious diseases such as parvovirus or feline leukemia. Opposing stimuli present in the animal from other conditions or disease processes may cause variation in the laboratory results. Stress, inflammation, dehydration, and fasting (starvation) can all influence laboratory values and are common conditions in animal cruelty cases.

Stress is a common cause of mature neutrophilia along with lymphopenia and eosinopenia. The expected stress-induced changes may not be seen on every laboratory results. In dogs, mild to moderate monocytosis may be seen. In cats, it is common to see neutrophilic leukocytosis in response to fear or excitement such as with struggling or exercise. This is because of the marginal pool of neutrophils that are shifted to the circulating pool. Cats have a much larger marginal pool than dogs, which can cause a significant physiological leukocytosis (three marginal neutrophils to every one circulating neutrophil). Cats also can have pronounced transient lymphocytosis in response to the same stimuli because of the lymphocytes' ability to divide and recirculate between blood and tissues (Latimer and Tvedten 1999).

Monocytosis is found in approximately 11 percent of hospitalized cats and 30 percent of dogs. Monocytes serve to replenish macrophages in tissues. Monocytosis may be seen in acute and chronic disease processes, although they are considered a later component of the inflammatory response. Stress can cause monocytosis. Severe stress is normally the cause of lymphopenia and eosinopenia. With monocytosis in the absence of lymphopenia and eosinopenia, inflammation or tissue destruction should be suspected (Latimer and Tvedten 1999).

Inflammation can cause leukocytosis, neutrophilia with or without a left shift, and toxic neutrophils (Burkhard and Meyer 1995). Acute inflammation (septic and nonseptic) usually causes neutrophilia. Chronic inflammation usually has minimal to absent left shift and minimal to absent leukocytosis. The leukogram may be normal with mild, chronic, or surface inflammation, such as with cystitis (Latimer and Tvedten 1999).

If an animal does not eat for 48 hours or longer, then ketogenesis occurs. Dogs and cats use ketones efficiently so ketoacidemia does not usually occur. If ketonuria or ketoacidemia is present, then diabetes mellitus or liver failure may be the underlying cause. The serum bilirubin, alanine transaminase (ALT), aspartate transaminase (ASP), and sulfobromophthalein retention time (BSP) may be increased because of liver gluconeogenesis. Blood urea nitrogen, urine specific gravity, glomerular filtration rate, and serum phosphorus may be decreased because of decreased protein consumption. Plasma potassium may be decreased because of the increased aldosterone secretion that occurs with food deprivation (Bartges and Osborne 1995). With prolonged starvation, there are several laboratory changes caused by the consumption of muscle protein to meet energy requirements (see Chapter 11).

Dehydration causes decreased glomerular filtration and the urine specific gravity may be increased. The animal may be azotemic because of dehydration. Total protein, sodium, chloride, and potassium may be increased because of dehydration.

Blood Loss Calculation

The amount of blood lost by an animal because of injury is an important measurement for a criminal investigation. This can be calculated from the animal's hematocrit or the environment (see Chapter 2). In response to acute blood loss, the body draws fluid into the blood vessels over time to maintain the blood pressure. The accuracy of the initial hematocrit depends on the time elapsed and the administration of resuscitative fluids. If the total protein is normal, then not enough time may have elapsed for the body to respond to the blood loss. A calculation of the volume of blood loss may be made using the current hematocrit, the normal blood volume, and the standard hematocrit for the species.

$$(\text{Normal Standard Hct} - \text{Current Hct}) \div \text{Normal Standard Hct} = \text{Fractional Blood Loss}$$

$$\text{Fractional Blood Loss} \times \text{Animal's Normal Blood Volume} = \text{Blood Volume Loss}$$

Parasites

When conducting an exam on a live or deceased animal, it is important to look for, identify, and address heartworms, intestinal parasites, or ectoparasites. Parasites are usually easily prevented and treated and are normally addressed with routine veterinary care, especially in young animals. They can cause stunted growth and disease, which may become life threatening. Several parasites have zoonotic potential posing a significant health risk. For each parasite, it is critical to document what the treatment for the infestation would have entailed and what preventative measures should have been taken. If possible, the veterinary records should be obtained and examined for any notations regarding recommendations of prevention or treatment of parasites.

Roundworms

Roundworms in dogs *(Toxocara canis* and *Toxascaris leonina)* and cats *(Toxocara cati* and *Toxascaris leonina)* are very common and are a potential zoonotic risk. They can become infected after directly ingesting the ova or through an intermediate host. The animal can also become infected though the mother either via transmammary or transplacental passage. The larvae can migrate through the tissue causing hepatic fibrosis, and pulmonary or even brain lesions. The worms live in the small intestine and cause inflammatory infiltrates in the wall of the intestine such as eosinophils. They may enter the stomach and sometimes are found in the vomitus. Roundworms may cause diarrhea, poor hair coat, poor weight gain, and stunted growth especially in young, growing animals. If they are severely stunted, they may never reach their normally expected size even with treatment. If there are a high number of roundworms they can cause obstruction of the bile duct or the small intestine (Willard 2003). The ova may be found on fecal examinations but in cases of tissue migration clinical signs may be present prior to ova production (Willard 2003). The eggs are extremely hardy and may remain in the environment for prolonged periods of time.

Whipworms

Whipworms *(Trichuris vulpis)* are found primarily in the eastern United States. They infect animals when the ova are ingested and subsequently they attach themselves to the mucosa of the colon and cecum. The ova can persist in the environment for long periods of time. They can infect dogs and cats, although whipworms are much less common in cats and do not seem to produce as severe symptoms as trichuriasis in dogs. Whipworms can cause mucosal inflammation, bleeding, and intestinal protein loss. They can cause a mild to severe colonic disease, including hematochezia and protein-losing enteropathy. In severe cases they may cause hyponatremia and hyperkalemia, which may be misinterpreted as indicative of hypoadrenocorticism. The hyponatremia may become severe enough to cause central nervous system signs such as seizures (Willard 2003). Whipworm ova are shed intermittently, require proper flotation solutions because of their density, and may be missed on fecal examination. They may be found on necropsy in the cecum or colon.

Hookworms

Hookworms (*Ancylostoma* spp. and *Uncinaria* spp.) are more common in dogs than cats and pose a zoonotic risk. The animal becomes infected through ingestion of the ova, transcolostral transmission, or newly hatched larvae may penetrate the skin. The adult worms attach to the small intestinal mucosa ingesting mucosal plugs or blood depending on the worm species (Willard 2003). They also may be found in the colon in severe infestation. Young infected animals may develop life-threatening blood loss or iron-deficiency anemia. They also may have melena, diarrhea, frank fecal blood, stunted growth, and/or failure to thrive (Willard 2003). If they are severely stunted, they may never reach their normally expected size even with treatment. Hookworm infestation should be strongly considered in any young animal that has iron-deficiency anemia without the presence of fleas. In older dogs that have other intestinal problems, hookworm infestation may contribute to the disease. They also may have prolonged clotting times in severe cases. Hookworm ova may be found on fecal exam. There have been rare occurrences in which 5–10-day-old puppies died because of exsanguination from massive transcolostral infection prior to ova production (Willard 2003).

Tapeworms

Tapeworms (*Dipylidium caninum* and *Taenia* spp.) can infect dogs and cats. They become infected through ingestion of an intermediate host such as fleas, lice, or wild animals. They may cause minimal symptoms, such as anal irritation from the passage of the segments. They may cause vomiting or intermittent loose stool, commonly with fresh blood. Tapeworms also may contribute to other gastrointestinal disease, such as inflammatory bowel disease. With heavy tapeworm burdens, they may cause intestinal obstruction, especially in younger or smaller animals. The parasites usually are diagnosed by visualization of the segments on the perineal area or on the outside of the feces. *Taenia* spp. ova may be seen on fecal exam. The eggs of *D. canis* are not usually seen unless the segment breaks apart.

Strongyloidiasis

The parasite *Strongyloides stercoralis* may be seen in puppies living in crowded conditions and is a zoonotic risk. Infected animals are usually systemically ill and have severe mucoid or hemorrhagic diarrhea. They also can develop verminous pneumonia if the parasites penetrate the lungs (Willard 2003). The parasite produces motile larvae that can penetrate skin and intestinal mucosa, causing re-infestation prior to defecation of the larvae within the feces. The larvae are detected in fresh feces by direct examination or Baermann sedimentation (Willard 2003).

Fleas

Fleas are ectoparasites that can cause severe skin disease, tapeworms from ingestion, life-threatening anemia, and act as a vector for blood parasites in both dogs and cats. With the development of safe veterinary topical flea control products, animals that go outside or live predominantly outside should not develop a flea infestation problem. Fleas also feed on human blood if there is not enough animal surface area or animal blood available. Fleas can drain enough blood from feeding to cause life-threatening anemia, especially in young or debilitated animals. They can cause severe skin allergy and secondary bacterial skin infections. Fleas are an intermediate host for tapeworms and if ingested cause tapeworm infestation. They also can carry blood parasites (e.g. *Mycoplasma hemofelis*), which may cause other diseases.

Heartworms

Heartworms *(Dirofilaria immitis)* can infect both dogs and cats causing significant disease. In dogs, they can develop pulmonary hypertension (cor pulmonale), occlusion of heart and pulmonary vessels (caval syndrome), emboli, and right-sided congestive heart failure. The dogs may be asymptomatic or exhibit signs of fatigue, exertional dyspnea, syncope, shortness of breath, coughing, or hemoptysis. They may have weight loss and have poor body condition. They may show signs of right-sided heart failure, such as jugular distention and ascites. In severe pulmonary arterial disease and thromboembolism, they can cause epistaxis, thrombocytopenia, disseminated intravascular coagulation, or hemoglobinuria. In some dogs, aberrant worm migration can cause other related signs to the area of migration such as hind limb lameness, paresthesia, and ischemic necrosis (Ware 2003).

It has only been recently recognized that heartworms pose a significant threat to cats, even though they are usually only infected with 1–10 heartworms. In cats, heartworms may cause lethargy, vomiting, coughing, dyspnea, syncope, or sudden death. In most cases, cats are completely asymptomatic or the signs are so subtle they often go unnoticed. Neurological signs may occur with aberrant worm migration, including seizures, mydriasis, blindness, dementia, hypersalivation, ataxia, and circling (Ware 2003).

Heartworm prevention has been a primary focus of the veterinary community for a very long time and there is an expected level of knowledge from the pet owner. If heartworms are found during a necropsy exam of a dog, it is important to count the number of heartworms present in the heart and vessels. Tissues of the lungs, vessels, heart, and liver should be submitted for pathology to document microscopic changes and damage possibly caused by the heartworms.

Forensic Necropsy

Overview

The difference between a necropsy and a forensic necropsy is in its objectives and relevance. In addition to determining the cause of death, the goal is to establish the manner of death (non-accidental, accidental, natural, undetermined), any contributory causes, and the time of death. Because of the medicolegal implications of the forensic necropsy, all findings and lack of findings must be documented. The lack of findings can aid in the determination of the causes of injury. The forensic necropsy exam is a process of documenting all injuries and the unremarkable findings, interpretation of how the injuries occurred, and the determination or exclusion of other contributory or causative factors. To fully integrate and properly interpret all the findings, consideration must be given to information provided about the scene from the investigators and all test results. It is important that the veterinarian know all the circumstances leading up to and surrounding the death prior to performing a necropsy. All interviews should be in a written report and provided to the veterinarian.

The forensic necropsy actually begins at the scene. There should be a diagram or photographic documentation of the scene, preferably both. At the scene the body should be touched and moved as little as possible to prevent destroying evidence and avoid contamination. Paper bags should be placed on the feet and the body preferably wrapped in a clean white sheet and then placed in a clean body bag or plastic bag for transport. The body should be placed under refrigeration and never frozen. Freezing destroys the microscopic architecture of the tissue making histopathology useless.

Full body radiographs, including the head, legs, and tail, should be performed on the animal. This is to look for fractures, internal abnormal findings, and other hidden evidence of injury. This is especially important in penetrating injuries and gunshot cases. There may be external evidence of bullet exit wounds that is actually caused by bone fragments or a piece of the bullet. With the use of semi-jacketed ammunition, the lead core may exit the body but the jacket will remain in the body, which is the forensically important piece of evidence.

Gross Necropsy

A complete necropsy must be performed in cases in which the cause of death is not known. The gross appearance of the animal and internal organs should be documented with photographs as previously stated and with written detailed descriptions (see Appendices 6–20). The body should have measurements taken from the muzzle to rear; height to the head, shoulders, and pelvis; and the width and height of the muzzle and head.

External Exam

The body should have been wrapped in a clean white sheet and/or body bag for transport. If radiographs are to be taken (to document gunshot wounds, fractures, and foreign material in stomach/intestines) they can be made while the animal is still in the body bag. Any bags or material that the body was wrapped in should be examined and saved. Photographs should be taken of the unopened bag, after the bag is opened and during the necropsy procedure to document any lesions or changes. The feet should have been covered with bags and secured to prevent loss and contamination of evidence. These bags should be removed for examination of the feet. Each bag should be labeled with the foot it was removed from, by whom, the date, and time. Each bag should be placed in a separate evidence bag and saved for laboratory analysis.

The external examination of the body should include careful examination for trace evidence (see Chapter 4), fibers, ligature markings, blood, parasites, fecal material, chemicals, oils, bruising, cuts, scrapes, and foreign bodies. The general body condition should be documented and degree of dehydration (if present) noted. The presence and location of rigor and lividity should be noted. Any missing body parts should be documented. The hair coat condition, areas of alopecia, crust formations, ectoparasites, contusions, and presence of swellings should be recorded. An otoscopic and eye exam should be conducted to look for evidence of trauma. Discharges from mouth, nose, rectum, prepuce, vagina, and ears should be examined and cultured. Any odors from the body (decomposition, motor oil, insecticides, feces, etc.) should be described. The temperature of the body should be recorded. If the body was previously frozen this should be noted in the record. Mucous membranes, mouth, ears, genitalia, rectum, and vulva should be examined for normal or abnormal color, ulcerations, prolapses, foreign objects, etc. Penetrating wounds should be probed and the extent or depth noted. Bones and extremities should be palpated for fractures or masses. Feet and nails should be examined for damage and particles of evidence collected. Any external parasites and larvae should be collected and preserved according to the instructions in Chapter 14.

Necropsy Technique

The necropsy should include an examination of all the internal organs with collection of samples for histopathology, microbiology, virology (FA testing), parasitology, clinical pathology, and toxicology. The body or specimen should be placed on its left side with the feet facing the veterinarian. An incision is made through the skin on the midline from the tip of the chin to the rectum, avoiding the penis. The skin is dissected away from the body, exposing the underlying subcutaneous tissue and muscle. The right front leg should be grasped and lifted. Cut all muscles between the subscapular area and the rib cage to free the limb and either lay the leg back on the table or remove it entirely from the body. Examine the prescapular and axillary lymph nodes for location, size, and color. The hind limbs can be cut at the coxofemoral articulations to allow them to lie flat on the table. The body should be examined for hemorrhages, fractures, body condition, fat atrophy, and amount of autolysis. Fractures, lacerations, puncture wounds, and any lesions should be photographed and measured.

A routine necropsy procedure should be followed. Reflect the skin from the body. To open the abdomen make a shallow incision through the abdominal muscles and peritoneum adjacent to the last rib. Lift the opening and continue to enlarge it to the xiphoid cartilage of the sternum. Continue to enlarge the opening dorsally and then caudally. Note any fluid, blood, or foreign objects in the abdomen. Examine the abdominal cavity for any abnormalities, such as organ displacements, torsions, color of internal organs, and size of organs. Note if the diaphragm is intact. Puncture the diaphragm and listen for the presence of negative pressure.

Next, cut deeply into the submandibular muscles close to the inner rims of the mandibles. Dissect around the tongue and retract the tongue and disarticulate the hyoid bones. Examine the tonsils, palate, and mouth. Lift the tongue backward toward the chest and dissect the trachea and esophagus back to the thoracic inlet. In cases of suspected trauma to the neck the tissue around the esophagus, trachea, and neck in general is examined thoroughly prior to removal of the tongue/trachea/esophagus as just described.

To remove the ribs use pruning shears or rib cutters by cutting along the costochondral junctions from the last to the first rib. Detach the wall of the rib cage by cutting along the neck of ribs to expose the internal thoracic organs. Note the position, color, texture, and size of the lungs and thoracic tissues. Palpate the lungs for any nodules or firmness. At this time samples can be taken or the organs can be removed to a necropsy table for individual examination. The esophagus and trachea should be opened and the mucosal surface examined. White foam (edema fluid), fluid, or aspirated food should be documented and sampled. Samples of all organs (trachea, esophagus, thyroids, lungs, heart, lymph nodes, stomach, pancreas, duodenum, ileum, jejunum, colon, adrenals, kidneys, urinary bladder, liver, ovaries/uterus/testicles, spleen, muscle, bone marrow, skin, and brain) should be placed in 10 percent buffered formalin. Remember to section completely through the tissue. For example, the kidney samples should include from the cortex down through the renal pelvis. The intestines should be opened to examine the contents and the mucosal surface. Abnormal areas of any organ should be sampled in addition to more normal adjacent areas. Remember to have adequate formalin in the containers for the amount of tissue for adequate preservation (one part tissue to 10 parts liquid).

The skin of the head should be dissected and reflected to examine for any evidence of trauma or wounds. The head can be disarticulated from the spinal column, thus allowing for removal of the dorsal portion of the skull prior to removal of the brain. It is usually best for a university necropsy service to perform the internal cranial exams. The laboratory should be contacted regarding submission of the head and/or brain.

Additional samples from any wounds, lungs, trachea, intestines, kidneys, liver, spleen, skin with fur attached, feces, and half the brain should be placed in individual containers to be held for cultures, toxicology, or further testing. Stomach contents and urine should be saved in glass or leakproof containers for toxicology. The femur can be cracked to allow the formalin to penetrate the tissues better during fixation. Remember to save a portion of the bone marrow frozen for possible fat analysis.

The history provided with the case may indicate that additional tissues should be taken. An example would be a death thought to be caused by strangulation in which tongue, larynx, neck muscle, and surrounding tissues should be saved in formalin after photographing. Additional samples of areas of possible bruising or imbibition should be placed into formalin to help distinguish between the two and help document evidence of trauma or healing, if present. If there is evidence of previous fractures noted by callus formations or more recent fractures, these should be examined and preserved for microscopic examination. Fractures should be examined to determine if they were antemortem or postmortem. This involves examination for tissue damage, hemorrhage, and trauma to the area. If adult heartworms are present, their numbers should be counted or estimated (if too numerous to count).

With a necropsy it is important to document both the normal and abnormal findings. Sample collection is needed to document any abuse but also to document any underlying conditions, such as heartworms, intestinal parasites, parvoviral enteritis, panleukopenia, cachexia, etc.

Antemortem vs. Postmortem Injury

To determine whether a wound was antemortem or postmortem requires gross and/or microscopic exam. Traditionally, the presence of hemorrhage is indicative that the heart was still beating when the injury occurred and indicates antemortem injury. However, there is the possibility of postmortem hemorrhage associated with postmortem trauma. In humans, this may be seen when the vitreous is withdrawn from the eye using a syringe and needle. If there is a sufficient survival time after the injury prior to death, it is possible to see evidence of an inflammatory response in the injured area with histopathology examination. In humans, this may take several hours (Di Maio and Di Maio 2001).

Histopathology of the wounds may reveal if there was vital reaction to the wounds, indicating antemortem trauma. The precise timing of the repair process is variable depending on the size of the wound and whether or not it becomes secondarily infected. However, usually within 24 hours neutrophils appear at the margins of the wound and fibrin clot. Within 24 to 48 hours there is proliferation and migration of epithelial cells to begin to fuse the incision. By day 3 the neutrophils generally have disappeared and been replaced by macrophages. Granulation tissue invades the wound and by day 5 has filled the wound. The surface epithelium is back to its normal thickness with a mature epidermal architecture with surface keratinization. During the second week there is continued proliferation of fibroblasts and collagen.

The analysis of enzyme activity at the wound site using histochemistry, enzymology, and biochemistry can help differentiate antemortem vs. postmortem injury in humans. Enzyme activity can be detected up to 5 days postmortem and also can be used to date the injury. In antemortem wounds, there is a zone of increased enzyme activity at the periphery that occurs over a set time interval for different enzymes. Other markers, such as DNA, C3 factor, catecholamines, and vasoactive amines have been used; histamine and serotonin are elevated in antemortem wounds (Di Maio and Di Maio 2001).

Therapeutic or Diagnostic Wounds

When an animal has been treated at a hospital prior to death, it is vital to get a history of the procedures that were performed, including any resuscitative measures.

Wounds that result from hospital procedures may be misinterpreted as injuries. The original wounds may have been obscured or obliterated by surgical procedures, they may have been used for chest tubes, or resuscitation may have caused additional injuries. It is important to find out if the animal was euthanized and the route used to administer the solution, as it could affect the necropsy finding. A full medical history is needed, including all medications administered and the time they were given. All tubes, intravenous lines, and drains should not be removed upon the death of the animal until a necropsy is performed.

Decomposition

Decomposition is a term used to refer to the processes of putrefaction and autolysis. A study of decomposition of small pigs was conducted in Virginia by the FBI's National Center for the Analysis of Violent Crime in 1998. Five small pigs, less than 30 pounds, were placed in different environments: surface deposit, no covering; surface deposit covered with tree branches and deadfall; enclosed in a roll of carpet; shallow grave of less than 1 foot; suspended by a rope from a tree approximately 2.5 feet above the ground. The pigs were deposited in late May and monitored for 75 days. The temperatures averaged from the 60s to the 80s and 90s Fahrenheit. Their observations found that pigs rapidly decompose. In all the pigs except the hanging pig, the soft tissue was almost completely consumed, leaving the skeletal components by day 12. The hanging pig was more protected by scavenging and insect activity. It was most exposed to the sun and wind, causing rapid desiccation and mummification and preserving the skeletal elements. The majority of scavenged skeletal elements were recovered within 15 feet of the original body location (Morton and Lord 2002).

The severely decomposed, skeletonized, or burnt body should be handled very carefully and samples taken for possible testing. The remaining body should be photographed, measured, weighed, and radiographed. Radiographs may reveal gunshots or broken bones. Depending on the decomposition, samples of kidney may reveal ethylene glycol poisoning. Stomach contents may still be positive for poisons. Examination of bones may reveal evidence of trauma. Samples should be saved for DNA testing (see Chapter 4).

Non-tissue Sample Collection

In humans there is an autopsy protocol for collection of fluid specimens from the body. Always use a clean needle and syringe. Place blood, stomach contents, urine, bile, and vitreous in glass containers. Plastic polymers can be leached out by these fluids, which can cause interference on gas chromatography; their peaks can mask certain compounds. Blood should be attempted to be collected from peripheral vessels for toxicology testing because of redistribution artifacts that are possible when taking blood from near the heart (Di Maio and Di Maio 2001). In descending order of preference the locations are: the femoral vessels, subclavian vessel, root of the aorta, pulmonary artery, superior vena cava, and heart. The blood should be placed in a glass tube (red top tube, purple top); if blood is to be analyzed for volatiles, the blood should be put in a tube with a Teflon-lined screw top because volatiles can diffuse through a rubber stopper. All the vitreous should be collected; all the urine (large quantities are needed for certain drug testing, i.e. steroid screens); and 10–20 ml of bile (Di Maio and Di Maio 2001). Always collect sample of fur of each color with roots to hold for DNA; take muscle and freeze for future DNA testing. The bone marrow can be tested for feline leukemia virus. The spleen and small intestine can be tested for parvovirus.

Vitreous

In humans, the vitreous of the eye may be analyzed for antemortem toxicology and certain disorders. The aqueous is commonly used in large animals. The vitreous is acellular, less susceptible to biochemical changes, and more resistant to decomposition than blood. In humans and dogs, the vitreous can be analyzed for electrolytes postmortem. The postmortem blood concentrations change because of cellular breakdown. Most antemortem electrolyte abnormalities are reflected in the vitreous. Elevated sodium and chloride may be seen with dehydration. The potassium levels are inaccurate for hyperkalemia because of the potassium released postmortem. The measurement of this potassium release is helpful sometimes in determining time of death (see Chapter 14). Hypokalemia may be reflected in the vitreous but this is uncommon because of the postmortem rise of potassium masking the antemortem hypokalemia. In addition, decomposition can lower the sodium and chloride levels. If the potassium level is 15 mEq/L or higher, then the concurrent sodium and chloride levels are of questionable value (Di Maio and Di Maio 2001).

The blood urea nitrogen and creatinine levels are reflected in the vitreous of humans. With normal renal function, elevated urea nitrogen, along with increased sodium and chloride, are indicative of antemortem dehydration. In uremia the vitreous urea is elevated as well (Di Maio and Di Maio 2001).

The vitreous glucose levels of humans have a wide range (0–180 mg/dl) and are significant if elevated. Vitreous bilirubin, alkaline phosphatase, SGOT, and calcium are of no value diagnostically (Di Maio and Di Maio 2001).

The vitreous is also useful for toxicological analysis in humans. The vitreous can be tested for a variety of drugs, including cocaine, morphine, propoxyphene, and tricyclic antidepressants (Di Maio and Di Maio 2001).

Mulla et al. showed that in humans there is no significant difference for potassium, sodium, chloride, or calcium levels between the same pair of eyes at the identical postmortem intervals for different subjects (Mulla 2005). It is recommended to analyze the vitreous as soon as possible because prolonged storage, either refrigerated or frozen, can affect the concentration of electrolytes. To collect the vitreous, use a 12-ml syringe and needle; perform a scleral puncture on the lateral canthus; and aspirate gently, avoiding tearing loose tissue fragments surrounding the vitreous chamber. Only use clear fluid for analysis and do it within 1 hour for the most accurate results. In the Mulla et al. study they centrifuged the sample at 2,050 g for 10 minutes. To analyze potassium, sodium, chloride, and calcium they used the Beckman Coulter LX 20 Automated Analyzer, which uses ion-selective electrode methodology (Mulla 2005).

Handling the Body after Examination

Before disposing of the body, remove all collars and hold as evidence even though pictures were taken. One never knows if further testing of the collar will be needed or an issue of identification arises for which the collar may be needed. Refrigerate but do not freeze the body until all samples are taken and results are in to make sure there is no need to examine the body further. Do not dispose of the body until the prosecutor authorizes or the investigation or the case is closed.

Special Considerations

Bodies in Bogs

Bog bodies refer to human and other mammalian remains found in wetland peat deposits. These are composed of a stagnant water source and microbial activity. The remains buried in bogs undergo different decay and changes than bodies in other environments. The epidermis is lost in wetland environments but the dermis is usually well preserved allowing visualization of any evidence of trauma. In addition to the outer integument, the keratin structures (nails and hair) usually are preserved as well. Collagen fibers are preserved in bog bodies. The brain may maintain its size and shape. The digestive tract may be found intact. Adipose tissue is found less commonly and the musculoskeletal system preservation is variable (Brothwell and Gill-Robinson 2002).

Bone Examination

The examination of bones may be required to identify the species, determine evidence of trauma, or possibly determine the cause of death. There are a variety of circumstances in which bone examination can be indicated such as cannibalism, traumatic injury, fire victims, and buried remains (see Chapter 2). There may be times when the species identification of the bones may be critical to the number of counts of animal cruelty with which a person is charged. Examination of human bones falls under several disciplines, such as forensic anthropology and archeology. There has been limited research on animals, primarily done in the course of applying their findings to humans. All bones, regardless of species, are similar in characteristics and responses to the environment, trauma, or modification of any kind. Veterinarians can learn from the research findings on humans and other species and apply this to examinations of dog and cat bones. The field of veterinary forensic research is ever expanding and data may be unpublished yet available from the researcher. It is important to take steps to examine and record all findings and then seek answers to unanswered questions.

For all animal cases, it should be anticipated that it may become important to identify the bones as belonging to a particular owner. Samples of the bones should be taken and held for potential DNA testing (see Chapter 4).

Pseudotrauma

It is important when evaluating bones that their excavation note the presence and location of roots in relation to the bones *in situ*. Roots can reach great depths, and acid-secreting roots can modify bone and dental enamel, causing abnormalities that can be misinterpreted as trauma. Small roots may travel through the medullary canals, splitting the shaft of bones as they expand. They may also grow, destroying articulations and occasionally penetrate the cortex of the bone. Fine rootlets may cover the surface, creating a lace-like pattern (Saul and Saul 2002). Roots may create openings in bones that may be misinterpreted as wounds caused by projectiles or other penetration trauma. Projectile entrance wounds into bone are typically smaller on the outer surface and larger on the inner surface. Exit wounds through bone usually cause the bone to bevel outward. Both entrance and exit wounds may have associated fracture patterns from the site of straight or curved lines, tapering, radiating, beveling, or concentric. Roots can cause weakening of the bone, causing more jagged and random fractures (Saul and Saul 2002). Erosions on the surface of the bone may be misinterpreted as incised defects. The grooves caused by roots usually are wavy and have rounded floors, whereas incised trauma usually has straight, often parallel grooves that are V-shaped (Saul and Saul 2002). In addition to insects and animal scavengers, roots may displace bones and artifacts. Insects and animals can create pseudotrauma and pseudopathology. Blood vessels on the surface of the bone may be misinterpreted as incised wounds. On close inspection blood vessel impressions have smooth channels and pores for branching vessels rather than the striae associated with incisive trauma (Saul and Saul 2002).

Trauma

When looking at bones, the veterinarian needs to try to determine antemortem or postmortem changes from perimortem. It is important to get a full history of the circumstances surrounding the death of the animal, the environment, and any known trauma that may have taken place. Perimortem changes or injuries, i.e. injuries that occurred at or immediately prior to death, can provide evidence regarding the circumstances surrounding the death, contributing cause of death, or weapon used. The vital reaction of bleeding from bone is a perimortem indicator and evidence of bone remodeling is indicative of antemortem injury. It is difficult to determine perimortem vs. postmortem damage to fresh or nearly fresh bone because of the moisture in the bone, which tends to respond to modification as if it were fresh (Sorg and Haglund 2002). As the bone loses moisture, is exposed to the elements, and undergoes changes caused by exposure, it becomes stained in the outer layers. At this stage postmortem vs. perimortem changes are more easily distinguished because the postmortem modifications usually disrupt the outer layers, exposing the unstained bone underneath.

Sharp Force Injury

Sharp force injury to bone can be perimortem resulting from stabbings or cuts, or postmortem, usually resulting from mutilation or dismemberment. Various tools are used to cause sharp injury, including knives and saws. Saw marks are usually postmortem, involving repetitive movements for dismemberment or mutilation. All marks on the bone should be analyzed for evidence of perimortem or postmortem injury. Usually evidence is best found in soft tissue but in cases of decomposed or skeletonized remains the bone examination may be the only source of clues. If there are cuts to the cartilaginous ends of the bone, there may be a pattern imprint related to the weapon. Any patterned injury should be preserved using casting material for tool mark comparison to any recovered weapon. Mikrosil is a rubber casting material that is inexpensive and easily used. It may be ordered from any criminal supply company in brown, which is the preferred color for tool mark examiners. Vital reaction on bone may be evidence of bone remodeling resulting from healing or bone staining from hemorrhage. Hinged, bent areas of bone indicate perimortem trauma such as elevations of slivers of bone (Saul and Saul 2002). Perimortem cuts into bone usually are the same color as the rest of the surface bone, whereas postmortem cuts usually are lighter in color than the rest of the bone. However, if the bone with postmortem cuts has been exposed to the elements for a period of time, both the surface and the cuts will be the same color such as those caused by scavengers (Symes et al. 2002).

Knives are the most common weapons in sharp-force trauma, although any instrument or tool with a sharp edge or point may be used. Knife wounds may be classed as knife-stab wounds (KSW) or knife-cut wounds (KCW). Knife-cut wounds are incisive wounds resulting from the actions of a slash, flick, tear, chop, or hack. Knives have at least one sharpened edge on a thin blade, sometimes terminating in a point, and a blade bevel (blade tapering). Other tools can be classified as knives, such as box cutters and razor blades. Blades from machines do not have a thin blade with edge beveling and tend to cause lacerations in soft tissue and possible scraping, incised injury, or fractures to the bone. The blunt side of the blade, or the spine, may cause shaving wounds to the bone. Knife stab wounds also may cause fractures (Symes et al. 2002). If a knife has a serrated edge it may cause a jagged pattern on one side of the cut bone.

Saws have teeth that cut a groove (kerf) into the bone that is defined as the walls and floor of the cut. There are different types of saws but the majority have flat-edged teeth so the cut is actually chiseling or shaving versus cutting when used. This creates a square cross-sectioned kerf floor that is larger than the blade width. Cross-cut saws have different teeth that create a W-shaped kerf floor. Saws are further characterized by the number of teeth per inch (TPI). The striae on the walls of the kerf provide information about the sides of the teeth, the shape, and the motion of the blade. The direction of the motion may be determined by examination of the kerf. There may be indicators of false starts and a breakaway spur that help indicate direction (Symes et al. 2002).

When examining bones, it must be considered that scavengers can cause similar marks that may be misinterpreted as sharp force trauma. During the processing of bones for forensic analysis, marks may be created on the bone by the tools used to remove the soft tissue of the bone. Scalpel blades are very thin and flimsy so they should be easy to distinguish from true knife cuts or stabs, but they must be addressed and documented.

Scavengers

Scavengers usually are drawn to a decomposing body as a food source. The types of animals may vary and include wolves, coyotes, dogs, foxes, opossum, birds, pigs, and rodents. It is important to avoid misinterpretation of tooth marks on bones as tool marks. It has been observed that the primary target on human remains for wolves, dogs, coyotes, and pigs seems to be the visceral contents of the body (Berryman 2002). The bones may have tooth marks of various kinds on the surface of the bone and some may be fractures. Carnivores tend to cause four different types of tooth mark artifacts: punctures, pits, scoring, and furrows. The tooth marks may be conical, which can be from the point of a knife also. Pigs tend to cause elongated and usually parallel scoring on the bone from their incisor teeth dragging along the surface, or turning the bone. They also may cause punctures to the bone. In addition to the viscera, pigs have been found to focus their scavenging on the face and throat of human remains (Berryman 2002).

Bone Modifying Effects of Water Environments

The aquatic environment can have an effect on the bones of bodies that have been placed in the water. Water that has significant current and heavy sediment can cause abrasions and round off any projections normally present on the bone. This may be caused by the sediment or the current causing the bone to abrade against other objects. These abrasions may obscure or obliterate indicators of trauma, including incisive and penetration signs. If the bones have been subjected to heavy currents where they have been forcefully pushed against solid objects, they may fracture. These signs of trauma may be difficult to differentiate from perimortem injury. Marine organisms may encrust the bones at and above the waterline. Based on the species and environment, it may be possible to establish a timeline for how long the bones have been in the water. Dissolution, which is the pitting and corrosion of the surface of the bone, may result from water environment of bioturbation, such as the erosions caused by gastropods (Haglund and Sorg 2002).

Fire Victims

In the bone analysis of fire victims, it is important to differentiate perimortem trauma from postmortem damage caused by heat and fire. The extremely high temperatures on the scene can alter non-osseous material such as glass, leather, insulation, and wood in such a way as to resemble bone. It is important to examine the bones *in situ* to determine their relationship to the fire and other evidence at the scene.

Color changes found in human bones can provide evidence of the fire temperature or duration. At temperatures <200°C the bones show a gradual darkening to dark brown; at 300°C they turn black; at >300°C the color shifts to tan and then to gray, depending on the environmental conditions. Bones burned in open air are gray by 600°C and develop a purple hue at 1,100°C. Bones burned surrounded by topsoil turn dark gray at 800°C to 900°C. Bones that are calcined in color indicate the bone was exposed to intense high temperatures for an extended period of time (Dirkmaat 2002). A fire temperature determination based on bone color changes should only be an approximation. The availability of oxygen and the insulating effects of muscle mass each play a larger role in the calcination process than the fire temperature (Correia and Beattie 2002).

References

Bartges, J.W., and C.A. Osborne. 1995. Influence of Fasting and Eating on Laboratory Values. In *Kirk's Current Veterinary Therapy XII Small Animal Practice*, ed. J.D. Bonagura, and R.W. Kirk, pp. 20–23. Philadelphia: W.B. Saunders.

Berryman, H.E. 2002. Disarticulation Pattern and Tooth Mark Artifacts Associated with Pig Scavenging of Human Remains: A Case Study. In *Advances in Forensic Taphonomy*, ed. W.D. Haglund, and M.H. Sorg, pp. 487–495. Boca Raton, FL: CRC Press.

Brothwell, D., and H. Gill-Robinson. 2002. Taphonomic and Forensic Aspects of Bog Bodies. In *Advances in Forensic Taphonomy*, ed. W.D. Haglund, and M.H. Sorg, pp. 119–132. Boca Raton, FL: CRC Press.

Burkhard, M.J., and D.J. Meyer. 1995. Causes and Effects of Interference with Clinical Laboratory Measurements and Examinations. In *Kirk's Current Veterinary Therapy XII Small Animal Practice*, ed. J.D. Bonagura, and R.W. Kirk, pp. 15–20. Philadelphia: W.B. Saunders.

Correia, P.M., and O. Beattie. 2002. A Critical Look at Methods for Recovering, Evaluating, and Interpreting Cremated Human Remains. In *Advances in Forensic Taphonomy*, ed. W.D. Haglund, and M.H. Sorg, pp. 435–450. Boca Raton, FL: CRC Press.

Di Maio, V.J., and D. Di Maio. 2001. *Forensic Pathology,* 2nd ed. Boca Raton, FL: CRC Press.

Dirkmaat, D.C. 2002. Recovery and Interpretation of the Fatal Fire Victim: The Role of Forensic Anthropology. In *Advances in Forensic Taphonomy*, ed. W.D. Haglund, and M.H. Sorg, pp. 451–472. Boca Raton, FL: CRC Press.

Haglund, W.D., and M.H. Sorg. 2002. Human Remains in Water Environments. In *Advances in Forensic Taphonomy*, ed. W.D. Haglund, and M.H. Sorg, pp. 201–218. Boca Raton, FL: CRC Press.

Latimer, K.S., and H. Tvedten. 1999. Leukocyte Disorders. In *Small Animal Clinical Diagnosis by Laboratory Methods*, 3rd ed. ed. M.D. Willard, H. Tvedten, and G.H. Turnwald, pp. 52–74. Philadelphia: W.B. Saunders.

Morton, R.J., and W.D. Lord. 2002. Detection and Recovery of Abducted and Murdered Children: Behavioral and Taphonomic Influences. In *Advances in Forensic Taphonomy*, ed. W.D. Haglund, and M.H. Sorg, pp. 151–171. Boca Raton, FL: CRC Press.

Mulla, A., K.L. Massey, and J. Kalra. 2005. Vitreous Humor Biochemical Constituents Evaluation of Between–Eye Differences. *The American Journal of Forensic Medicine and Pathology* 26(2):146–149.

Munro, H.M., and M.V. Thrusfield. 2001a. 'Battered Pets': Features That Raise Suspicion of Non-accidental Injury. *Journal of Small Animal Practice* 42:218–226.

Munro, H.M., and M.V. Thrusfield. 2001b. 'Battered Pets': Non-accidental Physical Injuries Found in Dogs and Cats. *Journal of Small Animal Practice* 42:279–290.

Reisman, R. 2004. Medical Evaluation and Documentation of Abuse in the Live Animal. In *Shelter Medicine for Veterinarians and Staff*, ed. L. Miller, and S. Zawistowski, pp. 453–487. Ames, IA: Blackwell Publishing.

Saul, J.M., and F.P. Saul. 2002. Forensics, Archaeology, and Taphonomy: The Symbiotic Relationship. In *Advances in Forensic Taphonomy*, ed. W.D. Haglund, and M.H. Sorg, pp. 71–97. Boca Raton, FL: CRC Press.

Searcy, G.P. 2001. The Hemopoietic System. In *Thomson's Special Veterinary Pathology*, 3rd ed., ed. M.D. McGavin, W.W. Carlton, J.F. Zachary, pp. 325–379. St. Louis: Mosby.

Sorg, M.H., and W.D. Haglund. 2002. Advancing Forensic Taphonomy: Purpose, Theory, and Process. In *Advances in Forensic Taphonomy*, ed. W.D. Haglund, and M.H. Sorg, pp. 3–29. Boca Raton, FL: CRC Press.

Symes, S.S., J.A. Williams, E.A. Murray, J.M. Hoffman, T.D. Holland, J.M. Saul, F.P. Saul, and E.J. Pople. 2002. Taphonomic Context of Sharp-Force Trauma in Suspected Cases of Human Mutilation and Dismemberment. In *Advances in Forensic Taphonomy*, ed. W.D. Haglund, and M.H. Sorg, pp. 403–434. Boca Raton, FL: CRC Press.

Ware, W.A. 2003. Heartworm Disease. In *Small Animal Internal Medicine*, ed. R.W. Nelson, and C.G. Couto, pp. 169–184. St. Louis: Mosby.

Willard, M.D. 2003. Disorders of the Intestinal Tract. In *Small Animal Internal Medicine*, ed. R.W. Nelson, and C.G. Couto, pp. 431–465. St. Louis: Mosby.

Chapter 4

Special Considerations in Animal Cruelty Cases

Trace Evidence

Overview

Edmond Locard (1877–1966) is considered the founder of forensic science. He developed the rule that "every contact leaves a trace," also known as the Locard Exchange Principle. This principle is based on the transfer theory that any time two or more surfaces come in contact with each other, there is a mutual exchange of trace matter between the surfaces. Although DNA answers the question of "who?", trace evidence can answer what, where, how, and when. Trace evidence comes in a variety of forms that are virtually limitless and require microscopic examination (Table 4.1). The key is that the trace evidence can be linked to a suspect, victim, scene, location, tool, weapon, or some other element of the crime.

The basis for trace evidence analysis is that persons or animals cannot visit a crime scene without leaving something of themselves behind or taking something with them. Evidence may be transferred by direct deposit or secondary transfer. Direct deposit is from direct contact with the source. Secondary transfer refers to a transfer of evidence through an intermediary person or object to an animal, person, object, or location. With secondary transfer, there is no direct contact between the source of the evidence and the surface from which the evidence is recovered. When examining an animal or the crime scene, the veterinarian and investigators are looking for evidence that can help recreate the event, link a suspect to a victim, a victim to the scene, or a suspect to a scene.

Trace Evidence on the Animal

There are some positive and negative attributes of an animal's body and behavior for retention and retrieval of trace evidence versus a human's. The animal's fur can hold embedded trace in the same manner as human hair and there is an entire body to which trace evidence can stick. However, depending on the density and length of the fur, the trace may be more easily dislodged and lost. Certain precautions should be taken to preserve any potential trace evidence on the animal. The persistence of trace is affected by the size and texture of the material being transferred, the surface on which it is retained, and how easily it may be removed. The ability to retrieve trace evidence is also affected by the length of time since the offense was

Table 4.1. Types of trace evidence.

Hair	Skin
Fur	Tape
Fiber	Tape residue
Paint	Fire debris
Chemicals	Fire accelerants
Gunshot residue	Glass
Soil	Feathers
Pollen	Plastic
Metal	Sand
Brick dust	Sawdust
Vegetation	Body fluids

committed and the activity of the suspect or victim. It should be noted that trace evidence can be found on the human body after a prolonged period of time and it can survive the environmental elements, including submersion in water. Trace has been found on the body of homicide victims weeks later, after heavy rains.

There are different considerations when looking for trace evidence on animals. The human nail has a pocket under which trace evidence may become trapped. In animals this is less likely unless the nail is frayed and the evidence is caught in the nail, the fur between the toes, or around the foot pads. Evidence on the feet can be lost easily, especially if the animal was mobile or licked the feet afterward.

It is important to consider the possible behavior of the animal during and after the assault. In response to injury, the victim may hide and/or roll around on the ground. Animals often lick at their injuries or bite at painful areas. During the assault, the animal may have responded defensively by biting or scratching the assailant. Alternatively, the suspect may have taken precautions to prevent this by using something to control the mouth and/or feet of the animal.

Collection and Analysis of Trace Evidence

It is important to have all information from the case prior to the examination of the animal. This includes what the suspect was wearing (if the information is available), any wounds on the suspect, what was present at the scene, and the different environments the animal may have been kept prior to examination. The investigator should provide the veterinarian with photographs to obtain most of this information, which helps focus the search for certain trace evidence. The veterinarian must consider all background information along with any hypothesis formed during the case assessment.

There are several other points to consider when assessing the significance of trace evidence. These include possible contamination, the transfer and retentive properties of the material, the degree of specificity and certainty attached to the identification of the material, commonness of the material, level of discrimination in material comparison, and one-way vs. two-way transfer (Houck 2001). The significance of any recovered trace evidence is based on all the information gathered from the investigation. It is important to have all this information for the laboratory to be able to decide which evidence to test and what tests to perform. It also can determine the order in which they analyze the evidence to prevent contamination. Any assessments made usually are subjective, with a high level of confidence supported by the overall data.

Proper steps should be taken to avoid contamination of evidence on the victim and at the crime scene. The veterinarian should avoid having contact with the suspect prior to examining the victim. When examining the animal, the veterinarian should wear a surgical cap, gown, mask, and gloves. The examining table should be cleaned thoroughly first and a clean sheet or white roll paper placed underneath the animal (see below).

The veterinarian must carefully examine the face, lips, teeth, legs, and feet for any obvious trace evidence. The body should be examined using a UV light source. UV light can cause certain types of evidence to fluoresce, such as bodily fluids and fibers (Fig. 4.1). An indirect light source, such as a flashlight held at an angle, can help identify especially small pieces of trace evidence. A magnifying device is useful to detect and collect evidence. The physical context of the trace evidence is paramount to the value of the results. It is important to first photograph the evidence before retrieval and document the description and location. Once removed from its original location it can never be put back exactly where it was.

All evidence should be photographed *in situ* prior to collection and packaging. To collect trace evidence, it is best to have special tools. Evidence collection tweezers are best to retrieve hair and fibers. These plastic tweezers have ridges on the tips that have increased contact with applied pressure, thus allowing a more secure grip on fine objects. Tissue, such as Kim Wipes, may be used to retrieve hair or fibers. There are evidence collection lifters with protective backers that can be used to pick up hair, fibers, dust, pollen, and other similar trace evidence. The lifter is similar to

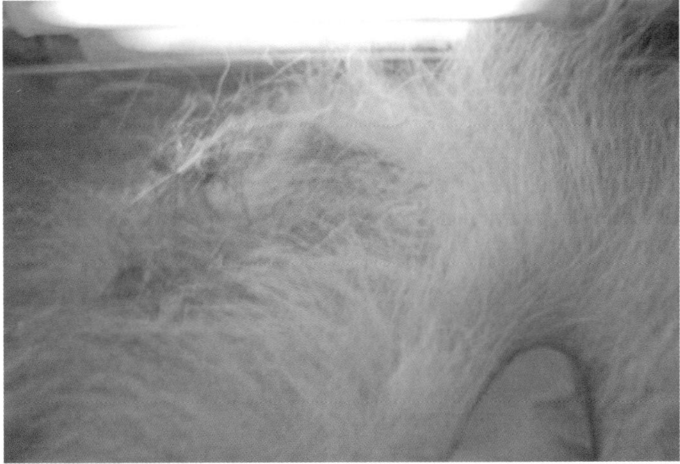

Fig. 4.1 UV light causing saliva on the fur to fluoresce. For color detail, please see color plate section.

clear tape with an adhesive side that is then pressed onto the evidence and then placed down on a vinyl cover, which is the backer. If lifters are not available, regular tape may be used and then placed on wax paper or something else with a similar slick covering. It is not recommended to fold the tape onto itself because this can cause damage to the evidence when the tape is pulled apart. Any trace evidence lifting tape should be stored in a separate container or protective packaging to prevent contamination.

Precautions should be taken not to lose trace evidence during the collection process, especially in outdoor situations, making sure wind or moving air is blocked from the processing area. Place any hair or fiber inside a paper envelope or plastic jar and label properly (see Chapter 3). All trace should be collected in separate containers. A control sample of the victim's fur should always be taken, one of each color and with the root intact, for potential comparison to other evidence related to the crime or found during the course of the investigation. Human hair is easily distinguished from non-human hair by examining the core that runs through the center of the shaft (medulla). Humans have a thin medulla and animals have a thick medulla. There are large data bases of the characteristics of animal fur that may be used for identification of fur evidence.

The animal has a huge body of fur in which trace evidence may become embedded. First the body should be inspected for any obvious evidence. Then the animal, live or deceased, should be placed on white roll paper that is taped down to the table. The animal should be combed in sections with a fine tooth comb. Any obvious trace evidence should be collected and placed in a paper envelope. Then all remaining debris on the paper should be collected and saved for laboratory analysis. Another option is to use a special evidence vacuum on the body. There are several kinds of vacuums that capture all the debris into a special filter assembly that is then sent for analysis. The nails on the animal's feet should be scraped with a scalpel or special evidence scraper over a tissue or jar to collect any potential trace evidence. In deceased animals it is best to remove the entire nail by disarticulation or cutting the nail off at the base.

In addition to fur, trace may be found on collars and leashes, bowls, toys, dog house, carriers, and anything else that can be linked to the animal, suspect, or crime. Any collar, leash, or tie-outs should be inspected for obvious trace evidence and then the item should be saved for further laboratory analysis.

When collecting tape evidence or other sticky material, it should be placed in a box lined with wax paper. Accelerants are more likely to be found by veterinarians examining a burn victim. Samples of the accelerant may be taken by swabbing the area or cutting off the fur. As with all swab samples, a control sample should be taken adjacent to the area of interest. Because accelerants evaporate quickly and are flammable, the sample should be placed in airtight non-porous containers such as non-coated paint cans or glass jars with non-plastic lids. Gunshot residue (GSR) is an important piece of evidence (see Chapter 8). It may be found in other areas than inside the wound created by the bullet. GSR may be found scattered on the body or a nearby object, or it may have ricocheted off an object. The GSR particles may be collected using lifting tape to determine their concentration and pattern, and for particle analysis.

Forensic Botany

Overview

Forensic botany refers to the forensic analysis of botanical evidence. This includes plant anatomy, plant growth and behavior, their reproductive cycles and population dynamics, and plant classification schemes to species identification. Because plant material is ubiquitous, it is often found on bodies or at crime scenes as trace evidence. The types of botanical evidence include seeds, grass stains, plant leaves, plant stems, fruit, petioles, roots, and pollen (see Forensic Palynology). Plant matter may be found in stomach contents or feces; or on fur, clothing, vegetation covering the body, or wood from a weapon. Plant material also can be associated with poisoning. This botanical evidence may be from direct contact with the plant or as secondary transfer from an object or body. Plant-derived evidence can be linked to specific locations and certain seasons. This can be used to verify an alibi, track movements of the suspect or body, aide in determination of time of death, or determine the primary crime scene in cases in which there is a secondary body dump site.

Plant DNA may be linked to a specific tree or plant. The same DNA testing performed on animal tissue may be performed on plant tissue, including mitochondrial DNA. In addition, DNA tests may be performed on specialized organelles called chloroplasts, which are more resistant to environmental insult (Budowle 2005).

Because plant matter is ubiquitous, it is important to recognize botanical evidence. The location of the evidence and the types of samples collected are dependent on the nature of the crime. It may be easier to recognize significant botanical evidence in indoor crime scenes. In outdoor or indoor scenes, botanical evidence should be compared to the surrounding plants to identify displaced leaves, seeds, or pollen that are foreign to the scene. There may be broken branches or leaves removed from a plant that may or may not be associated with the crime scene. Botanical evidence may be found surrounding the body, on a suspect, on the victim, or inside the body. The botanical evidence found may help with crime scene reconstruction based on the point of entry, travel path of perpetrator, area in which the crime occurred or site of body dump, and point of exit (Ladd and Lee 2005).

Collection of Evidence

The evidence location and condition must be documented prior to collection. Documentation should include weather conditions, photographs, sketches, diagrams, and written notes. The location of surrounding vegetation and their condition should be documented. Items such as broken branches, trampled areas, and fruit or flowering plants should be noted. A sketch should be made of the crime scene including all vegetation and a scale reference.

When collecting botanical evidence, it should be done by hand and in a manner to minimize contamination by using gloves, masks, and clean instruments or swabs. Collection should include whole plants, any fragments that may be used for a physical match, and any pieces on the body. Each sample should be packaged separately in a paper bag. Plant matter from stomach contents should be collected separately.

Any plant matter for microscopic analysis may be placed in 10 percent formalin. Fresh fecal matter that is to be analyzed for plant material should be collected in a plastic or glass jar and refrigerated. Dried feces should be placed in a paper bag.

For plant DNA testing, the size of the plant fragment can be a factor in the ability to obtain a DNA profile. A large quantity of the plant material should be recovered at the scene, taking care to prevent cross-contamination. The sample should be placed in a paper bag and stored in a freezer.

Forensic Palynology

Overview

Forensic palynology is the study of pollen, spores, and other acid-resistant microscopic plant bodies (known as palynomorphs) as it relates to matters of law. Pollen and spores are valuable forensically because of their microscopic size, are produced in vast numbers, can be identified to a plant taxon, and are highly resistant to decay (Milne et al. 2005). Pollen and spores are so morphologically complex that they can be linked to a specific plant type, site, region, or country. They are often called "the fingerprints of plants" (Milne et al. 2005). The value and significance of pollen and spore evidence are dependent on the case, types of pollen present, amount of pollen produced, prevalence of the particular pattern, and dispersal pattern. The same questions and linkages may be answered with pollen or spores as with all botanical evidence.

Because of their vast numbers and ubiquitous nature, pollen is often microscopically present on a body or object. Pollen may be found on shoes, clothing, fur, rope, carpet, and inside the nasal cavity or upper airways when inhaled. Submerged water plants also rely on pollination to reproduce. When a victim is associated with a body of water in which the submerged plants may be pollinating, the pollen may be valuable evidence.

Collection of Evidence

It is important to take appropriate samples, and anticipate that pollen and other botanical evidence may become significant later. Because pollen can be recovered from almost any surface that has been exposed to air, it is critical to prevent contamination during the collection and storage of samples. Sterile gloves should be used. All instruments should have been cleaned and stored in sealed, airtight containers prior to use. All samples should be placed in sterile, airtight containers and sealed immediately.

Control samples are needed from the scene (primary and secondary), as well as the places where the victim and suspect live or work. This supplies a baseline pollen record for later comparison to any recovered pollen of forensic interest (Milne et al. 2005). The control samples may be surface soil, mud, or water, including plant reference material associated with these areas. A minimum of 15–20 g of soil or mud samples should be collected in a glass or plastic container or sterile plastic bags. The collection of soil is done by 10–20 regularly spaced "pinch samples" (1/2–1 teaspoon) of the top 1 cm of soil by walking back and forth in a particular sampling area. All the samples are put together from that area in a container and shaken to mix. Several soils samples should be collected starting at 1–2 m^2 from the target area of the crime scene; then 50–100 m^2 for the locality sample; then 50–100 m away from the scene for a regional sample. Sample areas should include any entrance and exit points of entry to the crime scene. For water, a minimum of 0.5–1 L is sufficient (Milne et al. 2005).

Storage should be done to prevent contamination and prevent bacterial and fungal growth, which can feed on pollen and hinder analysis. Dry pollen samples can be stored at room temperature. Moist or damp samples should be refrigerated or frozen. With water and sludge samples, a small amount of alcohol or phenol should be added prior to refrigeration. Any water or soil samples may be frozen, which will not damage pollen or spores (Milne et al. 2005).

Surrounding plants and vegetation should be photographed and reference samples collected for identification. Any flowering plants should be collected. Smaller plants (<30 cm in height) may be collected intact; a 30-cm section of larger plants should be collected, leaving leaves on stems, flowers, or fruits. All plants should be placed in cardboard folders, large envelopes, or between newspaper or similar absorbent material. If plants are going to be stored for a short period, they may be placed in refrigeration. If the time period is going to be longer, the plants should be dried and pressed to preserve identifiable features (Milne et al. 2005).

DNA: Deoxyribonucleic Acid

Overview

Animal DNA has been proved to be as unique to the individual animal as for humans. Animals live in close contact with humans and animal-derived trace evidence is often found at a crime scene or on a suspect. This is crucial evidence that can link a suspect to a crime. The uniqueness of animal DNA has profound implications in all criminal cases because one in three criminals owns a cat and one in four owns a dog. This is similar to the general pet ownership statistics.

Research has shown that inbreeding in dogs does not affect the ability to match DNA to a particular animal (Halverson and Basten 2005). The results for cats show the same results. In response to a criminal case in Canada, testing was conducted on an island population of cats that were isolated and had significant inbreeding. Dr. Stephen O'Brien from the National Cancer Institute found that there was a 1:70,000,000 chance of another cat having the same genetic profile.

There are three categories of animal DNA evidence: the animal as victim, perpetrator, or witness. The animal as victim can occur in cases of animal abuse, theft of an animal, or identifying the remains of a lost pet. DNA from an animal may be matched to a weapon, toys, bedding, brushes, bowls, and other items related to the crime or animal. Situations in which the animal is a perpetrator are animal attacks, property damage caused by an animal, or an unrestrained animal causing an accident. DNA from the animal may be found on wounds, clothing, or property. In animal attacks, this testing is important to prevent innocent animals from being euthanized for aggressive behavior. The animal as a witness involves the animal's presence during the commission of a crime. The use of animal DNA has been used successively in several criminal cases to link a suspect with a crime. During the commission of the crime, there can be transfer of hair, saliva, blood, urine, or feces from the victim's animal to the suspect and/or crime scene and from the suspect's animal to the victim and/or crime scene.

Mitochondrial DNA (mtDNA) is often used when the sample of nuclear DNA is too small or degraded. The mtDNA is unique in that it is maternally inherited and shared by all along the maternal line. This mtDNA is shared with siblings and other litters born to the same mother, the mother's siblings, the mother's mom and her siblings, and so on. The mitochondria are more plentiful than nuclear DNA, making this test very important for cases in which there is a lack of usable nuclear DNA, especially when there has been an extensive decomposition of the remains.

Examination of the Animal

When examining a case of animal cruelty, one must consider what DNA evidence from the human may have been transferred to the animal. When the abuse required the proximity of a human to the animal, there will most likely have been a transfer of evidence. In addition, the animal may have bitten or scratched the assailant during the attack, retaining human DNA on the teeth or nails. If injured, the assailant may have deposited blood on the animal. It is important to consider all possible scenarios when examining an abuse victim.

The body of the animal should be examined for DNA evidence, including blood, hair, saliva, urine, and semen. A UV light should be used to examine the entire body including the feet. Any blood found should be swabbed for testing, especially if there are no obvious wounds on the animals. In knife stabbings, it is possible that the perpetrator slipped and cut his hand, leaving blood evidence on the animal. The buccal surfaces of the teeth and gums should be swabbed. In live animals, the nails should be clipped and/or scraped with a scalpel for possible skin cells from the attacker. With deceased animals, it is best to remove the entire nail (see Collection and Analysis of Trace Evidence). A control sample of the victim's DNA always should be collected for comparison testing.

Collection of DNA Evidence

General

Samples of DNA should be collected by veterinarians, law enforcement, or other authorities who can testify to the collection procedures. The DNA laboratory should be contacted prior to shipment of any samples to determine what tests will be needed, the priority of testing, and ensure that collection and submission procedures are followed. It is preferable to submit the original item of evidence for testing. Alternatively, swabs of the item may be taken when that is not possible. Clean latex or nitrile gloves should be worn during collection of DNA samples to avoid contamination.

There are four factors that affect the ability to obtain an interpretable DNA profile: sample quantity, sample degradation, sample purity, and ratio of major and minor contributors from DNA mixtures. It should be noted that usable DNA evidence has even been recovered from human fire victims. Each source of DNA requires special collection and submission procedures. Sources of DNA include fresh collected blood, dried blood stains, wet blood stains, buccal (cheek) swabs, bones, teeth, hair, feces, muscle, organs, hide, saliva, semen, and urine. In general, dry samples should be collected in a paper or manila envelope, sealed, and labeled according to proper chain of custody procedures (see Chapter 3). They should be stored at room temperature away from direct sunlight. Moist samples should be tightly sealed, labeled, and frozen.

It is crucial to collect a control sample prior to collecting the suspect sample. This reduces the chance of contamination from other materials. For this reason, the same solution must be used for both control and evidence samples when moistening the swabs. Only sterile swabs should be used for collecting evidence and each swab should be placed in a separate envelope. Care should be taken to avoid dirt or leaf material contamination, which can inhibit DNA analysis. For moist evidence, the area should be swabbed, allowed to air dry, and then placed in a paper envelope or special swab boxes. For dry samples, the swab should be moistened with sterile water or saline solution available from a drug store. The area should be carefully rubbed with the swab and then allowed to air dry.

Blood Evidence

Fresh blood collected by venipuncture should be placed into an EDTA or ACD tube, refrigerated, and shipped overnight to the laboratory. For dried blood stains, the entire object should be shipped if possible. It should be placed in a paper envelope and shipped in a non-plastic package at room temperature. Blood that is found frozen in snow or ice should be placed in a tightly sealed tube and kept frozen. For dried blood stains on absorbent material that cannot be shipped, the area should be cut from the material, placed in a paper envelope, and stored at room temperature. Swabs should be collected for blood stains on non-absorbent objects that cannot be shipped. Large wet blood stains should be swabbed. For smaller stains, the entire object should be submitted after allowing the sample to air dry.

Buccal Swabs

Buccal (cheek) swabs are a non-invasive method for collecting animal DNA samples. Swabs may be provided free by DNA laboratories. Food and water should be withheld for 20 minutes prior to sampling. The swab is placed inside the cheek and swirled 10 times collecting two swabs from each animal. The swab should be air dried briefly and returned to the provided wrapper, leaving the end of the wrapper open.

Teeth and Bone

Teeth are useful sources of DNA when the soft tissue is too degraded. The pulp of the teeth is well protected from decomposition. Viable DNA has been found in teeth up to 2 years postmortem. It is preferable to submit at least two molars in good condition without any cracks or chips. Do not clean or bleach the teeth. If there are no available teeth, then a 3- to 4-inch piece of long bone may be submitted. Do not clean or bleach the bone. Both teeth and bone samples that are wet should be wrapped to prevent fluid leakage during shipping.

Hair

Hair may be submitted for DNA testing. Pull out approximately 50 hairs from the animal, taking care to obtain the hair roots. Do not cut the hairs, and place the sample in a paper envelope. If the postmortem interval is greater than 24 hours, then hair samples should not be collected. Loose hairs found on the body, objects, or other surfaces may be collected individually and placed in paper envelopes or collected with trace lifting tape and placed in a paper envelope. Mitochondrial DNA testing can be used on hairs without roots.

Muscle, Organs, and Hide

Muscle, organs, and hide samples may be used for DNA unless it has been over 72 hours postmortem and/or the body has significantly decomposed. Spleen, muscle, and liver are good sources for DNA. The fresh tissue should be frozen in an airtight container and shipped overnight with a cold pack. Paraffin embedded tissue can be used for DNA. A 1-inch square piece of tissue should be submitted in a sealed container. Formalin fixed tissues possibly can be used if the tissues have fixed for up to 10 days.

Saliva, Semen, Feces, and Urine

Dried saliva, semen, and urine evidence may be swabbed, but it is preferred that the entire item be submitted. Fresh semen or urine should be placed in a leakproof container and frozen. At least 50 ml of urine are needed for DNA testing. Feces also can be used for DNA testing. Dried feces should be placed in a paper container. Wet feces should be collected in a leakproof container and immediately frozen.

Other Unique Identifiers of Animals

There are some other unique characteristics of animals that can be used to identify an individual animal. The most obvious identifiers are microchips and tattoos. All victims of animal cruelty should be scanned for a microchip, making sure to use a scanner that can read international chips. The body should be inspected for tattoos, which usually are located on the ears or caudal ventral abdomen. The nose print of the dog has been found to be as unique to that individual dog as a fingerprint is to a human. Footprints are not as usable unless there is something unique about the foot such as a deformity or missing toes. The pads of a cat are similar to a dog nose in that they are covered in creases and wrinkles. Future research may show that these pads may be used for identification of a particular cat. The dentition of animals has not been proved as particularly useful when used for comparison of bite marks. Recent research shows that they were unable to distinguish members of the same Family of animals by using the shape of the jaws or bite mark patterns (Murmann et al. 2006). Positive identification may be possible if a particular animal has a unique characteristic in the mouth such as a broken tooth.

Münchausen Syndrome by Proxy

Overview

Münchausen syndrome by proxy (MSBP) is a specific type of abusive syndrome perpetrated on children. The name Münchausen comes from a Baron von Münchausen, who was a reputed teller of exaggerated lies and who later became addicted to the attention from his tales. This syndrome is characterized by an adult providing falsification of illness in a proxy, the child, to deceive the medical professionals so they will believe the child is ill. In the veterinary setting the proxy is the animal. Based on fictitious symptoms, doctors may hospitalize a patient, run a myriad of tests to investigate the symptoms, and render treatment. The motive of the perpetrator is to gain sympathy and attention. In child abuse cases, a high proportion of these perpetrators have been abused as children (Munro and Thrusfield 2001).

One of the warning signs of MSBP in children is the sudden death or unusual illness of the family pet. The index of suspicion of MSBP in animals may be raised when the symptoms or signs are deliberately produced or invented by the owner; the owner initially denies falsifying or causing the symptoms or signs; or the symptoms are reduced or resolved when the pet is separated from the owner (Munro and Thrusfield 2001). There are three different stages of falsifying the illness. The first stage is "false illness story alone," which does not cause any direct harm but may cause unnecessary tests and treatments. The second stage is "false illness story plus fabrication of signs," which involves manipulating records or tampering with samples. The last stage is "induced illness," which involves causing physical harm to the animal, producing a myriad of clinical signs (Munro and Thrusfield 2001).

It is the very bizarre nature of the symptoms and the complexity of the problem that makes detecting MSBP difficult. There are several things to consider in these cases: the animal victim who is being abused; the owner, whose mental state may be unstable; and the relationship between the owner and the veterinarian, which may hinder the doctor's ability to recognize the symptoms. These owners may present themselves as very caring, nurturing, and believable while actually injuring the pet. They seem to find great emotional satisfaction when their pet is hospitalized, whereas most owners have anxiety related to this event. These owners believe that by hospitalizing their pet the doctors and hospital staff think that they are good owners. The perpetrators are often very calm when informed of the unusual medical symptoms and tests. They want diagnostic tests done and tend to be very involved with the care and treatment. They may excessively praise the staff. They may seem to have a medical background and seem knowledgeable about the pet's illness (Hanon 1991). It is important that the veterinarian does not become enmeshed with the perpetrator and then become easily manipulated. It is important to remember the perpetrator's entire motive is to receive attention and sympathy.

Symptoms

The symptoms of MSBP victims can be anything, depending on what was used to induce the illness. Because any number of things may be used to make the animal sick, the range and degree of symptoms are limited only by the imagination of the owner. One hallmark sign of MSBP for the veterinarian is when the results are very bizarre, do not fit with any clinical picture, are contradictory, or fall into the category of something an experienced veterinarian has never seen before. A study by Munro and Thrusfield found nine suspected cases of MSBP out of 448 reported cases of non-accidental injury. The features of these cases included attention-seeking behavior by the owner characterized by repeated requests for treatment; abnormal laboratory findings (electrolytes); recovery of the animal upon hospitalization (separation from the owner); interference with and breaking of an orthopedic IM pin; unexplained and suspicious circumstances of serial pet deaths in one home; serial incidents; fear of owner; frequent veterinarian changes; and admission of the deliberate injury by the owner (Munro and Thrusfield 2001).

Deliberate poisoning and suffocation then revival may be one of the forms of abuse used to induce the desired symptoms. The most common clinical signs in children include hematuria, hematemesis, seizures, central nervous system depression, apnea, failure to thrive, diarrhea, vomiting, fever, rashes, and hypertension (Munro and Thrusfield 2001). The perpetrator may add his or her personal blood or blood from uncooked meat to the urine, vomit, or even feces. Over-the-counter medications, veterinary prescriptions, the owner's personal prescriptions, salt, or chemicals may be administered to the animal, producing gastrointestinal signs, neurological signs, biochemical changes, or even death. The owner may interfere with equipment used for treatment in the hospital or sent home with the animal. If the perpetrator has access to a syringe, he or she may inject foreign substances under the skin, including bodily fluids such as feces. A feature in children MSBP cases is that the parent will shop around for physicians (Munro and Thrusfield 2001). One of the biggest clues that MSBP is the problem is the resolution of clinical signs once the pet has been removed from the owner for a period of time. The veterinarian must rule out that the environment or another individual in the home might be the source of the problem and not the owner.

Outcomes

Abuse by MSBP has high morbidity, high mortality, and high re-abuse in children. The long-term outcome is considered poor when the proxy remains with the caregiver inflicting the abuse. Of the nine cases reported in the Munro and Thrusfield study, three resulted in death and two required euthanasia. In addition, two of the cases had serial animal involvement over an extended period of time. When MSBP is suspected, the animal should be kept under constant watch and the owner should not be allowed alone with the patient. The goal has to be the safety of the victim. The perpetrator of MSBP may view the pet as a surrogate child. Although initially denying his or her actions, it may be possible to elicit a confession. Emphasis should be placed on the welfare of the animal and the possibility of a fatal outcome unless the doctor knows what was done to the animal (Hanon 1991).

Evidence

Evidence must be obtained to determine what the animal was being subjected to, administer correct treatment, and pursue criminal action. Because the perpetrators of MSBP may take advantage of any opportunity to continue the abuse and induce symptoms while the animal is examined or hospitalized, any place the owner had access to in the veterinary hospital needs to be searched for evidence. The offender may have taken certain items to use in the future, such as syringes, needles, and medications. Certain items should be collected as possible evidence and testing, including the sharps containers; trash can contents, which may contain syringes and needles or poisons; all IV lines and catheters; and all medication the owner had access to for the pet. All food and water in the cage should be inspected for evidence of foreign material, such as powders or tablet fragments; all of the food and water should be saved for toxicology tests. Any samples taken from an animal that is currently in the hospital should be collected and checked for foreign material.

Stress

Overview

Stress may be defined as an abnormal or extreme adjustment in physiology and/or behavior in response to prolonged or intense aversive stimuli (Griffin and Hume 2006). To recognize stress, the veterinarian must have an understanding and appreciation of the physical, psychological, and behavioral needs of the animal. These needs are affected and determined by the species, gender, reproductive status, age, and environment. They include proper space, ability to escape to a safe area, light, proper bedding, environmental enrichment, sanitary environment, proper food, and potable water.

An animal's response to stress is usually to develop coping behaviors such as hiding or escaping. The animal's ability to cope varies with the individual animal and type of stressor. The unpredictability of the stressor may induce chronic fear and anxiety. Depending on the severity of the stressor and the animal's coping ability, the animal may adapt over time and the stress response may no longer be activated (Griffin and Hume 2006).

The psychological impact of stress on housed cats is primarily caused by the lack of opportunity for active behavioral coping responses. The impact of the stressor is directly related to the degree the cat can exert a behavioral response to the stimulus. The most severe stress response is when the stressor is perceived as uncontrollable or inescapable (Griffin and Hume 2006). This is especially important in hoarding situations and whenever cats are housed with unfamiliar dogs.

Several factors affect the stress response, including novelty, severity, predictability, chronicity, and duration (Griffin and Hume 2006). The animal's prior experiences, socialization, personality, and genetics affect the individual stress response. Multiple stressors can have a cumulative effect. The physiological effects of stress are compounded by poor nutrition (Griffin and Hume 2006).

Physical Manifestations

Acute stress causes the release of epinephrine and norepinephrine through the activation of the sympathetic branch of the autonomic nervous system. This catecholamine release can be triggered by several different stimuli in dogs and cats. However, in cats, apprehension is the most potent stimulus for its release (Griffin and Hume 2006). Triggers for apprehension can be anything unfamiliar to a cat presented in any form, including visual, auditory, and olfactory stimuli.

Persistent stress causes the activation of the hypothalamic-pituitary-adrenal (HPA) response pathway causing glucocorticoid secretion. Under chronic stress, the glucocorticoid secretion reduces over time and the animal actually becomes more sensitized to new stressors. When a chronically stressed animal is stimulated by a new stressor, the HPA system responds. Chronic activation of these pathways can have deleterious effects on the body, including insulin resistance, mental depression, increased susceptibility to infection, peptic ulcers, decreased reproductive capacity, promotion of dehydration, and sudden death (Griffin and Hume 2006). The pathology of disease of the urinary bladder, gingiva, lung, gastrointestinal tract, and skin may be affected by the increased endothelial and epithelial permeability caused by the stress response pathways (Griffin and Hume 2006). The metabolism may be altered because of chronic stress, resulting in weight loss, lack of normal growth, and abnormal behavior that may be harmful to the animal (Griffin and Hume 2006).

Suffering

Overview

In most states, animal cruelty laws are based on the suffering of the animal. It is the degree of this suffering that may decide on how a suspect is charged, felony or misdemeanor. Suffering also has an impact on the punishment issued for a crime by a judge or jury. As veterinarians we are considered the experts on the animal's condition, including pain and suffering. A time estimate is needed for injury and the pain present because this all goes directly to suffering.

Some states have language in their animal cruelty laws stating that any injury or suffering must be physical in nature for someone to be charged with animal cruelty. Because the laws are constantly changing and issues of non-physical suffering may be allowed, at least for punishment consideration, it is important to recognize that suffering does not always come in the form of physical suffering, such as pain. Veterinarians need to recognize suffering in the form of boredom, distress, and emotional maltreatment.

Suffering has been defined as different unpleasant states that one would avoid or remove themselves from if they could (Dawkins 2005). Suffering also has been defined as an unpleasant state of mind that disrupts the quality of life. This mental state is associated with unpleasant experiences, including pain, malaise, distress, injury, and emotional numbness (Gregory 2004). This state must be either severe or prolonged. The list of causes of suffering include: hot, cold, lack of food, lack of water, confinement, space restriction, lack of social companions, lack of stimulation, injury, and disease (Dawkins 2005). There are physiological and behavioral manifestations of suffering as well: increased corticosteroid levels (stress), respiratory rate, heart rate, or blood pressure; vocalizing; and the sudden release of urine or bowels (fear reaction). These findings have to be put in context with the situation, as some of these same responses can result from pleasurable experiences.

Animals may have severe or prolonged experiences of fear, pain, hunger, boredom, thirst, and so on. To further define suffering, one needs to look for evidence that the animal is trying to or would take steps to change the situation, either by escaping or to gain access to something they want or need (Dawkins 2005). One can then compare the animal's behavior after removal from the situation to show the true suffering. It should be noted if the animal is too weak to exhibit the behavior of escape or avoidance or seek change.

Learned helplessness may occur in animals that have been subjected to prolonged abuse. Learned helplessness refers to a condition in which the animal will not escape from a negative situation even when able to do so. This occurs in animals that have been subjected to prolonged abuse without any opportunity to escape. They "learn" that they are "helpless" to change their situation. Eventually, when presented with an opportunity to escape, the animal will not do so.

Boredom

Animals have an innate need to interact with their environment, explore, and play. Confinement and lack of stimulation lead to another form of suffering, boredom, which has physical and psychological impacts on the animal. Prolonged confinement can lead to behaviors of self-mutilation, aggression to other animals, tenseness, restless, agitation; licking, sucking, or chewing at cage surfaces; coprophagy; over-grooming; or fur pulling (Wemelsfelder 2005). To recognize boredom, one must understand that the criteria are fluid and changing. The degree of boredom for an animal is most evident when one observes the behavior after the environment is changed to enriched conditions.

Distress

Consideration should be given to the distress of animals as a form of suffering. Franklin D. McMillan has offered this definition:

> Distress may be conceived as the unpleasant affective state, akin to or the same as anguish, resulting from an inability to control or otherwise cope with or adapt to the unpleasant affect generated by altered or threatened homeostasis (McMillan 2005a, p. 105).

Examples of distress are boredom, pain, thirst, hunger, loneliness, fear, and any function of how an animal copes with the unpleasant affect. The term *affect* refers to any feeling, emotional or physical in origin. Evidence of unpleasant emotions in animals are fear, phobias, anxiety, separation anxiety, loneliness, boredom, frustration, anger, grief, helplessness, hopelessness, and depression (McMillan 2005a).

Emotional Maltreatment

Emotional maltreatment refers to the link between emotional states and physical health. Emotions can cause distress, anguish, and suffering. Long-term problems associated with emotional maltreatment may be separation anxiety, decreased learning, depression, difficulty with social interactions, or even physical manifestations of illness (McMillan 2005b).

Because the idea of maltreatment in animals is analogous to children, the terminology associated with child maltreatment may be used. The US Department of Health, Education, and Welfare defines maltreatment as actions or inactions that are neglectful, abusive, or otherwise threatening to an individual's welfare (McMillan 2005b). Note that the term *maltreatment* includes both neglect and abuse. Maltreatment should be looked at from the perspective of the victim, the animal, in which the animal is harmed or at risk of harm.

Traditionally, neglect is considered to be a passive act or act of omission by the caregiver to provide basic physical and emotional needs of a dependent being (McMillan 2005b). Most animal cruelty laws include neglect as a form of animal abuse. It is estimated that greater than 80 percent of cruelty cases are classified as neglect. Customarily, neglect has been characterized by a lack of intent. Rather, neglect is considered a result of ignorance or poor judgment. However, a *reasonable person* standard should be applied to the situation. This refers to what a reasonable person would think and do in the given situation. For example, when someone does not provide food or fresh water for an animal, a reasonable person knows that the result will be death from starvation and/or dehydration.

Sometimes proving intent by the abuser is required to meet the animal cruelty statute in certain states. Physical and emotional abuse is considered an active maltreatment characterized by intent to harm. These overt acts or acts of omission also are characterized by the caregiver's knowledge that the action or inaction will result in harm to the animal (McMillan 2005b).

There are four categories of maltreatment: emotional neglect, physical neglect, emotional abuse, and physical abuse. There can be crossover of neglect to abuse depending on the caregiver's intent as well as local and state laws.

Emotional Neglect

The emotional needs of animals include social companionship and mental stimulation. The mental stimulation required depends on the age, sex, species, and specific traits of the animal (McMillan 2005b). The physical needs of animals include food, water, shelter, temperature regulation, oxygen, health care, and exercise. Failure to meet both emotional and physical needs of an animal will result in harm to the animal. An emotional need may be defined as any need that is signaled by an emotional affect (McMillan 2005b). Emotional needs of most animals include the following:

- Control: the ability to exert meaningful change to situations, especially those of an unpleasant nature
- Ability and resources to cope with aversive events
- Sufficient living space

- Mental stimulation
- Safety, security, and protection from danger
- Social companionship for social animals
- Adequate predictability and stability to life events (McMillan 2005b, p 172)

It is an accepted fact that dogs are pack animals and need social companionship. Recent research on cats confirms that they are social animals as well. Studies show that cats form close social bonds between siblings and their mother. It also was found that given an option, cats prefer to live in colonies with other cats rather than living alone.

Emotional Abuse

Emotional abuse may be defined as the deliberate infliction of emotional distress on another individual (McMillan 2005b). It includes acts of commission or omission that have caused or may cause serious behavioral, cognitive, emotional, or mental disorders (McMillan 2005b). The following categories of emotional abuse used for children may be applied to animals:

- Rejecting: emotional deprivation
- Terrorizing: deprivation of safety and security; hostility; creation of a "climate of fear"
- Taunting: causing frustration or anguish
- Isolation: deprivation of social interaction and companionship
- Abandonment: termination of care, or desertion
- Overpressuring: excessive demand to perform or achieve (McMillan 2005b)

Physical Abuse

Physical abuse can cause emotional maltreatment if it causes emotional distress. There is evidence that emotional maltreatment produces harm that is often worse than physical abuse. This is seen in children with long-term effects resulting from emotional maltreatment; there have been similar findings in dogs (McMillan 2005b). The harm depends on the animal's coping ability to the event. In animals, the long-term consequences may be seen as behavioral problems under otherwise normal conditions, similar to post-traumatic stress syndrome in humans.

Pain

It is important to recognize pain and the manifestations of pain in animal cruelty cases. Sometimes, it may be the only symptom found. Pain contributes to the animal's suffering and it is critical to document it in the records and report. Pain is something with which a judge and jury can understand and empathize, regardless of whether or not they own pets. It is a vital piece of information for the prosecution of animal abuse cases. Animals can be stoic and instinctively hide signs of pain, which makes their symptoms more subtle but their injuries no less painful.

Table 4.2. Signs of pain.

Cats/Dogs	Cats	Dogs
Increased RR	Purr, groom	Whine, whimper
Increased BP	Growl, hide	Timid, aggressive
Increased HR	Squint eyes	Fixed stare
Blanched mucous membranes (vasoconstriction)	No change of body position	Arched posture
Muscle splinting (thoracic pain)	Laying sternal, balled up	Restlessness
Stress leukogram	Decreased human interaction	
Catabolism		
Change in vocalization		
Attention seeking		
Guarding of painful areas		
Lick, chew, paw at painful area		
Change in voiding behavior		
Change in grooming behavior		

Source: Tranquilli, W.J., K.A. Grimm, and L.A. Lamont. 2004. *Pain Management for the Small Animal Practitioner.* Jackson, MS: Teton NewMedia.

Veterinarians often downplay the amount of pain an animal is in and fail to recognize and treat it. Often, the most dramatic symptom found after the fact is the change in an animal's behavior, appetite, or demeanor when the pain is alleviated. The clinical signs of pain may differ based on the species and breed of the animal. Chronic or pathological pain causes a decrease in appetite and/or drinking; decreased healing; increased risk of infection; and change in sleep patterns, behavior, and mobility or movement of the animal, all of which are adverse outcomes (Table 4.2).

References

Budowle, B. 2005. Foreword. In *Forensic Botany: Principles and Applications to Criminal Casework*, ed. H.M. Coyle, pp. vii–ix. Boca Raton, FL: CRC Press.

Dawkins, M.S. 2005. The Science of Suffering. In *Mental Health and Well-Being of Animals*, ed. F.D. Millan, pp. 47–56. Ames, IA: Blackwell Publishing.

Gregory, N.G. 2004. *Physiology and Behaviour of Animal Suffering.* Oxford, UK: Blackwell Science.

Griffin, B., and K.R. Hume. 2006. Recognition and Management of Stress in Housed Cats. In *Consultations in Feline Internal Medicine*, ed. J.R. August, pp. 717–734. St. Louis: Elsevier Saunders.

Halverson, J., and C. Basten. 2005. A PCR Multiplex and Database for Forensic DNA Identification of Dogs. In *Journal of Forensic Sciences* 50(2):352–363.

Hanon, K.A. 1991. Child Abuse: Münchausen's Syndrome by Proxy. *FBI Law Enforcement Bulletin.*

Houck, M.M. 2001. *Mute Witnesses: Trace Evidence Analysis.* San Diego: Academic Press.

Ladd, C., and H.C. Lee. 2005. The Use of Biological and Botanical Evidence in Criminal Investigations. In *Forensic Botany: Principles and Applications to Criminal Casework*, ed. H.M. Coyle, pp. 97–115. Boca Raton, FL: CRC Press.

Millan, F.D. 2005a. Stress, Distress, and Emotion: Distinctions and Implications for Mental Well-Being. In *Mental Health and Well-Being of Animals*, ed. F.D. Millan, pp. 93–112. Ames, IA: Blackwell Publishing.

Millan, F.D. 2005b. Emotional Maltreatment of Animals. In *Mental Health and Well-Being of Animals*, ed. F.D. Millan, pp. 167–180. Ames, IA: Blackwell Publishing.

Milne, L.A., V.M. Bryant Jr., and D.C. Mildenhall, 2005. Forensic Palynology. In *Forensic Botany: Principles and Applications to Criminal Casework*, ed. H.M. Coyle, pp. 217–252. Boca Raton, FL: CRC Press.

Munro, H.M., and M.V. Thrusfield. 2001. Battered Pets: Münchausen Syndrome by Proxy (Factitious Illness by Proxy). *Journal of Small Animal Practice* 42:385–389.

Murmann, D.C., P.C. Brumit, B.A. Schrader, and D.R. Senn. 2006. A Comparison of Animal Jaws and Bite Mark Patterns. In *Journal of Forensic Sciences* 51(4):846–860.

Tranquilli, W.J., K.A. Grimm, and L.A. Lamont. 2004. *Pain Management for the Small Animal Practitioner*. Jackson, MS: Teton NewMedia.

Wemelsfelder, F. 2005. Animal Boredom: Understanding the Tedium of Confined Lives. In *Mental Health and Well-Being of Animals*, ed. F.D. Millan, pp. 79–92. Ames, IA: Blackwell Publishing.

Willard, M.D. 2003. Disorders of the Stomach. In *Small Animal Internal Medicine*, ed. R.W. Nelson, and C.G. Couto, pp. 418–430. St. Louis: Mosby.

Chapter 5
Patterns of Non-accidental Injury: Non-penetrating Injuries

Overview of Blunt Force Trauma

Blunt force trauma can be the result of accidental or non-accidental causes. It is important to examine the entire animal for clues as to the incident and sequence of events. There may be evidence of repetitive abuse such as older bruises or healing fractures. External signs of bruising in animals may not be present even with significant internal injuries.

The injuries caused by blunt force trauma depend on the amount of energy delivered and transferred to the body, how it is delivered, and the body's reaction to the forces. Factors involved are the amount of force delivered, time over which the force is delivered, region struck, extent of the body surface over which the force is delivered, and nature of the weapon (Di Maio and Di Maio, 2001). When a weapon breaks or is deformed on impact, the energy delivered to the body is reduced because part of the energy was used in the break or deformation of the weapon. The severity of the injury may be reduced if the body moves with the blow, which increases the time over which the energy is delivered. Regardless of the amount of force, the larger the area over which the energy is delivered, the less severe the injury. A weapon with a broader surface will inflict less injury than a narrower weapon. If there is an object at the end of the weapon, all the energy will be concentrated at the end, creating a more severe injury. A blow to a flat portion of the body dissipates energy over a larger area than a blow to a rounder portion of the body, such as the head.

When examining a victim of blunt force trauma, there should be consideration and determination of the force required to cause the injury. This determination can be made by comparing the injuries with what is seen in other accidental or non-accidental cases. For example, the injuries sustained in known hit-by-car (HBC) victims or high-rise syndrome cases that one has seen may be used for comparison. Consultations with colleagues, especially those who work in emergency medicine, may be needed to draw on their experience. It is important to use analogies in court to explain the amount of force required to cause such injuries.

Abrasions

Overview

Abrasions involve injury to the epidermis resulting from compression and destruction of the epidermal layers or friction against a rough surface. Antemortem abrasions are red to reddish-brown in animals. In humans, postmortem abrasions are yellow, translucent, and have a parchment-like appearance (Di Maio and Di Maio 2001). Abrasions may be caused by blunt force trauma from a weapon, dragging, or crushing and tearing of the skin. Abrasions may have gross or microscopic debris embedded in the wound related to the object that caused the injury or the area in which the injury occurred. The three categories of abrasions are scrape or brush abrasions, impact, and patterned abrasions (Di Maio and Di Maio 2001).

Scrape/Brush Abrasions

Scrape or brush abrasions are created when a blunt object scrapes off the superficial layers of the skin, sometimes exposing the deeper dermal layers and causing fluid leakage from the vessels. This causes a serosanguineous fluid covering on the abrasion. When the area is incised, there usually is no hemorrhage in the underlying soft tissue, indicating the injury is confined to the epidermis. Grating or sliding abrasions are caused when the body slides across a surface such as a pavement. Ligatures, nooses, and dragging a body across a rough surface cause scrape abrasions. It is theoretically possible to find a bunching of epidermis at one end of the abrasion indicating direction of movement, but this is not commonly seen in humans (Di Maio and Di Maio 2001).

Impact Abrasions

Impact abrasions are crushing injuries caused when the blunt force impacts perpendicular to the skin. This may occur from a weapon or a fall. Impact abrasions usually affect the skin over bony prominences in which there is less underlying protective tissue.

Patterned Abrasions

A patterned abrasion shows the imprint of the weapon or surface that caused the abrasion. This may be seen with ligature injuries that leave a patterned imprint revealing the type of ligature used. In humans, intermediary material on the body such as clothing may leave an imprint from the crushing force of the weapon used.

Artifacts

Postmortem artifacts may be misinterpreted as abrasions. Insect feeding postmortem may be mistaken for abrasions (see Figure 14.2). The drying of areas of skin may resemble abrasions. Careful examination should allow the differentiation between true abrasions and artifacts.

Dating Abrasions

In humans, the dating of abrasions is possible with histological examination by documenting the stages of healing. The first stage is scab formation. The deposit of serum, red cells, and fibrin indicate survival after the injury. Infiltration of neutrophils in a perivascular formation may start in 2 hours but is clearly visible in 4–6 hours, indicating the injury is 4–6 hours old. Under the area of epithelial injury, a zone of infiltrating neutrophils in the bed of the scab is present by 8 hours. A surface zone of fibrin and red cells, followed by a zone of infiltrating neutrophils, and then a layer of damaged abnormally staining collagen appear by 12 hours. In impact abrasions, the surface zone is comprised of crushed epithelium (Di Maio and Di Maio 2001).

Epithelial regeneration marks the second stage of healing. The regeneration comes from the margins of the abrasion and the surviving hair follicles. In scrape abrasions, this growth of epithelium may appear in as little as 30 hours. In most other abrasions, it is visible by 72 hours (Di Maio and Di Maio 2001).

The third stage of healing is subepidermal granulation, which occurs only after epithelial covering of the abrasion is complete. Perivascular infiltration and chronic inflammatory cells are present. It becomes prominent during days 5 to 8. During days 9 to 12, changes in the overlying epithelium are most prominent as it forms keratin and becomes progressively hyperplastic. Collagen fibers may begin to appear (Di Maio and Di Maio 2001).

The fourth and final stage of healing is regression, which starts around the 12th day. The epithelium is remodeled, becoming thinner and atrophic. The collagen fibers become more prominent. The vascularity of the dermis decreases, and a definitive basement membrane develops (Di Maio and Di Maio 2001).

Bruising/Contusions

Overview

A contusion or bruise is an area of hemorrhage caused by blunt force trauma that ruptures the blood vessels. The size and severity of the contusion depends on the blunt force applied and the vascularity of the tissue. Because animals have a reduced blood supply to their skin compared with humans, external bruising is not as commonly seen on the surface of the skin. When it is seen in animals, it is usually caused by severe force that may not only cause bleeding in the skin but also in the underlying tissue structures. Other causes for apparent bruising include a variety of clotting disorders. In addition, the apparent surface bruise may actually result from bleeding that has followed the path of least resistance through tissue from a deeper or adjacent area of injury such as a fracture.

Contusions also may be present in the internal organs and internal body walls. The appearance of bruising may be delayed for several hours, especially if it is located in an anatomical site in which there is reduced blood supply. Therefore, continued monitoring of the live animal is essential to detect bruising. The absence of a bruise does not indicate the absence of blunt force trauma. A live animal may have suffered severe blunt force trauma but not have any external signs except for tenderness in the injured areas, which may be difficult to discern. In these cases as with all suspected cases of abuse, radiographs and blood work may reveal evidence of acute and chronic injuries.

Postmortem Findings

Postmortem exam can reveal the true extent of the bruising, which is usually quite a bit larger than what was apparent on the surface. The fur may need to be shaved to look for bruising. It is possible to see bruising even in dark-pigmented skin. Bruising may take minutes to several hours to form in animals and may fade quickly depending on the extent of damage. Photographs must be taken of the bruising pattern hourly as they form to capture the full representation. It is possible that early on the bruise may be more reflective of what caused the bruise and as bleeding continues, especially from the deeper tissue, the pattern may become obscured. The skin should be reflected over the entire body to look for subcutaneous or deeper tissue bruising.

At first appearance, contusions may be grossly difficult to differentiate from postmortem lividity (see Chapter 14). A contusion involves hemorrhage into the soft tissue and the blood cannot be wiped or squeezed out when incised. This is not the case in areas of lividity (Di Maio and Di Maio 2001). Over time, decomposition can make it extremely difficult to differentiate antemortem bruising and lividity. Hemolysis of the red blood cells creates diffuse discoloration of the soft tissue. The blood within the vessels and the erythrocyte leakage caused by the breakdown of the blood vessels from decomposition hemolyze. The erythrocytes in the soft tissue from antemortem bruising also hemolyze, making it impossible to distinguish from an area of livor mortis.

Patterned Bruising

A patterned contusion may be seen that reflects the shape and sometimes details of the object that was used to cause the bruise (Fig. 5.1). Asymmetry to the bruise may be a clue because bleeding follows the path of least resistance. Depending on the area of skin and gravity, it tends to flow from the center outward, forming irregular or blurred lines. If the contusion was caused by a weapon, it may be possible to find evidence of the tool in a bruising pattern or indentation of the skin, tissue, or even bone. If a flat object is used, there may be two parallel lines of bruising. If a rod was used, the contusion pattern is linear in shape. Rods and similar objects also can cause skin lacerations if used with enough force or if the skin is more susceptible to tearing, such as with young or geriatric animals (see Figure 6.1). The imprint of a shoe or fingertips may be seen from grabbing or holding the animal. Bruising may extend beyond the site of impact, obscuring the pattern created by the object.

It is important to find out if investigators have a suspected weapon that was used in the incident. A weapon may be identified or discovered later in the investigation, so it is important to preserve any evidence that may be linked to the offending ob-

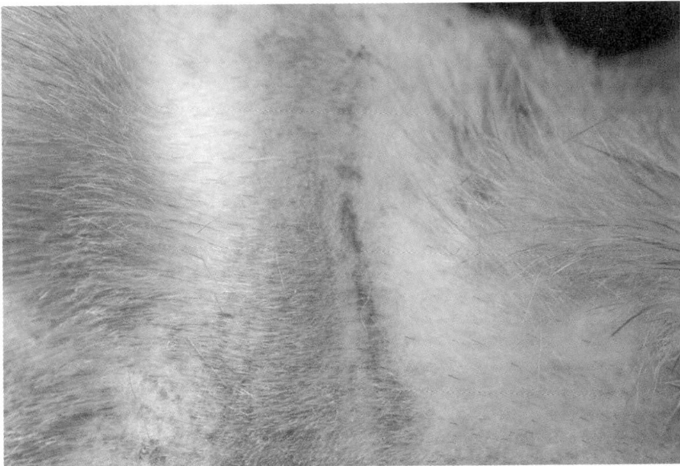

Figure 5.1 Interrupted bruising pattern caused by chain collar *(right)* and bruising from nylon collar below *(left)*. For color detail, please see color plate section.

ject for later comparison or confirmation. The patterns and indentation of the skin may fade or resolve very quickly, so it is important to take photographs immediately. A photographic scale must be placed next to the contusion for a forensic specialist to use the photograph for later comparison with a suspected weapon. For any indentations, a cast should be taken. Mikrosil is a rubber casting material that is inexpensive and easily used for this purpose. It may be ordered from any forensic supply company. It comes in a variety of colors, although brown is the preferred color for tool mark examiners.

Dating Bruising

The dating of contusions by histology has not been found to be possible in humans (Di Maio and Di Maio 2001). The healing of a bruise is dependent on the number of bruises in the area, vasculature of the injured area, amount of subcutaneous tissue and fat, type and severity of the force that caused the bruise, and any underlying disease that may impair local tissue reactions. Contusions undergo color changes over time because of the breakdown of hemoglobin, but the color change and time for change are variable. In animals, bruising initially may appear red, purple, or dark blue. As time progresses the bruise may fade and turn brown. At best, one can say the bruise appears recent or is older (Di Maio and Di Maio 2001).

It is possible to cause contusions postmortem if a severe enough blunt force is directed at the body within a few hours after death. This causes rupture of capillaries and forces blood into the surrounding tissue. Antemortem contusions that occur immediately prior to death may not have had enough time to show a vital reaction detectable by histology. If the contusion occurred antemortem with enough time for the body to mount a response, evidence of a vital reaction may be seen with microscopic examination of the injury.

Fractures

Direct Force

Fractures may be caused directly or indirectly by blunt force trauma. When a long bone is struck, it tends to bend, causing a fracture in the opposite side of the bone where there is greatest tension on the convex aspect of the bend. With significant force, crushing of the concave side of the bone can occur. Focal or crushing fractures can occur because of blunt force trauma depending on the amount of force and size of the area to which it is directed. A focal fracture results from a small force applied to a small area, usually causing a transverse fracture. The overlying tissue often has minor injuries such as contusions, abrasions, or lacerations. In the lower leg areas, where two bones are present, usually only one bone is fractured (Di Maio and Di Maio 2001).

With larger forces, a crush fracture may be produced and the overlying tissue injury usually is extensive. A variety of fractures can result from a severe impact, including oblique, transverse, comminuted, spiral, longitudinal split, segmental, tension wedge, and compression wedge. A tension wedge fracture occurs when the fracture begins at the opposite side and then radiates back at a 90-degree angle, creating the wedge. The point of the wedge indicates the direction of the force, and the base indicates the points of impact. On radiographs, tension wedge fractures may appear to be oblique fractures (Di Maio and Di Maio 2001).

The pelvic ring creates great stability of the pelvis. It requires immense force to disrupt this ring and cause fractures. Disruption of one part of the ring usually causes disruption in another part because of their strong connections.

Indirect Force

Indirect fractures are caused by the application of force distant from the fracture site. Bone is weaker to tension forces than compression forces. The classifications of indirect fractures are traction; angulation; rotational; vertical compression; angulation and compression; and angulation, rotation, and compression. In traction fractures the bone is pulled apart by traction. In angulation fractures the bone is bent, creating compression on the concave surface and tension on the convex surface, and causing it to snap. The resulting fracture usually is transverse. Rotational fractures are spiral fractures produced when bone is twisted. The direction of the spiral indicates the direction of the torque that caused the fracture. Vertical compression fractures are produced when the shaft of the long bone is driven into the cancellous end. This causes an oblique fracture of the long bone and may cause a T- or Y-shaped fracture of the end of the bone. Angulation and compression fractures have a transverse and oblique component caused by the two forces. In angulation, rotation, and compression fractures the angulation and rotation forces together produce an oblique fracture, while the compression increases the tendency toward fracture (Di Maio and Di Maio 2001).

Evidence of Long-term Abuse

The presence of multiple fractures in different stages of healing is highly indicative of repetitive abuse. There may or may not be bruising on the skin. If the fracture is acute, there will be hemorrhage from the marrow and adjacent tissue injury in the immediate vicinity of the fracture site and into the surrounding tissue. The rate of healing callus formation depends on several factors: the age of the animal, amount of displacement of the fracture site, and stability or amount of movement at the fracture site. Production of a callus begins with the external callus produced by the periosteum and the internal callus produced by the endosteum. Periosteal proliferation may be underway within 24 hours of injury. Mineralization can begin in 3 days, but this early fibrocartilaginous callus may not be visible in radiographs for 2 weeks. It may be palpated as a hard thickening but it must be differentiated from a resolving hematoma. On postmortem exam a gross and microscopic exam of the fracture area should be conducted to determine the stage of callus formation. At best, a time estimate for the fracture may be given as acute, recent, or older.

Hit-by-Car/Motor Vehicle Accident Injuries

HBC victims have characteristic injuries related to the incident. The impact of the vehicle to the body can cause several injuries depending on where the animal was hit, if the animal rolled under the car, how far it was flung, and where it landed. In addition to the blunt force injuries, the animal will have frayed nails, dirt or debris embedded in the fur or mouth, and abrasions. These are usually drag or sliding abrasions located on more than one area of the body. They are almost always found lateral on one side of the body and medial on the other side.

Primary impact injuries are caused by the first impact of the vehicle to the victim. After this, the victim may be thrown under, flung to the side or up onto the car, causing secondary impact injuries. The animal may have further injury from the undercarriage or wheels of the vehicle, and blunt force trauma from landing on the ground or on top of the vehicle. This may include head trauma, additional fractures, abrasions, debris, or glass from the site of injury embedded into the fur or wounds. If the animal had a secondary impact with the vehicle, then the final contact with the ground causes tertiary injuries. If the animal is lying on the ground and run over by a vehicle, then these types of impact injuries are not present. Instead, the expected injuries are crushing and/or flaying of the body where the vehicle contacted it.

Fall Injuries

When evaluating victims of falls, it is important to consider how the animal fell, the distance, the mass of the animal, and the animal species. In addition, it is important to know how the animal landed and if the animal could have landed on any objects. All the information regarding the fall is crucial to properly analyze and interpret the cause of the injuries.

With injuries caused by falls, it is important to consider that it was not accidental but possibly the animal was thrown or dropped by a human. If the animal accidentally fell, one would expect the animal to have frayed nails from frantically clawing at the edges before or during the fall, depending on the circumstances and surrounding surfaces. This may or may not be present in accidental falls. However, it is important to consider that the fall may have been non-accidental if the nails appear normal.

The animal should be examined for other injuries that may be inconsistent with the fall and are more indicative that the injuries occurred prior to the fall. To know what injuries to expect, it is important to know how and on what the animal landed. A fractured lower spine is not expected in a cat that accidentally fell off a one-story balcony to the asphalt. In suspected animal cruelty cases the animal always should be examined for evidence of repetitive abuse.

High rise syndrome is a term given to a complex of injuries associated with cats that have fallen from a significant height, usually 2–32 floors. The triad of injuries associated with this syndrome is epistaxis, fracture of the hard palate, and pneumothorax. Findings also can include pulmonary contusions, limb fractures, and possible bladder rupture resulting from the acute increase of intra-abdominal pressure. The hard palate fracture or split is caused by the force of the lower canines being thrust upward between the upper dental arcade.

Swinging/Dragging Injuries

It is not uncommon for animal abuse to involve swinging or dragging the animal, either by the tail or a limb(s), causing multiple injuries. Features of the resulting injuries may include abrasions, avulsion injuries (see Chapter 6), fractures, dislocations, ligament injuries, and muscle tearing. Bruising and fractures may occur when the animal is swung against an object or beaten. Dislocations of the limb joints or tearing of the limb attachments may be seen. If the scapula is completely avulsed from the thoracic wall, the scapula will protrude dorsally, higher than the opposite scapula, when the animal bears weight on that limb. Dislocation of the elbow joint, without fracture to the anconeal process, is caused by pulling and twisting the lower arm. This can indicate the animal was either swung or was hanging by that leg.

The tail of an animal is a favorite place for abusers to grab the animal. This can cause separation of the coccygeal vertebrae, usually closer to the pelvis than distally. Fractures of the vertebrae may be seen if the tail was forcefully jerked upward or to the side, or if the tail was stepped on. Contusions may be seen around the site of injury or, with injuries close to the pelvis, the hemorrhage may dissect down around the perineal region (see Figure 3.1).

Abrasions from dragging an animal usually are more circular and located over the points of the body that had contact with the ground. These abrasions usually contain embedded debris from the surface over which the body was dragged and should be collected as evidence. It is important to try to determine if the animal was alive when the injuries were sustained. All wounds should be inspected for evidence of healing or infection and submitted for histopathology in deceased animals.

Head Trauma

Overview

Traumatic injury to the head causes direct and immediate damage that is primarily mechanical in nature. These primary injuries may vary because of the force of the blow and the cause of the injury. Blunt force head trauma may result from a kick, fall, motor vehicle accident, animal fight, punch, or weapon, or be caused by the animal being thrown or swung against a structure or object. Other injuries may be found such as spinal cord injury.

The degree of brain injury depends on the acceleration, deceleration, and rotational impact forces that may cause shearing injury of the nerve fibers or diffuse axonal injury (Braund 2003). It also depends on the characteristics of the impacting object or surface, amount of force, and age of the animal. Often, the animal lacks evidence of external trauma to the head yet has severe brain injury.

Head injuries may include fractures, bone fragments embedded within the brain tissue, edema, ischemic laminar necrosis of the cerebral cortex, lacerations, contusions, hemorrhage within the brain parenchyma with focal or multifocal necrosis, and intracranial hemorrhage. There may be epidural, subdural, subarachnoid, and intraparenchymal hemorrhages (Fenner 1995). There are also species differences related to the type of head injuries sustained from blunt trauma. Head trauma injuries in cats usually involve mandibular symphyseal fractures, hard palate separation, and other maxillary injuries.

Blunt force trauma to the head may cause damage to the central nervous system (CNS) or peripheral nervous system (PNS) or both. The animals that sustain CNS damage are defined as having craniocerebral trauma (CCT) and may have reversible or irreversible injuries. Patients with PNS injury usually have a better prognosis of survival and less chance of serious sequelae than those with CNS injury (Fenner 1995). Victims of head trauma should be evaluated carefully to document injuries, determine cause of injuries, determine prognosis in live victims, and institute appropriate treatment.

Impact Injuries

Head injuries may be categorized as impact injuries or acceleration/deceleration injuries. Impact injuries are caused when the head strikes an object or surface, or the head is struck by an object. The surface or weapon that is relatively soft and yielding will absorb a large proportion of the impacting energy by way of deformation as compared with a hard unyielding surface or weapon. Impact injuries can cause soft-tissue injuries, fractures, brain contusions, epidural hematomas, and intracerebral hemorrhage. Impact soft-tissue injuries include abrasions, contusions, and lacerations. These injuries may reflect the weapon or surface that struck the head (see Patterned Abrasions and Bruising). Unlike humans, lacerations to the scalp of a dog or cat do not tend to bleed profusely.

Fractures

Impact injuries can cause skull fractures, which may or may not have concurrent brain injury. Skull fractures and fragments may cause lacerations and penetrating wounds of the brain without lacerations of the overlying skin. The fracture produced depends on several factors including the fur covering, thickness of the skin, thickness and configuration of the skull, and elasticity of the bone at the point of impact. It also depends on the object's shape, weight, and consistency that impacts the head along with the velocity with which the blow was delivered or the head struck the object (Di Maio and Di Maio 2001).

When a broad, flat object impacts the head, the skull flattens at the point of impact to conform to the surface. The flattened area bends inward, and the adjacent and more distant areas bend outward. This can cause fractures distant from the point of impact. In the area of sharp curves, linear fractures occur at the site of the outbending. Then the inbended area tries to rebound back, causing the fracture line to extend toward the area of impact as well as in the opposite direction. This fracture line may not completely extend to the area of impact or may extend through it. A low-velocity impact with a large area of contact between the head and the object may cause simple linear fractures (Di Maio and Di Maio 2001).

Circular fractures, either complete or incomplete, may be seen with higher velocity and force. Stellate fractures are caused by an even higher velocity and force, causing a depression in the bone at the site of impact. This area of severe inbending causes fractures on the inner surface that radiate outward from the impact site. The outbending areas fracture and radiate back toward the area of impact joining the inbending fractures. There may be circular fractures at the outbended area. They may be incomplete, stopping at a linear fracture, and indicating that the linear fracture preceded the circular. If the linear fracture stops at the circular, it indicates the linear fracture occurred after the circular fracture (Di Maio and Di Maio 2001).

Blows to different parts of the head can produce different effects. If the head is struck with a large amount of force by an object that has small surface area it can cause a depressed skull fracture, sometimes with fragmentation. This also can be caused when the skull is impacted in a small area by a large amount of force. There are no large deformations of the skull distant from the impact associated with this type of fracture such as linear fractures. Basilar fractures are caused by blows to the base of the skull. Hinge fractures are transverse fractures that completely bisect the base of the skull, creating a "hinge." These are usually caused by impacts on the side of the head and occasionally from the front of the mandible (Di Maio and Di Maio 2001).

Ring fractures are circular fractures that surround the foramen magnum at the base of the skull. They are caused by the head being driven down onto the vertebral column or the column being driven into the base of the skull. If the suture lines are not completely fused in the skull, then fracture lines can follow along these lines. These are called diastatic fractures. A contrecoup injury occurs in the area opposite the site of impact. A coup injury occurs at the site of impact. Contrecoup fractures are located at the opposite point of impact and are associated with contrecoup brain injury, primarily seen in human deaths caused by falls (Di Maio and Di Maio 2001).

Brain Contusions

Brain contusions may be produced by impact injuries to the head. They are typically more severe when associated with skull fractures. Brains with diffuse axonal injury usually have less severe contusions. It is possible to have severe open skull fractures with massive brain lacerations or evisceration without any contusions. Contusions are composed of hemorrhage and usually are associated with necrosis of the brain tissue. It is possible to have necrosis with minimal to no associated hemorrhage. The amount of hemorrhage depends on the type and size of vessel involved. Brain contusions usually are multiple, densely arranged, and streak-like in appearance. Overlying subarachnoid hemorrhage may be present (Di Maio and Di Maio 2001).

There are six types of contusions: coup, contrecoup, fracture, intermediary coup, gliding, and herniation. Coup contusions are located at the site of impact. They are caused by the inbending of the bone rebounding back, causing tensile force injury to the brain. Contrecoup contusions are located opposite to the point of impact and are caused by the brain rebounding back from the skull after impact. It is possible to see both coup (from the direct impact) and contrecoup contusions, but contrecoup injury is more extensive than the coup. This may be seen in head injuries caused by a fall. A blow to the head usually produces coup contusions, although it is possible to see associated but less extensive contrecoup contusions (Di Maio and Di Maio 2001).

Fracture contusions are caused by skull fractures. They may or may not be at the site of impact because fractures can occur distant from this point. Intermediary coup contusions are located in the deeper structures of the brain and follow the line of impact. Gliding contusions are areas of focal hemorrhages in the dorsal surface of the cerebral hemispheres, specifically involving the cortex and underlying white matter. They are usually associated with diffuse axonal injury and are not associated with the direction and site of impact. Herniation contusions are caused by brain herniation and are also independent of the direction and site of impact (Di Maio and Di Maio 2001).

Epidural Hematomas

Epidermal hematomas are caused by the primary impact and are usually associated with skull fractures. The skull is bent inward on impact, causing stripping of the dura and laceration of the meningeal vessels. They are usually unilateral and have a thick, disk-shaped appearance. Death from an epidermal hematoma is caused by brain displacement and compression of the brainstem (Di Maio and Di Maio 2001).

Subarachnoid Hemorrhage

Subarachnoid hemorrhage is the common injury of head trauma in humans. It can range from minor to severe and be focal or diffuse. Hemorrhage is of mostly venous origin and is usually diffuse over the cerebral hemispheres. There may be some pooling of blood on the ventral surface of the brain. Massive brain injury, including lacerations, may be present with little to no subarachnoid hemorrhage because of vessel spasm. Some artifactual hemorrhage may be caused on necropsy when removing the skull cap diffusing blood into the dependent portion of the subarachnoid space. Subarachnoid hemorrhage also can be produced by decomposition because of lysis of blood cells, breakdown of the vessels, and leakage into the subarachnoid space (Di Maio and Di Maio 2001).

Lacerations of the internal carotid, vertebral, or carotid arteries can produce subarachnoid hemorrhage over the base of the brain. The carotid artery may be damaged within the cranium in conjunction with skull fractures. It also may be damaged in the neck with cervical fractures or hyperextension injury. The vertebral arteries can be injured because of blunt force trauma to the neck (see below). This can cause subarachnoid hemorrhage to the base of the brain or thrombosis within the artery, causing infarction to the brain (Di Maio and Di Maio 2001).

Brain Swelling

Swelling of the brain can occur because of severe head trauma. This may be focal or diffuse. The swelling is results from vasodilation causing an increase in intravascular cerebral blood volume, cerebral edema, or both. This swelling causes a space-occupying mass effect. If the swelling becomes severe, herniation of the brain, brainstem hemorrhage, infarction, and necrosis can result.

Subdural Hygromas

A subdural hygroma may be seen when brain trauma causes the effusion of spinal fluid to the subdural space. This fluid may be blood tinged. The accumulation of spinal fluid can cause the same space-occupying effects of a subdural hematoma (Di Maio and Di Maio 2001).

Acceleration/Deceleration Injuries

Acceleration or deceleration injuries result from the sudden movement of the head, immediately after the injury, imparting shearing and tensile forces to the brain and creating intracranial pressure gradients. One type of injury produced is subdural hematomas, which are caused by the tearing of the subdural bridging veins. The second type of injury is diffuse axonal injury, which is secondary to injury of the axons (Di Maio and Di Maio 2001).

An impact to the head can produce linear or rotational (angular) acceleration, or a combination of both. Linear acceleration is caused by the force passing through the center of the head, which causes the head to accelerate in a straight line. When the impact force does not pass through the center of the head it causes rotational or angular acceleration. This causes the head to rotate about its center (Di Maio and Di Maio 2001). In theory, acceleration or deceleration injuries do not require an impact but virtually all are associated with an initiating impact force (Di Maio and Di Maio 2001).

Blunt force trauma to the head can cause intracerebral hemorrhage. This hemorrhage is located within the cerebral parenchyma and does not involve the surface of the brain. These areas are a collection of blood and usually well demarcated. Intracerebral hemorrhage is caused by acceleration/deceleration forces that are usually associated with gliding contusions and diffuse axonal injury (Di Maio and Di Maio 2001).

Diffuse Axonal Injury

Diffuse axonal injury is caused by sudden acceleration or deceleration of the head usually started by an impact to the head. The severity of injury depends on the force, the time over which the acceleration or deceleration occurs, and the direction of the movement. Experiments in humans have shown that motion to the side of the head causes severe injuries versus those in the forward or backward motion cause milder injuries (Di Maio and Di Maio 2001).

The longer the time period over which acceleration or deceleration occurs, the more likely it is to see diffuse axonal injury versus subdural hematomas. This is seen when the time impact is prolonged. Injuries can range from mild to severe (even death). There may only be physiological dysfunction without disruption of the axons at low acceleration or deceleration. When there is reversible physiological disruption it is known as a concussion (Fenner 1995). With increasing force, there is increasing physiological and structural disruption of axons. The cell membranes are damaged, which may be reversible in some cells (Di Maio and Di Maio 2001).

Histologically, diffuse axonal injury is seen as axonal swelling, initially dilated, then club shaped, then finally round balls called "retraction balls" (Di Maio and Di Maio 2001).

Subdural Hematomas

Subdural hematomas often are not associated with skull fractures. There may or may not be cerebral contusions or grossly obvious brain injury. They are caused by a head impact to a hard surface, which causes the brain to accelerate. This produces stretching and tearing of the bridging veins that drain the surface of the cerebral hemispheres into the sinus. Subdural hematomas are more likely than diffuse axonal injury to occur, the more rapid the acceleration or deceleration and the shorter the time for the acceleration or deceleration. There is no association of the location of skull fractures to the location or presence of a subdural hematoma. Typically these hematomas are more lethal because the same acceleration and deceleration forces producing diffuse axonal injury to the cerebral parenchyma. They also may cause brain displacement, possible cerebral edema, and compression of the brainstem (Di Maio and Di Maio 2001).

Shaken Baby Syndrome

The violent shaking of infants can cause major damage of the brain. This shaking causes the head to flop back and forth, producing extensive intracranial (often subdural) and retinal hemorrhages. The injuries result from the indirect acceleration and deceleration traction stresses from the whiplash action. The violent forces can produce stretching of axons in the cerebral white matter strong enough to shear off the axons. These ends then retract into globoid shapes, known as retraction balls. The cause of the retinal hemorrhages is not known but is believed to result from increased retinal venous pressure, extravasation of subarachnoid blood, and traction caused by angular deceleration of the retinal vessels at the vitreoretinal interface (Di Maio and Di Maio 2001).

In several reported cases of shaken baby syndrome, evidence has been found of impact trauma to the head. This has caused some pathologists to change the terminology to shaken impact syndrome. In these cases, the retinal and intracranial hemorrhage is caused by the shaking; then the head is impacted against a hard surface, causing further intracranial bleeding, contusions, and possible fractures. One would reason that the same forces should cause cervical fractures and/or spinal cord damage, but that has not been found in human cases. Di Maio and Di Maio believe that head injuries reported to be the consequence of shaking actually result from impact force to the head (Di Maio and Di Maio 2001).

Examination of Head Trauma Victims

Overview

Examination of suspected head injuries should be thorough. Sometimes the animal has no outward signs of trauma or neurological dysfunction. The only indicators of head trauma may be found in the eyes, ears, nose, or mouth. The skull should be palpated for fractures. Skull radiographs and full body radiographs should be taken to document the injuries to detect occult injuries. The outcome of head trauma injuries is affected by location and severity of the head injury and progression of injury resulting from edema and ischemia.

Ocular Injuries

Ocular injuries are primarily caused by blunt force trauma to the head causing closed trauma to the eye. Sometimes, the only injury in head trauma is to the eye. It is important to do a complete eye exam, including fluorescein stains of the cornea, anterior chamber exam, fundic exam, and measurement of the intraocular pressure. Trauma to the head may present as hemorrhage in the conjunctiva, nictitating membrane, sclera, or the periorbital tissues. There may be anterior uveitis present with hyphema, hypopyon, or fibrin clots. Evidence of anterior uveitis may not be as obvious after the acute event and the fibrin and blood may have clotted and sunk to the ventral anterior chamber. There may be traumatic luxation of the lens. Retinal hemorrhage or retinal detachment may be found. Retinal scarring may be seen from previous retinal injury. It is important that other causes of the exam findings be ruled-out, such as clotting disorders, hypertension, and other causes of anterior uveitis. Special attention should be paid to unilateral injuries because they are more supportive of a blow to the head versus a general systemic problem.

Traumatic proptosis occurs when the globe of the eye is displaced rostrally from the orbit because of blunt force trauma. It requires substantial force to induce proptosis in cats and non-brachycephalic dogs (Ramsey 2000). Usually concurrent injuries are found, including severe craniofacial, CNS, and intraocular trauma.

In dogs, the most common problems with traumatic proptosis include strabismus, chemosis, exposure keratitis, corneal ulceration, and hyphema. In cats, they include corneal perforation, hyphema, and facial fractures (Ramsey 2000). Debris may be embedded in the globe or surrounding tissues, which is important forensic evidence. A traumatic proptosis in a cat or non-brachycephalic dog has a poor prognosis for vision. It is uncommon for cats to regain vision after replacement of the proptosed eye. Other poor prognostic indicators include optic nerve transaction, no visible pupil, extensive hyphema, facial fractures, and avulsion of three or more extraocular muscles (Ramsey 2000).

Ear Injuries

Injury to the ear may be the only evidence found in blunt force trauma to the head. Petechiae may be found on the surface of the pinna or the base of the ear (Fig. 5.2). The tympanic membrane may be ruptured with evidence of bleeding. Frank hemorrhage may be found in the ear canal. Bleeding from the inner ear may be associated with intracranial hemorrhages in dogs and cats (Braund 2003). There may be evidence of petechiae within the lining of the ear canal. This finding is unique to animal victims of head trauma. As with ocular injuries, the asymmetry of injury can provide clues as to the underlying cause.

Nasal and Oral Injuries

The nasal area may be injured from blunt or sharp force trauma. Epistaxis is invariably present. Because of the presence of blood clots and subsequent edema, obstruction of the nasal cavity may develop, forcing open-mouthed breathing. This may last for several days until the swelling subsides. Fractures of the nasal bone and maxillary bone may be present, which reduces the patency of the nasal cavity. Subsequent secondary infection and necrosis of the conchae may develop over time. Fracture of the hard palate and the palatine symphyses can be seen because of blunt force trauma or a fall from a significant height. These injuries are caused by the lower canines being forced upward between the maxillary dental arcades. Edema and hemorrhage of the palatine mucosa may obscure the cleft until tissue necrosis develops several days later (Bedford 1995).

Examination of the oral cavity may reveal injuries related to head trauma. These include injuries to the palate, teeth fractures, tongue lacerations, and contusions of

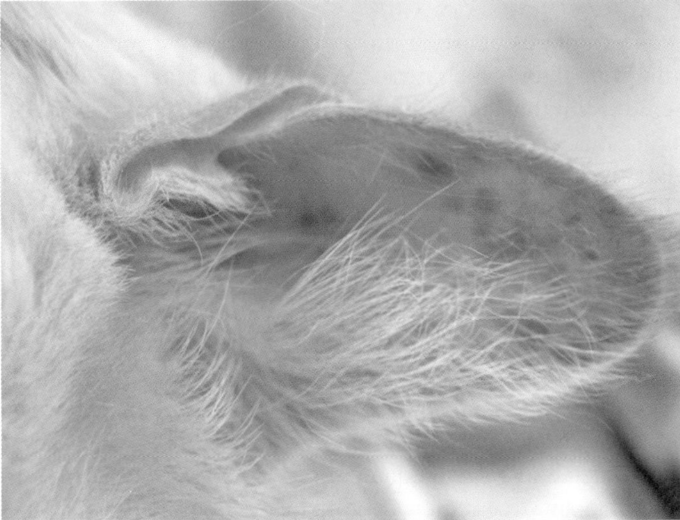

Fig. 5.2 Petechiae on the ear pinna caused by blunt force trauma to the head. For color detail, please see color plate section.

the surrounding skin and mucosa. Blood may be found secondary to oral injuries or from nasal injury draining into the back of the mouth.

Neurological Assessment

It is important to classify the CNS injury based on the location of the affected area in the brain. This can help determine the prognosis, for example in brainstem injury patients, who have a poor prognosis even with treatment.

The animal's level of consciousness and whether it is abnormal or normal should be noted. A coma lasting 48 hours or longer is considered a grave prognostic sign (Braund 2003). It is very important to note if there is a change in the level of consciousness over a period of time. Deteriorating clinical signs indicate progressive brain swelling or possible brain herniation (Braund 2003). The animal may appear awake but does not respond properly to the environment, indicating an abnormal level of consciousness that indicates cerebral injury. An animal that is in a stupor or coma has an abnormal level of consciousness, which is indicative of either cerebral or brainstem injury.

The eyes should be examined for pupillary light responses (PLRs), pupil size and symmetry, physiological nystagmus (doll's eye maneuver), and ocular injury. When interpreting eye test results it is important to rule out injury to the optic nerve. With optic nerve injury, normal physiological nystagmus should be present. There may be abnormal pupil size in either cerebral or brainstem damage. In cerebral injuries, the animal has small pupils with normal PLRs and normal physiological nystagmus. In brainstem injuries the animal can have small or large pupils, abnormal or absent physiological nystagmus, and usually abnormal PLRs. In cerebellar injuries there may be abnormal pupil size but there is usually normal consciousness and normal physiological nystagmus (Fenner 1986). Animals that are stuporous or comatose with dilated pupils have a poor prognosis (Braund 2003).

Peripheral nerve injury must be ruled out in suspected cerebellar injuries. The posture of the animal and response to stimuli may help determine the location of the injuries. In rostral brainstem injuries, the animal may have episodes of decerebrate posturing that can appear similar to the opisthotonic posturing caused by cerebellar injury. The level of consciousness helps differentiate the site of injury because in brainstem injury the animal is in a stupor or coma (Fenner 1986). Lastly, the cranial nerves and spinal reflexes should be examined to determine sites of injury and whether there are multiple locations.

The primary brain injury actually sets off a cascade of secondary biochemical events that can exacerbate the neurological problems known as secondary injuries. These changes can occur within hours to days after the primary event. These injuries are believed to be caused by progressive ischemic brain injury and are affected by several factors, including decreased blood flow autoregulation, altered cerebral metabolism, inadequate cerebral perfusion pressure, hemorrhage, increased cytokine and free radical production, increased excitotoxins, depletion of neuronal adenosine triphosphatase (ATP) levels, decreased intracellular magnesium levels, intracellular accumulation of calcium and sodium leading to astrocytic swelling, and cytotoxic edema (Braund 2003). The result of these events is increased intracranial pressure and progressive damage to the brain parenchyma. In addition, some secondary events are thought to be related to the activation of the sympathetic nervous system, causing a further increase of intracranial pressure (ICP), systemic hypertension, myocardial necrosis, cardiac arrhythmias, increased nutritional requirements, and non-cardiogenic pulmonary edema (Fenner 1995).

Respiratory distress associated with head trauma may be caused by indirect injury to the soft tissues of the neck. The blow to the head causes rapid acceleration of the skull, resulting in tearing of the soft tissues of the neck, the hyoid apparatus or larynx, and cervical spine fracture or subluxation (Braund 2003). Systemic hypotension or hypovolemia exacerbates the autolytic processes in the brain, resulting in further parenchymal damage and edema with a resultant rise in ICP (Dewey 2005). In human patients with severe head trauma, mortality is doubled with concurrent secondary injuries of hypoxia and hypotension (Braund 2003).

The increased ICP is caused by intracranial hemorrhage and brain edema. The high ICP is further compounded by the decreased cerebral blood flow because of the compressed dural veins. If not ameliorated, increased ICP may cause brain herniation and also may result in secondary spinal cord myelomalacia (Dewey 2005). Brain edema may be caused by cytotoxic edema, which accumulates primarily in neurons and astrocytes because of cellular hypoxia. Vasogenic edema, which affects primarily the white matter, may be another component of brain edema. This type of edema is extracellular and is caused by leakage across the injured blood-brain barrier. The increased ICP also causes CNS hypoxia. The hypoxic animal then may develop hypercarbia, which in turn increases the ICP even more. Seizures are common in CCT patients and may be seen early on or develop later because of the brain injury (Fenner 1995).

Neck and Spinal Injuries

Neck Injuries

The pharyngeal area, larynx, and trachea may be an area of trauma resulting from bite wounds from an animal attacker, strangulation, blunt or sharp force trauma, or the animal being grabbed by the throat. The pharyngeal injuries may include edema of the pharynx and surrounding tissue, hematoma, laceration, or fracture of the hyoid bone. If the hyoid bone is fractured in a surviving animal, the symptoms may be painful swallowing (Venker-van Haagen 1995). Laryngeal injuries may lead to life-threatening edema, causing upper airway obstruction. The cartilage can be damaged, causing further narrowing of the airway. Lacerations of the larynx can result in emphysema into the surrounding tissues (Venker-van Haagen 1995). In tracheal injuries there may be tears in the tracheal wall or fractures of the tracheal rings. Subcutaneous emphysema is the primary result of these injuries, although depending on the location of the trauma, pneumomediastinum, peritracheal, or intermuscular emphysema may develop (Brayley and Ettinger 1995).

Spinal Injuries Caused by Head Trauma

Blunt force trauma to the head can cause cervical vertebrae injuries. Atlanto-occipital dislocation is caused by the separation of the craniocervical ligament attachments. They may or may not have osseous injury to the vertebra and may have associated ventral brain lacerations. On the axis, C2, a fracture of the neural arch between the superior and inferior articular processes is called the hangman's fracture. It is caused by axial loading forces with flexion or extension. Atlantoaxial dislocations are more difficult to detect (Di Maio and Di Maio 2001).

Hyperextension of the head of an animal may be caused by an accident or a human exerting force on the body or head to cause the hyperextension. This could be done if the perpetrator grabs the head and swings or flings the animal, or if the animal is thrown or kicked with enough force to cause hyperextension upon landing.

With severe hyperextension, there may be injury to the brainstem. This can vary from tears and hemorrhage to complete avulsion. Subarachnoid hemorrhage is found normally. In humans, these injuries usually are associated with fractures of the upper cervical vertebrae and the base of the skull. Lacerations of the brainstem can occur without cervical or cranial fractures and usually are associated with subarachnoid hemorrhage around the brainstem (Di Maio and Di Maio 2001).

Hyperextension of the head of an animal can result in traumatic atlantoaxial luxations. This can occur in all breeds of dogs and cats and is a result of the rupture of the atlantoaxial ligaments or fracture of the dens at its junction with the axis (LeCouteur and Child 1995). Clinical signs usually are acute and are associated with the incident; they may be delayed in onset as well. In three reported cases of injuries to dogs, two presented with mild neurological deficits and cervical pain, and one had vestibular abnormalities and tetraparesis (LeCouteur and Child 1995). The clinical signs can vary and include sensitivity to the head, cervical pain, tetraparesis, and tetraplegia. This type of injury can cause spinal cord trauma leading to hemorrhage and edema to the brain, causing dysphagia, facial paralysis, vestibular deficits, opisthotonos, or respiratory paralysis and death (LeCouteur and Child 1995).

Spinal Injuries

Spinal injuries may be associated with blunt force trauma caused by motor vehicle accidents, physical blows, fights, or falls. The injuries may cause vertebral fractures, luxations, subluxations, dural tearing, or disk extrusion resulting in spinal cord concussion, compression, laceration, or distraction (Braund 2003). Reports of subluxation injuries at C5-C6 associated with dog fighting injuries indicate a possible anatomical predisposition for subluxation at this level (Braund 2003).

Fractures of the axis appear to be more common than other cervical vertebrae (Braund 2003). There is direct primary injury to the spinal cord resulting from mechanical disruption of the nerve pathways followed by secondary injury caused by ischemia, edema, hypoxia, and multiple biochemical deleterious events, including reduced spinal blood flow. The end result is membrane destruction, ischemia, edema, cell death, and possibly permanent neurological dysfunction (Braund 2003).

A complete neurological exam must be performed to determine the level of spinal injury. This exam should be reported over time to detect progression of damage and deteriorating neurological function. Radiographs should be taken to document the presence of fractures, luxations, or subluxations. It is important to rule out congenital deformities, underlying nutritional factors, or metabolic disorders.

Chest Injuries

Blunt force or sharp force trauma to the thorax can result in bone fractures, hemothorax, myocardial trauma, lung injury, tracheobronchial fractures or avulsions, damage to the major vessels, pneumomediastinum, pneumothorax, or diaphragmatic rupture. Injuries to the lungs include contusions, hematomas, lacerations, lung torsions, or lung collapse. If the surface of the lung at the site of impact does not absorb the full force of the blow, the energy can be transferred to the opposite side, usually fixed, causing contrecoup contusions (Di Maio and Di Maio 2001). Pulmonary contusions may take as long as 24 hours to develop radiographically.

The chest wall may have rib fractures, flail chest, sternal fractures, thoracic spine, or vertebrae fractures. Because of the pliability in some animals' chests resulting from age and/or conformation, significant damage to the intrathoracic structures can occur without fractures of the ribs or sternum. Rib fractures may damage the internal chest structures during the compressive blow, and then rebound back into position. Rib fractures may lacerate or puncture the lungs, vessels, or heart (Figs. 5.3, 5.4). Myocardial injuries include contusions, lacerations, hemorrhage, pericardial effusions, cardiac tamponade, or myocardial necrosis. The primary clinical signs of injury, which may not develop for 12–24 hours, are ST-T abnormalities on the electrocardiogram and cardiac arrhythmias (Sisson and Thomas 1995). Severe grinding force to the chest can cause multiple fractures and mangling of the lungs.

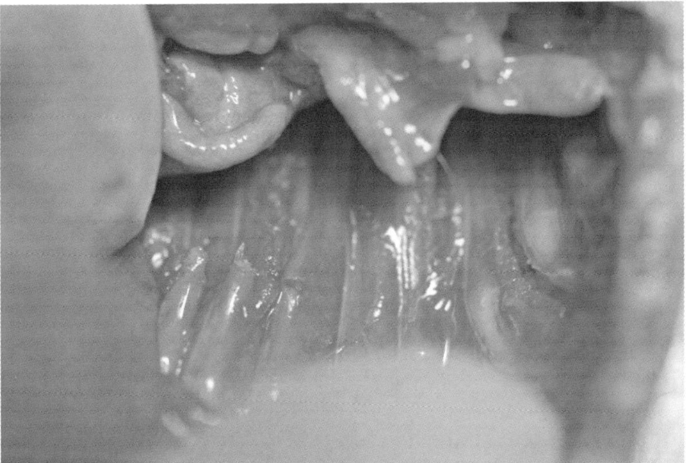

Fig. 5.3 Multiple rib fractures caused by blunt force trauma. For color detail, please see color plate section.

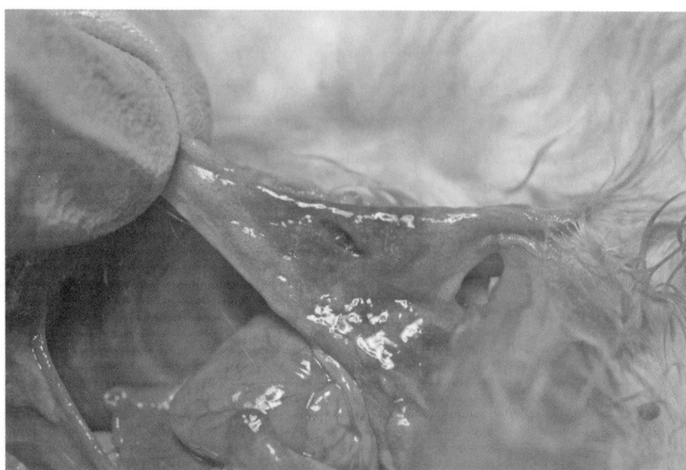

Fig. 5.4 Lung lacerations and contusions secondary to the rib fractures seen in Figure 5.3. For color detail, please see color plate section.

Abdominal Injuries

Abdominal injuries may be caused by blunt force trauma from blows to the abdomen, crushing injury, dog bites, or falls. In child abuse, abdominal injuries are the second most common cause of death, which may be caused by the delay in recognition of the injury and initiation of treatment. Because bruising is not obvious in animals and their symptoms of pain and injury are often hidden, the same may be true in animals.

The abdominal walls are lax and compressible, which readily transmit the force from a blow to the internal viscera. The injuries owing to blunt force to the abdomen depend on the organ affected. The absence of external injury does not exclude the possibility of injury, which is sometimes massive, to the abdominal organs. Blunt force trauma to the abdomen may cause rupture of hollow organs (gastrointestinal tract, bladder, and uterus), fractures or tears of solid organs, diaphragmatic tears, abdominal wall tears, hemorrhage within organs, free hemorrhage, and leakage of organ contents into the peritoneal cavity. Pancreatitis may be seen secondary to blunt force trauma to the abdomen. Hemorrhagic pleural effusions may be caused by abdominal trauma. Urinary tract trauma (bladder, urethra, ureter, and kidneys) may be seen because of compressive forces or fractures of the pelvis or os penis. Major vessels may be injured and organs may be avulsed from their attachments. The omentum may be bruised, torn, or major vessels damaged. Subcapsular hematomas may be present on the liver or spleen. The rupture of hollow organs usually occurs when the organs are distended with food (stomach) or urine (bladder) at the time of the blow (Di Maio and Di Maio 2001).

Ligature Injuries

It is not uncommon for ligatures to be used as a form of abuse or to control the victim. The types of injuries seen depend on the type of ligature, compression forces of the ligature, and length of time the ligature was on the animal. Animals may have ligatures around their mouth, legs, genitalia, or tail. Ligatures cause compression and constriction of the skin and vessels, creating tissue swelling and edema. The ligature may cut through the skin into the underlying tissue depending on the type of ligature, amount of constriction and compression, movement of the animal, and time elapsed.

When examining the animal, the ligature should be carefully removed to preserve all potential trace evidence. Any knots or twisted ends should be preserved intact and the ligature cut on the opposite side. Often the joined areas of the ligature have trace evidence or skin cells related to the perpetrator.

If the ligature is no longer present, the wound should be carefully examined for embedded trace evidence related to the ligature. The wound may have a pattern that is indicative of the type of ligature used. Patterned injures are those that mirror the object that caused them. This pattern should be thoroughly photographed with a photographic scale in each photo.

The depth and width of the wound should be measured. Cultures should be taken of any infection. A time estimate should be given for the ligature to have been on the animal. This is possible by evaluating the granulation tissue. In general, a granulation bed forms in approximately 1 week and granulation tissue continues to grow at a rate of 1 mm/day, slowing as the lesion ages to 1 cm/month (Reisman 2004).

References

Bedford, P.G.C. 1995. Diseases of the Nose. In *Textbook of Veterinary Internal Medicine: Diseases of the Dog and Cat*, vol. 1, 4th ed., ed. S.J. Ettinger, and E.C. Feldman, pp. 551–567. Philadelphia: W.B. Saunders.

Braund, K.G. 2003. Traumatic Disorders. In *Clinical Neurology in Small Animals: Localization, Diagnosis and Treatment*, ed. K.G. Braund. Ithaca, NY: International Veterinary Information Service (www.ivis.org).

Brayley, K.A., and S.J. Ettinger. 1995. Diseases of the Trachea. In *Textbook of Veterinary Internal Medicine: Diseases of the Dog and Cat*, vol. 1, 4th ed., ed. S.J. Ettinger, and E.C. Feldman, pp. 754–766. Philadelphia: W.B. Saunders.

Dewey, C.W. 2005. Emergency Treatment of Head/Spinal Trauma. In *Proceedings of the Eleventh International Veterinary Emergency and Critical Care Symposium.* Atlanta, GA, September 7–11, 2005. pp. 493–497.

Di Maio, V.J., and D. Di Maio. 2001. *Forensic Pathology,* 2nd ed. Boca Raton, FL: CRC Press.

Fenner, W.R. 1986. Head Trauma and Nervous System Injury. In *Current Veterinary Therapy IX Small Animal Practice*, ed. R.W. Kirk, pp. 830–836. Philadelphia: W.B. Saunders.

Fenner, W.R. 1995. Diseases of the Brain. In *Textbook of Veterinary Internal Medicine: Diseases of the Dog and Cat*, vol. 1, 4th ed., ed. S.J. Ettinger, and E.C. Feldman, pp. 578–629. Philadelphia: W.B. Saunders.

LeCouteur, R.A., and G. Child. 1995. Diseases of the Spinal Cord. In *Textbook of Veterinary Internal Medicine: Diseases of the Dog and Cat*, vol. 1, 4th ed., ed. S.J. Ettinger, and E.C. Feldman, pp. 629–696. Philadelphia: W.B. Saunders.

Ramsey, D.T. 2000. Exophthalmos. In *Kirk's Current Veterinary Therapy XIII Small Animal Practice*, ed. J.D. Bongura, pp. 1086–1089. Philadelphia: W.B. Saunders.

Reisman, R. 2004. Medical Evaluation and Documentation of Abuse in the Live Animal. In *Shelter Medicine for Veterinarians and Staff*, ed. L. Miller, and S. Zawistowski, pp. 453–487. Ames, IA: Blackwell Publishing.

Sisson, D.D., and W.P. Thomas. 1995. Myocardial Diseases. In *Textbook of Veterinary Internal Medicine: Diseases of the Dog and Cat*, vol. 1, 4th ed., ed. S.J. Ettinger, and E.C. Feldman, pp. 995–1032. Philadelphia: W.B. Saunders.

Taylor, S.M. 2003. Abnormalities of Mentation, Loss of Vision, and Pupillary Abnormalities. In *Small Animal Internal Medicine*, ed. R.W. Nelson, and C.G. Couto, pp. 983–990. St. Louis: Mosby.

Venker-van Haagen, A.J. 1995. Diseases of the Throat. In *Textbook of Veterinary Internal Medicine Diseases of the Dog and Cat*, vol. 1, 4th ed., ed. S.J. Ettinger, and E.C. Feldman, pp. 567–575. Philadelphia: W.B. Saunders.

Chapter 6
Patterns of Non-accidental Injury: Penetrating Injuries

Introduction

Forensic classification of penetrating injuries, excluding gunshot wounds and other projectiles, are lacerations (split wounds), incised wounds (cuts), and stab wounds. It is important to know if law enforcement has the instrument or weapon suspected to have caused the injury or death of the animal. When evaluating penetrating injuries, the veterinarian must consider that the investigators will eventually have the weapon and take steps to ensure that evidence is collected from the animal for comparison.

Lacerations

A laceration is a tear in tissue caused by a crushing or shearing force (Fig. 6.1). This can occur on the skin or internal organs. Skin lacerations may be caused by blunt force directed by an object, a fall, or an impact from a vehicle. The margins of skin lacerations tend to be bruised, abraded, and irregular. The laceration may have a pattern that mirrors the offending object. Long, thin objects tend to produce linear lacerations but may produce one that is Y-shaped. The wound should be examined for deeply embedded material related to the object used.

Lacerations usually are present in areas where the skin is fixed and more easily stretched and torn. The underlying blood vessels and nerves are stronger than the skin forming a visible "bridge" of the underlying tissue. This bridging differentiates a laceration from an incisive wound (Di Maio and Di Maio 2001). A laceration resulting from an impact that contacted the body at an angle may have undermining of one side of the laceration, indicating the direction of the blow. The opposite side of the laceration is beveled and abraded (Di Maio and Di Maio 2001).

If the object was heavy and had a sharp edge, the wound may appear to be incised. Careful examination will reveal some margin abrasion and deeper tissue bridging. The use of a dull knife may cause injuries that appear grossly similar to lacerations. The use of a dissecting microscopic can help differentiate it from a

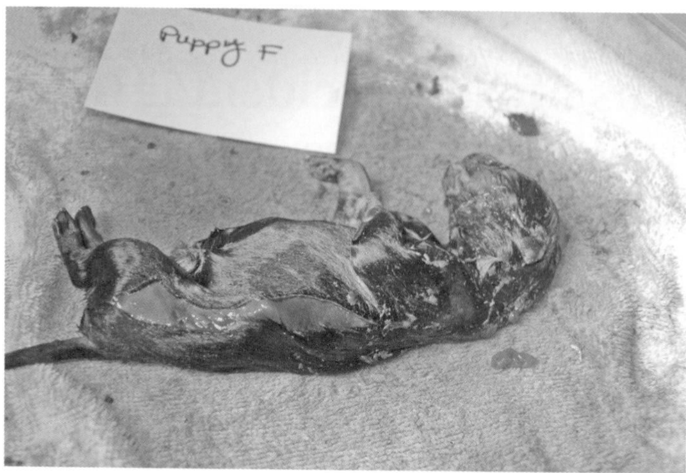

Fig. 6.1 Laceration on puppy caused by blunt force trauma using a barbell weight. For color detail, please see color plate section.

laceration. Decomposition can make differentiation from lacerations and incisive wounds impossible (Di Maio and Di Maio 2001).

Avulsion Injuries

Avulsion injuries to the external body involve a blunt force impacting the body at a tangential or oblique angle ripping skin and soft tissue off the underlying bone and fascia (Di Maio and Di Maio 2001). Avulsion also can occur with internal organs that are partially or completely torn from their attachments. Shearing forces also can cause the underlying soft tissue, connective tissue, and fascia to be avulsed from the overlying skin and subcutaneous tissue. The skin can appear normal except for a pocket of blood or blood-tinged fluid underneath. This can occur when an animal is picked up by the scruff of the neck and shaken.

Shearing and degloving injuries of the limbs or other areas of the body are commonly seen resulting from motor vehicle accidents or dragging injuries. They also may be caused by ligatures or any other means that can compress, twist, or otherwise strip the overlying tissue. These injuries may be simple lacerations or more extensive with severe loss of skin and the underlying soft tissue damaging the associated bones and joints. These wounds, by the very nature of their cause, are contaminated. Embedded in these wounds is a significant amount of foreign material that is forensically important. This wealth of trace evidence may link the victim to a crime scene or a suspect. Trace evidence includes dirt, debris, glass, and fibers.

The non-vital tissue becomes necrotic within 48 hours after the trauma (Beardsley 2000). In animals with these injuries it is critical to do a complete physical exam for other forensic evidence and additional injuries. It is has been reported that 70 percent of dogs with shearing and degloving injuries had concurrent injuries, including fractures, skin lacerations, and cardiopulmonary problems (Beardsley 2000).

Stab Wounds

Overview

Stab wounds are characterized by the depth of the wound exceeding the length of the wound. They may be caused by a variety of sharp pointed instruments, including knives, scissors, screwdrivers, pens, forks, broken glass, and ice picks. The most common weapon used is a knife, primarily a single-edged blade, which also can produce incising wounds with the sharp blade.

The force needed to cause the entrance wound depends on the sharpness of the instrument and the thickness of the skin. Some knives, even single-edged knives, have a sharp edge on both sides of the point, making entrance into the skin easier. Once the tip of the knife penetrates the skin, the rest of the blade slides easily into the body. The depth and length of the stab wound can indicate the amount of force used. A deeper wound than the length of the blade indicates great force was used when inflicting the stab wound.

Documentation

When examining a victim of stab wounds it is necessary to assign a number to each wound and record the location of the wounds. This should be done in two ways. One way is to use a diagram of a dog or cat showing the shape and location of the wounds, and assigning a number to each wound (see Appendices 14–15). The second way is to record the location by measurements to the nearest landmark on the body such as the midline, the spine, or a specific nipple. The wounds should be identified with the corresponding number on the drawing and the appearance fully described. When examining stab wounds it is important to take measurements of the width and depth of the wound. Photographs should be taken of each wound with a photographic scale next to the wound. The length of a stab wound does not necessarily correlate with the width of the knife. It can be greater than the width if the blade is drawn against the skin as it penetrates the skin or is withdrawn, thereby enlarging the wound. The elasticity or laxity of the skin can change the wound appearance, either increasing or decreasing the size.

The depth of the wound depends on the force, amount of penetration, and whether the blade met increased tissue resistance such as contact with bone. The depth may be equal, less, or greater than the length of the knife. If the knife is plunged into the body with great force, it may penetrate deeper than the length of the blade. It is difficult to make a determination of the blade length with only one stab wound. By measuring the depth of multiple wounds it is possible to provide an estimation of the length of the blade. One must be careful in measuring the depth because probing the wound can create false tracks. Examination of internal injuries and measuring from this site to the entrance wound can provide the wound depth.

Interpretation of Stab Wound Appearances

Knife Wounds

The appearance of the stab wound depends on the skin properties, the nature of the blade and knife, the movement of the victim, and the movement of the blade in the wound. With sharp knives, the wound is sharp and regular. If the weapon or part of the weapon is blunt or dull, the wound appears abraded and contused or jagged and contused. If the knife blade enters at an oblique angle, the wound can have a beveled margin on one side with tissue undermining on the other, indicating the direction the knife entered the body.

To understand knife wound appearances it is important to know the different parts of the knife. First there is the handle, which is composed of the grip, followed by a guard or cross guard. The guard is to protect the person's hand from slipping onto the blade and cutting him- or herself. The bottom of the blade is called the ricasso and is blunt on both sides. On a single-edged blade the sharp side is called the edge and the opposite blunt side is called the back of the blade. Where the sharp edge ends along the length of the blade is called the spine. The end of the knife blade is called the point; there may be a sharp edge on both sides of the point (Di Maio and Di Maio 2001).

The appearance of a stab wound depends on what part of the knife penetrates or contacts the skin and how deeply it is thrust into the body. It is not always possible to determine if the weapon was single- or double-edged from examination of a single wound. With multiple stab wounds, there is more likelihood of making that determination. With a single-edged knife, a stab wound has a point at one end. With a double-edged knife, there are points at both ends of the stab wound. It is possible for a single-edged blade to have points at both ends. This can occur if the knife is pulled downward after the point penetrates the skin, which keeps the squared-off back of the knife from contacting the skin. It also may occur if the point also has a cutting edge on the back and the knife is pulled down even slightly, in which case the back of the blade will not contact the skin.

It is also difficult to determine if the blade edge is smooth or serrated unless marks or imprints around the wound or on the skin reveal the configuration of the blade edge surface. If there is full penetration of the knife, the guard may leave an imprint on the skin. The ricasso can cause both ends of the wound to be square because of the blunt edges (Di Maio and Di Maio 2001). Superficial wounds may be made if the assailant was repetitively attempting to stab the animal and was unable to initially fully penetrate with the knife or was unable to control the animal.

The shape of the wound is also affected by the properties of the skin. If the skin is stretched when the stab wound is made, it may appear more broad and shorter when the skin relaxes. The Langer's lines also have an effect on the appearance of stab wounds. These are skin tension lines that have different orientations depending on the region of the body. If a stab wound is made perpendicular to the Langer's lines, it will tend to pull apart the edges of the wound. If it is made parallel to these lines, it will create narrow and more slit-like wounds. If a stab wound is made oblique to the Langer's lines it will appear asymmetrical or semicircular (Di Maio and Di Maio 2001). The edges of gaping wounds should be apposed with scotch tape to determine the wound length and approximate the knife width.

When the knife is withdrawn from the body, it may be twisted by the perpetrator or the victim may move, creating a secondary exit path. This can create a Y- or L-shaped wound if there is substantial movement. If there is only slight movement it can create a V-shaped notch or "fork" at the cutting end of the wound instead of a point (Di Maio and Di Maio 2001).

In single-edged blades the opposite end may be square-shaped from the back of the blade. This end also may look forked because of tears by the back of the blade. If the ricasso penetrates the wound, then both ends may be squared off and may or may not have tears resembling a forked area. These tears can be differentiated from the cutting edge because they are not as clean and sharp and usually are only found in the superficial skin layers (Di Maio and Di Maio 2001).

The imprint of the guard may be found on the skin if there is full penetration of the knife with sufficient force. If the knife is plunged straight and perpendicular to the skin, the mark from the guard is symmetrical. If the knife enters at an angle from the right, the mark is to the right of the wound. If the knife enters at a downward angle, the mark is above the stab wound. If the knife enters at an upward angle, the mark is below the wound (Di Maio and Di Maio 2001).

Miscellaneous Instruments

Stab wounds made with other instruments may reflect the unique characteristics and configuration of the weapon. Wounds made with ice picks are less common because they are no longer commonly used in households. Ice pick wounds can be easily missed and are sometimes mistaken for gunshot wounds caused by shotgun pellets or .22 caliber bullets. A fork may be used for stabbing, although it is very hard for the prongs of a kitchen fork to penetrate the skin. The perforations seen with fork stabbings correspond to the number of tines or prongs on the weapon and are evenly spaced. The wounds made by scissors depend on if the blades are open or closed. If the scissor blades are open, then two stab wounds are produced. If the blades are closed, the wound produced is caused by splitting the skin versus cutting. The stab wound created is linear and has abraded edges. If the screw holding the scissor blades together protrudes out, it can create an angular laceration in the middle along one edge of the wound (Di Maio and Di Maio 2001).

When screwdrivers are used in stabbing, the wound can show the characteristics of the type of screwdriver. A Phillips screwdriver produces a circular wound with abraded margins and four equally spaced cuts. A slit-like wound is produced by a flat-blade screwdriver with squared ends and abraded margins. This wound can be difficult to differentiate from one caused by a dull knife blade that is plunged up to the guard. Broken bottles may be used as weapons and tend to create sharp and ragged wounds. They tend to be in clusters with a variety sizes, shapes, and depths (Di Maio and Di Maio 2001).

Arrows

Wounds caused by arrows or crossbow bolts are considered stab wounds. There are often severe internal injuries and bone fractures. The arrowhead configuration determines the appearance of the wounds. In target arrows, the end is pointed and conical.

These produce circular entrance wounds similar to gunshot wounds. In hunting arrows, the ends have two to five knife-like edges. In the four-edged arrows, the wounds are X-shaped or cross-like and the edges appear incised without evidence of abrasions (Di Maio and Di Maio 2001). Impaling injuries may be seen either because of accidental falls or purposeful manipulation of the animal. It is important to get witness statements as to when the animal was last seen alive. All effort should be made to determine if the impaling took place antemortem or postmortem.

Determining the Sequence of Events: Effects of Blood Loss

After being stabbed, the victim may be able to move for a substantial distance, depending on the injuries sustained. A blood trail may be found at the scene that leads to the site of the assault. If the animal is stabbed multiple times, the last stab wound may appear bloodless if there was substantial bleeding from the other wounds. This also can make it difficult to determine if the wound was antemortem or postmortem and the determination may be perimortem, as the animal died before a tissue reaction could develop.

With a deceased animal there may be minimum drainage of blood from the wounds depending on the injuries. When the body is moved blood may escape through the wounds. There may be substantial internal blood if a large vessel located in the dependent part of the body was severed, allowing drainage from other vessels postmortem (Di Maio and Di Maio 2001). If the body has been immersed in water for a prolonged period of time, the blood from the wounds can be leached out by the water. This can give the wound the appearance it was postmortem versus antemortem.

Considerations in Removal of the Object

As with all penetrating injuries, care should be taken not to remove the foreign object in a live animal without proper preparation for treatment. The object is often causing compression and preventing hemorrhage. Withdrawal of the object may not only allow life-threatening hemorrhage, it may also cause more tissue damage. When the weapon is removed, care should be taken not to smudge potential fingerprints or destroy other forensic evidence. If a knife is embedded, the handle should be grabbed by the sides adjacent to the skin to avoid touching the portion of the handle where the assailant's hand and fingers likely had contact (Di Maio and Di Maio 2001).

Determination of the Weapon

Making a determination of the type of weapon used in stabbings should be done with extreme caution. The most information that can be given is usually an approximation of the blade width and length and whether it was a single- or double-edged blade. The determination of smooth versus serrated can be made only if there are marks on the skin revealing a serrated blade; this is rare. The guard pattern imprinted on the skin may be matched to a particular type of knife. Injuries to bones may leave an imprint pattern that may be matched to a weapon (see below). A weapon only can be matched to the wounds if a piece of the blade or weapon broke off in the body. This may be the tip of the knife when it penetrates bone. The recovered tip may be matched conclusively to a weapon by a forensic tool examiner using tool mark comparison.

All potential weapons recovered from a crime scene should be tested for blood and tissue, both human and animal. Initially, the suspected weapon may not be found at the scene but discovered later in the investigation. It should be anticipated that a weapon and/or suspect will be found and DNA samples should be taken from the animal to use for comparison testing. Also it should be noted that the assailant may slip and cut him- or herself during the assault, potentially leaving his or her blood on the animal's body or at the scene. All blood found on the animal and at the scene should be sampled separately and saved for testing.

Evaluation of Injuries

Stab wounds may inflict severe damage to the internal structures of the body. The cause of death depends on the injuries but often results from exsanguination. In the chest, there may be lacerations of the major blood vessels, lungs, heart, diaphragm, trachea, or the esophagus. Rib fractures, hemothorax, and pneumothorax may be found. In the heart, the ventricular muscle can contract slowing or terminating bleeding (Di Maio and Di Maio 2001). Stab wounds to the abdomen can cause lacerations of the organs or major blood vessels. If the intestinal tract is lacerated, death may be secondary to peritonitis.

Stab wounds to the neck can produce exsanguination, air embolism, trachea laceration, or asphyxia caused by soft tissue hemorrhage compressing the trachea and vessels of the neck. Arterial thrombosis is possible. Radiographs of the chest may reveal air embolus. Stab wounds to the head penetrating to the brain are uncommon and usually are through the eye or temporal region in humans (Di Maio and Di Maio 2001). These stab wounds can produce intracerebral, subarachnoid, and/or subdural hemorrhage. Stab wounds to the spine may occur and either cause fractures or spinal cord injury. The extremities may be stabbed, causing muscle, ligament, joint, or major vessel damage. Fractures are possible in the extremities, especially with arrows.

The ends of injured bone and especially cartilage may contain weapon patterns. With any penetration injury, the weapon used may leave tool marks on bone or cartilage. A cast should be taken of any indentation to preserve any tool marks for comparison to the offending weapon. Mikrosil is a rubber casting material that is inexpensive and easily used. It may be ordered from any forensic supply company. Brown is the preferred color for tool mark examiners (see Chapter 3).

Incised-Stab Wounds

An incised-stab wound is found when a stab wound changes to an incised wound. The stab is made first, but instead of withdrawing the blade, it is pulled along the body, cutting through tissue and creating a wound that is longer than it is deep. The only way to determine the direction is if there are markings at one end indicating where the blade was withdrawn (Di Maio and Di Maio 2001).

Incised Wounds

General Appearance

Incised wounds, also called *cuts,* are created by sharp-edged instruments or weapons, including knives, glass, or metal implements. The wound produced has a length greater than its depth. In contrast to stabbings, the length and depth of the wound do not correlate to the type of weapon used. Incised wounds should not be confused with lacerations. The edges are typically sharp and clean with no abrasions, contusions, or tissue bridging in the base of the wound. Lacerations have abraded ragged edges with tissue bridging. Instruments that have dull, irregular, or nicked cutting edge can produce incisive wounds that are abraded, irregular, or contused because of the pressure required to cut with that particular weapon. However, no tissue bridging is found in the depth of the wound.

Incised wounds typically are superficial at the beginning, become deeper, and then ending superficially. When a blade is held at an oblique angle, the wound has a beveled or undermined edge. When the blade is held at an extreme angle a skin flap is created. If the blade cuts along wrinkles of skin instead of a flat area, a straight line of interrupted cuts is seen when the skin is flattened where the blade cut just the tops of the wrinkle folds. If the blade draws the skin up into irregular folds as it cuts, the wounds may appear irregular or zigzag when the skin is flattened (Di Maio and Di Maio 2001).

Edges of incised wounds tend to gap open. The amount of the gap is determined on the orientation of the wound to the Langer's lines. An incised wound that is perpendicular or oblique to the Langer's lines gaps further than one that is parallel to the lines. The elastic fibers pull the skin apart and evert the edges (Di Maio and Di Maio 2001). Clear scotch tape can be used to appose edges together to get accurate measurements of the length. This also allows evaluation of the edges to try and determine the type of blade used. Documentation of incised wounds should be done the same as for stab wounds, including drawings, written descriptions, and photographs.

Superficial Incised Wounds (Hesitation Marks)

Superficial incisive wounds may be found adjacent to the deeper incisive wounds. In the past, classification of these incised marks in human cases has been termed *hesitation marks*. It has been suggested that these marks do not necessarily denote a hesitation or lack of intent by the perpetrator, but may instead show a repetitive attempt to perform the act (the cut) better each time. By assigning the term of hesitation, it gives a misleading description of the events that took place (Symes et al. 2002). These superficial marks also could be caused by the victim struggling during the attack.

Interpretation of Neck Wounds

Incised wounds of the neck may be produced from behind or in front of the body. If done from behind, the wound characteristics may reflect the initial cut from the end, indicating if the individual was right- or left-handed. In human homicides, the wound starts shallow and higher on the left side of the victim, extends deeper, then shallow again, terminating lower on the right side. If done from the front, a right-handed assailant creates incisive marks on the left side of the victim's neck, and the opposite for a left-handed assailant. Horizontal incisive wounds to the neck may be made from the front if the assailant makes swipes or slashes to the neck. Deep incisive wounds penetrating to the vertebral column are possible and are inflicted from behind the victim (Di Maio and Di Maio 2001).

Fatal Wounds

Death from incisive wounds often results from exsanguination. Death from neck incisive wounds may result from exsanguination or massive air embolus, which may be detected in chest radiographs (Di Maio and Di Maio 2001). If the body has been immersed in water for a prolonged period of time, the blood from the wounds can be leached out by the water. This can give the wound the appearance that it was postmortem versus antemortem.

Chop Wounds

Chop wounds are caused by heavy instruments with a cutting edge such as machetes, axes, and meat cleavers. These wounds appear incisive and have underlying damage to the bone, either fractures or a deep groove from the cutting edge. When the weapon is pulled out of the bone, it may be necessary to give it a sharp twist, which breaks off the adjacent bone or creates fractures. If the instrument strikes at an angle it may chop off disks of bone. The wounds may have both lacerations and incisive characteristics when there are crushing and cutting forces from the weapon. As with all penetrating injuries, the presence of hemorrhage into the surrounding soft tissue indicates the injury was antemortem. The immersion of the body in water can leach out the blood, giving the appearance of postmortem injury.

The weapon used can leave unique tool mark striations on the bone. Evaluations of the hacking trauma caused by machetes, axes, and meat cleavers have been conducted. Hacking blows to bone have at least one smooth, flat side. If the blow was directed at an angle, there is fracturing of the opposite side. Meat cleavers create clean, narrow wounds without fractures. Microscopically they create sharp, distinct thin, fine striations in the bone. Machetes produce wider, less-clean wounds with fractures in the bed of the cut and small fragmented bone at the entrance site. Microscopically they produce more pronounced striations than cleavers but they are coarse and less distinct. Crushing, fragmented wounds with fractures are produced by axes. Microscopically, they create no striations in the wounds of bone (Di Maio and Di Maio 2001).

Therapeutic or Diagnostic Wounds

When an animal has been treated at a hospital prior to death, it is vital to get a history of the procedures that were performed, including any resuscitative measures. Wounds that result from hospital procedures may be misinterpreted as related to the initial injuries. The original wounds may have been obscured or obliterated by surgical procedures, they may have been used for chest tubes, or resuscitation may have caused additional injuries or hemorrhage. All tubes, intravenous lines, and drains should not be removed upon death of the animal until a necropsy is performed.

Mutilation

Mutilation of a live or deceased animal may be seen. Oftentimes, these cases are caused by predators, such as foxes and coyotes. They also may be pranks using already deceased animals. Some cases are the result of animal cruelty. In all cases, it is imperative to determine if the animal was alive or deceased at the time of injury and the body should be examined for evidence of predation.

Predation is usually easily determined by close examination of the body. The edges of the wounds are often irregular with evidence of crushing and tearing. Puncture marks may be found. The bone injuries are often characterized by crushing and splintering. The bone injuries usually are seen on the sides and ends of the bones. The claws of the victim may contain embedded fur from the attacking animal.

Mutilation by humans may involve the cutting and removal of body parts such as the head, ears, and tails. These may be complete or partial with only a portion of the ear or tail removed. In Atlanta, a neighborhood began noticing that the stray cats all had injuries to their ears and tails. Investigators discovered that a man was taking the cats and mutilating their ears and tails in his apartment, taking pictures and keeping a log of each act.

The toenails may be pulled off as a form of torture versus accidental traumatic avulsion. The body may be partially or completely skinned. There may be decapitation or dismemberment of the body. The characteristics of the wounds to the skin and bones can help determine what type of weapon was used (see Chapter 3). The presence of hemorrhage and histology of the tissue can help determine antemortem versus postmortem injuries. If there are only distal body parts found without the proximal main part of the body, a determination of whether the animal was alive or dead at the time of mutilation cannot be made. The part of the body that was still connected to the torso will reveal any vital reaction if the animal was alive. Tissue samples should be taken for potential DNA comparison.

Ritualistic Crimes

Ritualistic crimes involve ceremonial acts that are often related to behavior patterns based on a belief in some occult ideology. These crimes can be not only disturbing, but also frustrating because of the general unfamiliarity with these practices. There are several groups that perform rituals that involve animal sacrifice and sometimes mutilation. These include Satanism, Voodoo, Santeria, and Palo Mayombe. The common factor of all these groups is the use of blood in their rituals. They believe that blood contains the life force energy and power.

The evidence found at the crime scene is the key to determining what group is involved. The use of blood is more significant than any other evidence found at the scene. Animal mutilation is one of the common crimes associated with ritualistic violence. Some groups use chickens, birds, and goats for their animal sacrifice; however, some use domestic animals such as cats and dogs. These groups include Satanism, Vampirism, and Palo Mayombe. The scene should be evaluated for symbols, symbolic objects, candles, calendars, the type of animal mutilation, and the species of animal used. These findings determine the belief system that committed the act.

Satanism

There are several Satanism categories that are linked with animal crimes and additional criminal activity. The Traditional/Intergenerational Satanist engages in blood rituals, animal and human sacrifice, sexual abuse, kidnapping, child pornography, arson, and ritual murder involving mutilation and cannibalism. The Self-Styled Satanist is linked with child molestation, animal mutilation, and homicide. The Youth Subculture Satanists engage in animal mutilation, vandalism, arson, school violence, grave desecration, and sometimes homicide. Their crimes tend to escalate over time. The Modern Satanists believe that violence is part of human nature and that ritualistic sacrifice is necessary to defer violence. They perform animal sacrifice and have been linked to human sacrifice (Perlmutter 2004).

Vampirism

The vampirism culture engages in blood rituals, role-playing games, and sadomasochism that can escalate to murder. The purpose of their ritual of blood letting and drinking is to acquire energy from the blood source. Some use animal blood if it is fresh. They also attribute magical qualities to the blood, believing they will acquire the strength and qualities of their victim. Vampirism has been linked with child molestation, vandalism, animal mutilation, and murder.

Palo Mayombe

Palo Mayombe is the dark side of the Santeria religion. Santeria and Palo Mayombe are a syncretic religion composed of two or more belief systems. They are Afro-Caribbean faiths formed from the Catholicism that was imposed on African slaves. The Africans tried to hide their beliefs by assigning a Catholic saint image to each of their gods. All syncretic religions incorporate the practice of magic and belief in the supernatural.

Palo Mayombe rituals center around the spirits of the dead; their purpose is to manipulate or threaten a person. Both religions perform animal sacrifice, using special *orisha* candles and other items in their rituals. A blood offering is part of their

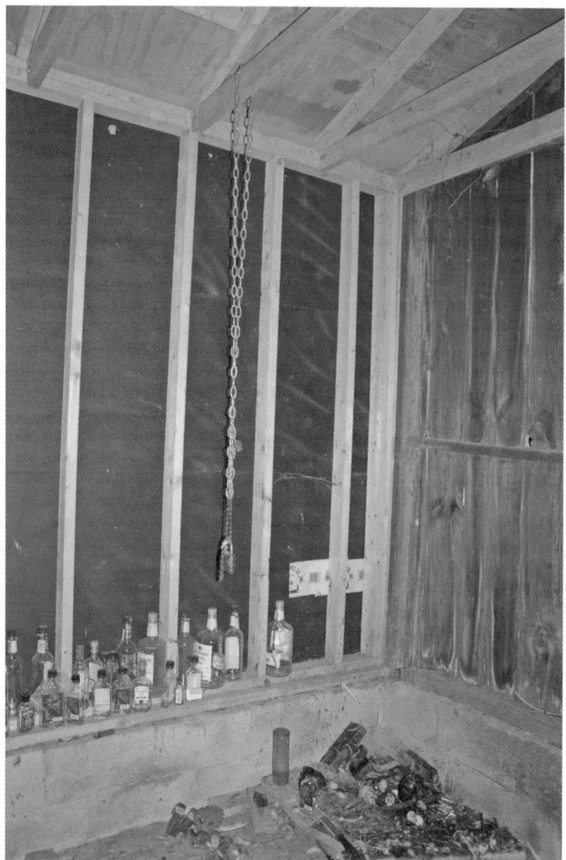

Fig. 6.2 Palo Mayombe ritual site with bottles of alcohol, candles, and a chain to hold the animals while dripping blood on the altar. For color detail, please see color plate section.

ritual to "feed" their orisha (god) and usually is associated with a larger problem or event. In Santeria, the animals commonly used are goats, roosters, and other birds. The animal is normally killed by slicing the throat or breaking the neck. Evidence of animal torture or mutilation is indicative of Palo Mayombe, another occult religion, or a non-religious act of cruelty. Animal sacrifice involving cats, dogs, or large animals such as cows are more commonly associated with Palo Mayombe, Satanism, other occult groups, or disturbed individuals.

The animal sacrifice usually involves removing the head from the body. The body may then be stuffed with food and other items. The head, and sometimes the body, are then disposed of in public areas such as beaches, railroad tracks, cemeteries, road intersections, or other locations that may have magical significance. With Palo Mayombe, the animal's body may be left at the entrance to a person's home or business.

There may be human bones at the scene of a Palo Mayombe ritual site. Bottles of alcohol are commonly found around the ceremonial site. There is a sacred con-

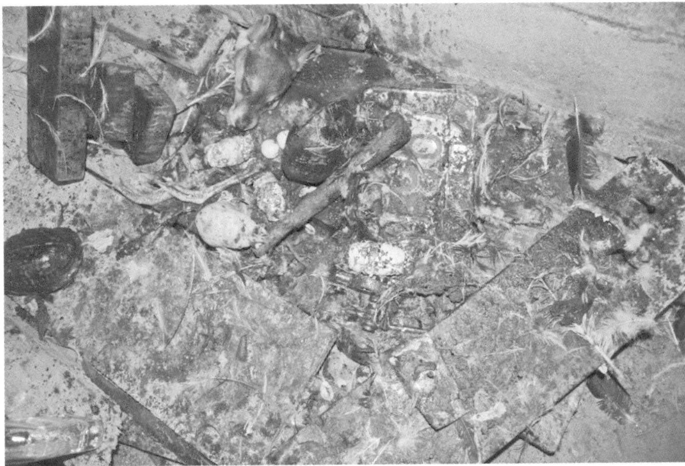

Fig. 6.3 Palo Mayombe inner altar containing bird feet, turtle shells, sea shells, eggs, feathers, animal bones, toy cars, pictures, license plate, and the head of a puppy. For color detail, please see color plate section.

tainer or cauldron containing a variety of herbs, human bones, sticks, stones, and animal bones or carcasses. This cauldron is "fed" with blood. It is common to find the blood drained from the body of the animal (Figs. 6.2, 6.3).

Crime Scene Investigation for Ritualistic Crimes

Evidence that is crucial to the investigation is anything that can establish time lines or ownership of the animals, or demonstrate that the animal was alive at the time of sacrifice. Any animal body or body parts should be collected for examination and to collect DNA samples. The animal should be examined for any evidence of antemortem injury and appropriate tissue samples taken. Any antemortem reaction only occurs in the parts of the body that were still attached to the cardiovascular system at the time of injury. The scene should be examined for containers used to hold the live animals during the ritual, such as carriers or bags. In addition, ropes or chains may have been used to suspend the animal over the ritual site.

In addition to written documentation, photographs taken of the scene should include all the names on the candles and any calendars. There may be bones of previously sacrificed animals. Blood spatter is always present, requiring careful documentation for analysis. Samples of all blood should be collected for DNA testing. Any knives found should be collected and tested.

References

Beardsley, S.L. 2000. Shearing and Degloving Wounds on the Extremities of Dogs and Cats. In *Kirk's Current Veterinary Therapy XIII Small Animal Practice*, ed. J.D. Bonagura, pp. 1032–1035. Philadelphia: W.B. Saunders.

Di Maio, V.J., and D. Di Maio. 2001. *Forensic Pathology,* 2nd ed. Boca Raton, FL: CRC Press.

Perlmutter, D. 2004. *Investigating Religious Terrorism and Ritualistic Crimes.* Boca Raton, FL: CRC Press.

Symes, S.A., J.A. Williams, E.A. Murray, J.M. Hoffman, T.D. Holland, J.M. Saul, F.P. Saul, and E.J. Pople. 2002. Taphonomic Context of Sharp-Force Trauma in Suspected Cases of Human Mutilation and Dismemberment. In *Advances in Forensic Taphonomy*, ed. W.D. Haglund, and M.H. Sorg, pp. 403–434. Boca Raton, FL: CRC Press.

Chapter 7

Patterns of Non-accidental Injury: Burns

Interpreting Burn Patterns

The suspicion of deliberate infliction of burns on an animal is raised when the history offered by the owner does not match the presentation of the burn, the environment, or the behavior of the animal. Some owners may blame the animal laying too close to a hot object as the cause of the burn. Although it is possible for an animal to sustain a thermal burn injury before registering the pain it is causing, the burn pattern may not match a contact burn. In animals with unexplained eschar the possibility of some kind of burn should be considered and investigated.

The appearance of the burn provides several clues as to its cause. Burns are usually a patterned injury that reflects the cause of the injury. Proper interpretation of the burn patterns can reveal the exact nature of events that may support or refute the history and help direct the investigation. A determination of where the burn started on the body may be made when there are more severe burns confluent with more superficial burns. Splash or spill burns have trickle-like burns where the offending liquid ran down the body. These trickle-like areas are usually more superficial than the place where the liquid first contacted the body. A burn pattern that is evenly distributed with the same degree of injury is indicative of an even rate of burn. This can result from a flash fire or chemical agent. The location of the burn can indicate whether the burn could have been accidental versus intentional. When an animal is set on fire and the fur burns for a short period of time there may not be large areas of burns to the underlying skin. Instead, there may be a wide distribution of isolated circular burns on the skin where the fur acted as a wick for the fire to reach the skin. There may be a larger burn area on the skin where the fire was initially ignited on the body (Figs. 7.1, 7.2).

Collection of Evidence

Evidence pertaining to a fire includes any substances and or devices that were used to cause the fire or produce the burn and related injuries. The accelerant, chemical, or liquid that caused the burn may be on the animal or nearby objects. There may be an odor associated with the injured area that may indicate the cause of the burn. It is imperative to take samples in all burn injuries. The burn and adjacent tissue

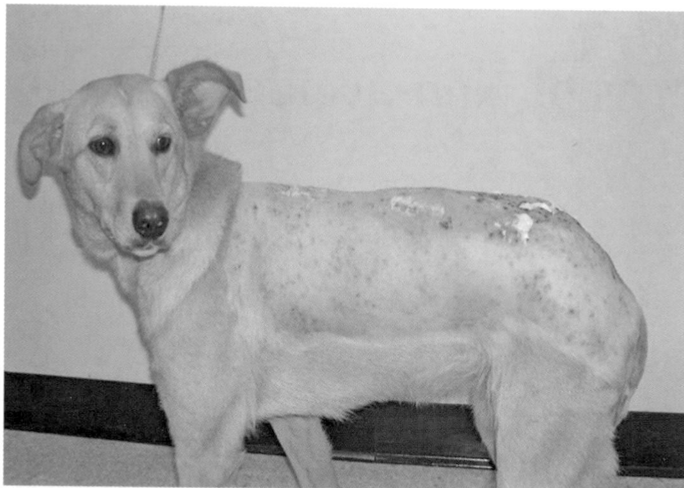

Fig. 7.1 This dog was seen running down the street with her back on fire. The fur was shaved revealing a symmetrical burn pattern on the sides of the torso and caudal pelvis. For color detail, please see color plate section.

should be swabbed for accelerants or chemicals. Samples of the fur and skin should be taken for residue testing. The soil beneath the animal and adjacent to it should be collected along with any bedding. The device used to ignite the fire may be a cigarette lighter, matches, or blow torch and may contain residue of the accelerant on the surface. When collecting evidence related to a fire it is important to use proper

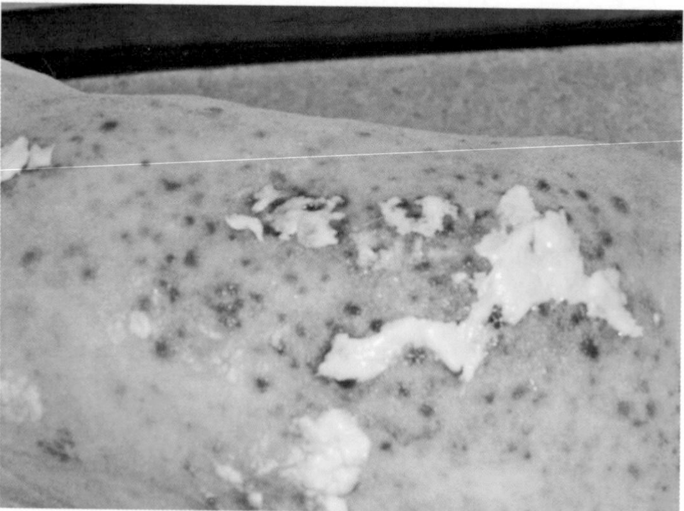

Fig. 7.2 Close-up of dog from Figure 7.1 revealing a few larger and deeper burn areas that have been treated with burn cream. The majority of the body is covered with small, circular burns because the fur acts as a wick for the fire to burn down to the skin. For color detail, please see color plate section.

containers. Accelerants are volatile substances and may escape through plastic. The best way to preserve this evidence is by placing it in a clean, uncoated paint can or a special container for arson evidence.

Burn Classification

The severity of each burn must be determined. This can be done using a classification system based on the degree or depth of the burn and total body surface area affected (Table 7.1). The severity of the burn is also determined based on the location. Burns affecting the face, eyes, ears, perineum, and feet are considered more severe because of the potential for serious disfigurement, loss of function, and severity of the pain associated with burns in these areas. The evaluation of the burn may be hindered by the hair coat, which prevents full visualization of the injured skin. Further complicating matters is the fact that skin is slow to heat and slow to cool. Thermal damage continues after the animal is removed from the source of the heat (Saxon and Kirby 1992). It is prudent to overestimate the burn severity than underestimate it.

Percentage of Total Body Surface Area

The burn must further be classified by the percentage of total body surface area (TBSA) involved. The TBSA may be quickly determined using the rule of nines. This rule assigns a certain body surface area percentage to each area of the body. Each forelimb accounts for 9 percent each; each hind limb is 18 percent; head and neck together is 9 percent; the dorsal and ventral thorax is 18 percent; and the dorsal and ventral abdomen is 18 percent (Saxon and Kirby 1992) and the perineum is 1 percent. Another method is to measure the burned area in centimeters and compare the body surface area in meters. The body weight in kilograms can be converted to body surface area in meters using the standard conversion table of body weight to total body surface area. It has been recommended in the past that animals suffering from burns involving over 50 percent of their body be humanely euthanized. However, in human burn cases there are increased survival rates in patients

Table 7.1. Burn classification.

Classification	Skin Layer	Pain	Signs
Superficial	Epidermis	+++	Erythema, desquamation
Partial-superficial	Partial epidermis, mid-dermis	++	Erythema, subcutaneous edema
Partial-deep	Total epidermis, partial dermis	++	Severe inflammation, dry surface, does not blanch
Full	Epidermis, dermis	–	Leathery (eschar), dry surface, blanched

Source: Saxon, W.D. and R. Kirby. 1992. Treatment of Acute Burn Injury and Smoke Inhalation. In *Current Veterinary Therapy XI Small Animal Practice*, ed. R.W. Kirk and J.D. Bonagura, pp. 146–154. Philadelphia: W.B. Saunders.

with over 85 percent of their body involved because of improvements in treatment and wound management techniques.

Degrees of Burn

First-degree burns are superficial burns that affect only the epidermis. They are characterized by pain, erythema, and desquamation, and are thickened. Erythema is less in animals than in humans with first-degree burns because of the lack of superficial vascular plexus. Healing occurs within 5 days and most often without scarring. Usually they are not included in burn surface calculation unless they exceed 25 percent of the body surface area (Jutkowitz 2005).

Second-degree burns include superficial and deep partial-thickness burns that involve the epidermis and one-half of the dermis. Superficial partial-thickness burns are painful, blistered, and blanch when pressure is applied (Hedlund 2002). The upper layers of the subcutaneous fat are still present. There is subcutaneous edema present, notable inflammation, and the hair is intact. The burn may appear moist, red, or mottled (Jutkowitz 2005). These burns usually heal in 2–3 weeks with mild scarring. Deep partial-thickness burns may appear moist, blistered, or dried. The wounds may have a red-mottled appearance, they do not blanch, and hair is easily epilated. They are slow to heal and are associated with serious scarring and loss of function (Jutkowitz 2005). Second-degree burns may vary in areas to third-degree burns changing in appearance. In the first 24 hours there is progressive damage resulting from heat injury, and the release of vasoactive substances, prostaglandins, and proteolytic enzymes, causing further edema and tissue destruction. If appropriate therapy is not started or secondary bacterial infection occurs this burn may progress to a third-degree burn (Hedlund 2002).

Third-degree burns are full-thickness burns characterized by a dark brown, leathery eschar and are dry with white or charred coloration (Fig. 7.3). In these burns there is full destruction of all the skin structures, sometimes extending to the subcutaneous tissue, and the hair easily epilates. There is much less pain than the other burns because the nerves have been destroyed. Healing occurs by contraction, epithelialization, and granulation or by surgical intervention. There is subcutaneous edema and necrosis resulting from superficial vascular thrombosis and deep vascular permeability (Hedlund 2002).

Damage to the underlying muscle or bone may occur and is considered a fourth-degree burn. These burns are associated with severe tissue necrosis and subsequent systemic illness (Jutkowitz 2005).

Systemic Effects of Burns

Burns may cause severe systemic problems, especially in animals with large burn surface areas. Severe burns are characterized by burns involving greater than 20 percent of the total body surface area (Jutkowitz 2005). Victims of burns often are in shock and develop multiple organ failure because of the loss of fluid and resultant hypovolemia, fluid shifts, electrolyte imbalances, protein loss, myocardial depression, raised peripheral vascular resistance, and increased blood viscosity. Some

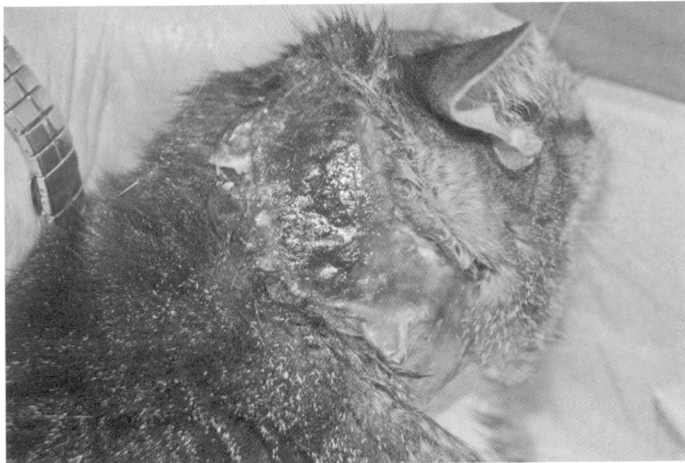

Fig. 7.3 Eschar burn on the neck of a cat caused by a heat lamp. For color detail, please see color plate section.

animals develop further complications, including sepsis, immunosuppression, renal failure, liver failure, anemia, cardiac abnormalities, and disseminated intravascular coagulation (Hedlund 2002). In burn patients, sepsis is a major contributor to death. The source of infection comes from the wounds, respiratory infection, and catheter sites. In addition, the gastrointestinal mucosal barrier is compromised, allowing endotoxins and bacteria to penetrate the blood stream contributing to multi-organ failure (Jutkowitz 2005).

General Histopathological Findings in Burns

Thermal burns often cause deeper injury than chemical burns. Some thermal and chemical burns may be clinically indistinguishable unless residue of the chemical is present on the hair coat or skin. Electrical and microwave radiation can cause lesions that are histopathologically indistinguishable. Areas of erythema without ulceration are the best sites for skin biopsy. Microscopically there is coagulation necrosis of the epidermis, which often extends through the epidermis to the hair follicles. Second-degree burns involve the adnexal glands as well. The dermal collagen is usually less necrotic than the epithelial structures. Third-degree chemical and thermal burns are characterized by full-thickness obliterative acellular necrosis of all dermal structures extending to the panniculus or deeper subcutaneous tissue.

Thermal Burns

General Findings

Thermal burns may be caused by fires, heating pads, ovens, hair dryers, hot liquid, steam, microwave ovens, heat lamps, space heaters, or radiators. Thermal damage produced by clothes dryers or hot gases are similar to injuries seen in fire victims (covered later in this chapter). Thermal burns may be produced by contact or near-contact to the heat source. Several factors affect the extent of the injury, including the temperature of the heat source, length of contact, and conductance of the tissue. Thermal burns from contact with a hot object may not be easily recognized after the injury. It may be a few days before anything abnormal is noticed. The fur may appear matted down and moist with eventual loss of hair and skin (Hedlund 2002).

The skin of the animal does not disseminate heat as the human skin does because of the lack of a plentiful superficial vascular plexus. In a burn wound in which the heat source had direct contact there is coagulation, cellular protein denaturation, and blood vessel coagulation (Hedlund 2002). There is plasma loss and tissue edema in the burn wound. Local tissue ischemia is apparent within 3–5 days (Smith 1995). There is a transition area that divides the devitalized tissue from healthy tissue. This area has potentially reversible tissue damage, reduced blood flow, and intravascular sludging. Because of the release of vasoactive substances there may be continued dermal ischemia, tissue edema, dessication, and secondary bacterial invasion. This transition zone is surrounded by hyperemic tissue. Eschar is the residue of coagulated skin elements composed of tough, denatured collagen fibers that form a strong protective covering of the wound. Comparatively, scabs are not as protective and are composed of dead skin cells, blood cells, and fibrin.

Initially, it may be difficult to assess the depth of a burn requiring repeated evaluation during the first 24 hours. Eschar covering can make determination of the wound depth difficult to assess. When raised and bent to reveal the underlying tissue, the eschar splits in first- and second-degree burns. In third-degree burns the eschar may or may not split and if it does, the split may extend down to the subcutaneous tissue. Bacterial invasion under the eschar occurs within 4 to 5 days (Hedlund 2002).

Radiant Heat Burns

Radiant heat burns are near-contact burns caused by the heat waves produced from a hot surface such as a flame, heat lamp, fire, oven, or radiator. Depending on the temperature, burns can occur in seconds. Conventional ovens that operate through radiant heat cook from the outside of the body in. Radiant heat causes maximum injury to the outside of the body. Initially, the skin may appear erythematous and blistered with possible skin slippage in areas. At first, the hair may be intact. If there is prolonged exposure the skin can become leathery with eventual charring (Di Maio and Di Maio 2001).

Microwave Ovens

Microwaves produce heat through molecular agitation, primarily through water. The larger the water content of the tissue, the greater the heat that is produced. Because muscle tissue contains more water than fat, it sustains more thermal injury (Di Maio and Di Maio 2001). The amount of damage also depends on the length of time the body is in the microwave oven and the strength of the microwaves produced. Microwaves produce heat directly to the internal tissue. The external body may sustain partial- to full-thickness burns that tend to be well demarcated without charring (Di Maio and Di Maio 2001). This may be more likely located in the thinner, peripheral tissue, such as the ears. The greatest injury is to the internal body. Burns are based on the water distribution in the tissues. Biopsies may show sparing of different tissues giving a sandwich-type appearance. For example, skin burns may show sparing of the subcutaneous fat and burns of the underlying muscle (Di Maio and Di Maio 2001).

Cigarette Burns

Cigarette burns may be found in abused children; these burn patterns and injuries are well documented. In acute burns the area is red, circular, 0.5–1.0 cm in diameter, and possibly wedge shaped if the cigarette was applied at an oblique angle. When there is a deliberate burn they are often full thickness, creating a crater. Older burns may be circular and sunken with thin scar tissue on the surface. Whereas accidental cigarette burns tend to be superficial and usually more eccentric. This is because of the brief brush with the hot ash from the cigarette (Munro and Thrusfield 2001). It is important to rule out other possible skin lesions when examining these areas. A biopsy of the lesions should help determine the cause.

Scalding Burns

Scalding burns are caused by contact with a hot liquid. They may be produced by immersion, spill or splashing, or exposure to superheated steam. Water heaters in most houses and apartments are set at 140°F. Full-thickness burns can occur in just a few seconds at this temperature. In animals, scalding can occur when the fluid temperature is >48.8°C or 120°F (Sinclair and Lockwood 2006). In humans, the time and temperature of water required to cause epidermal damage and full-thickness burns has been documented (Table 7.2).

In splash or spill burns, the fluid cools as it flows down the body. The burn is more severe where the fluid has initial contact with the skin, becoming more superficial where the fluid trickles down. Superheated steam causes severe scald-like burns. If the steam is inhaled there are laryngeal and tracheal burns with possibly nasal and deeper airway injury. There may be massive edema in the larynx causing occlusion of the airway and asphyxia (Di Maio and Di Maio 2001).

Table 7.2. Water temperature and scalding burns time in humans.

Temp (°F)	Threshold for Epidermal Injury	Full-Thickness Burns
120	290 sec	600 sec
125	50 sec	120 sec
130	15 sec	30 sec
140	2.6 sec	~7 sec
150	<1 sec	2.3 sec

Source: Di Maio, V.J., and D. Di Maio. 2001. *Forensic Pathology*, 2nd ed., p. 349. Boca Raton, FL: CRC Press.

Chemical Burns

Overview

Burns resulting from chemicals that are strong acids or alkalis cause severe tissue damage by interfering with cell metabolism or denaturing proteins. These burns may be external, internal, or a combination of both. Because thermal and chemical burns produce the same injury, the burn must be examined carefully to determine the cause.

Tissue damage occurs through different mechanisms of action with chemical burns. Chemicals that are oxidizing cause injury by coagulation of protein (chromic acid, hypochlorite, and potassium permanganate); dehydrating chemicals desiccate the tissues (sulfuric and hydrochloric acids); denaturizing chemicals fix or stabilize tissue through the formation of salts (picric acid, tannic acid, acetic acid, formic acid, and hydrofluoric acid); corrosive agents denature proteins causing erosion and ulceration (sodium-containing drain and oven cleaners, and phenol disinfectants); vesicants cause the release of tissue histamine and serotonin resulting in blisters (dimethylsulfoxide, cantharides, halogenated hydrocarbons, and gasoline) (Hedlund 2002).

General Findings

The degree of injury depends on several factors, including the type of chemical and its action, volume of chemical in contact with the body, strength of the chemical, length of contact time, penetration of the chemical, and whether or not the animal ingested any of the offending agent. Injuries can range from superficial to third-degree burns.

Chemicals that have contact with the eye can cause severe corneal damage, including full-thickness perforation and corneal necrosis. With chemical burns heat is often generated because of the chemical reactions causing thermal injury (Hedlund 2002). The ingestion of chemicals by an animal may be caused by accidental exposure, licking the chemical off the body because of accidental or intentional chemical burns, or intentional feeding of the harmful chemicals. Chemical burns caused by ingestion may be found on the tongue, palate, gums, oropharynx, along the esophagus, and in the stomach depending on how the agent was ingested and the amount.

Some chemical agents can cause systemic poisoning in addition to chemical burns. These include phenol, yellow phosphorus, and ammonium sulfide. Phenol can cause acute tubular necrosis and phosphorus can cause kidney and liver necrosis (Di Maio and Di Maio 2001). Common compounds can produce chemical burns with prolonged contact. Cement is a very strong alkaline compound with a pH of 12.5–14. Hydrocarbons, such as gasoline, can produce partial-thickness burns with prolonged contact. They have an irritating effect and high lipid solubility, which permits dissolution of fatty tissue (Di Maio and Di Maio 2001).

A wide variety of chemicals have been associated with animal abuse, including battery acid. Lye, which is sodium hydroxide, has been used intentionally on animals to cause burns. Lye is found in drain clog treatments and is used in methamphetamine manufacturing. The perpetrator may mix lye with flour or pancake mix to allow it to adhere more effectively to the body of the animal (Sinclair and Lockwood 2006). If lye is ingested it can produce transmural necrosis of the esophagus with just 1 second of contact. Gastric necrosis is common with the use of liquid lye and may be accompanied by perforation of the small intestine (Di Maio and Di Maio 2001).

Electrical Burns

Overview

Electrical burns occur when the body has contact with an electrical current with or without an exit point. The damage caused is because of the current, voltage, heat generated, and amount of time the victim is in contact with electricity. Current refers to the quantity of electricity passing through the wire and is measured in milliamperes (mA). The current is actually electrons flowing through the wire and the number of electrons increases with corresponding increase in current. Amperage is the most important factor in electrocution injuries. It is directly related to the voltage and indirectly related to the resistance. The longer current passes through the body, the greater the damage produced. Exposure to a lower current for a long period of time causes more damage than if exposed to a higher current for a shorter period. Voltage of electricity is another factor in electrocution. This is what causes more electricity to flow through the wire, analogous to water pressure. The higher the voltage, the higher the amount of electricity that passes through. Heat is also generated by the electrical current, producing thermal injury.

Upon entering the body, electrical current travels the shortest route from the point of contact to the point of grounding. The tissue resistance to electrical current in order of greatest to least is bone, fat, tendon, skin, muscle, blood, and nerves. Current flows along the path of least resistance such as blood vessels, nerves, and wet tissue. The current concentrates in tissues with greater resistance, such as bone, causing greater thermal injury. Oral exposure to electrical current is particularly damaging because the wet oral tissues are in direct contact with the bone (Hedlund 2002).

General Findings

Victims of electrocution are often found still in contact with the item that caused the injury. In animals, this is most commonly an electrical cord into which the animal has bitten. In animal cruelty cases, electricity may be used to torture or attempt to kill an animal. The injured animal is often found in a tonic state because of the contraction of striated muscles. In humans, these contractions can be severe enough to cause bone fractures (Di Maio and Di Maio 2001). Vomiting and defecation can occur with generalized tonoclonic activity. This state resolves in the surviving animal once the source of the electricity is removed from the body. The animal may be weak and ataxic afterward. Pulmonary edema may develop secondary to electrocution.

Oral burns can be found on the lips, palate, tongue, and gums, and oronasal fistulas may be present or develop later. Electrical burns cause the release of vasoactive substances and vascular thrombosis, resulting in tissue necrosis. The tissue may appear charred, tan, or pale gray. Tissue edema develops 1 to 2 days after the injury, although the extent of all the injuries may take 2 to 3 weeks to fully develop (Hedlund 2002). Local tissue ischemia may be apparent in 3–5 days (Smith 1995).

In victims of low-voltage electrocution, burns may be found around the area where there was electrical contact (the entry point) and the point of grounding (the exit point). These burns also may be completely absent if the point of contact was over a large broad area that had minimal resistance. The burn size generally is small and may be characterized by a chalky white lesion with a central crater and raised borders, or an area of erythematous blistering. The burn sites may have yellowish or black discoloration produced by heat. Microscopically, there is a Swiss cheese appearance to the epidermis. There may be minute particles of metal deposited in the burn from the conducting surface. There is no way to differentiate antemortem versus postmortem burns (Di Maio and Di Maio 2001).

With high-voltage electrocution, the burns may be extremely severe with charring of the body. Third-degree burns may develop at the contact site. There may be numerous individual and confluent third-degree burns. Multiple small burns may be produced by the arcing of the current. If the current is transmitted indirectly through another object the burns may be large and irregular. They are chalky white with a central crater and raised borders. The heat produces yellowish or black discoloration around the burn sites. There may be massive tissue destruction with very high voltage, including loss of extremities and organ rupture (Di Maio and Di Maio 2001).

Death owing to electrocution is usually caused by cardiac arrest. In lower amperage, electrocution causes muscle tremors to painful muscle contractions. As the amperage increases, loss of consciousness, ventricular fibrillation, and death can occur. Electrocution also can produce contracture of all the muscles, causing respiratory paralysis and death. Evidence of pulmonary edema may be found. The heat that is generated by electrocution may cause profound and massive tissue damage (Hedlund 2002). With high-voltage electrocution, there may be thermal damage to the respiratory center of the brainstem, causing respiratory arrest (Di Maio and Di Maio 2001).

Lightning Electrocution

Lightning electrocution may result from a direct strike or a side-flash strike. There are usually entrance and exit burns from the current. There may be cutaneous burns that microscopically show the epidermis separated from the papillary dermis. There may be singed fur and the tympanic membrane may be ruptured. If the animal survives, pulmonary edema may be present. Human survivors have pathognomonic skin injury called Lichtenberg figures. These lesions appear fern-like and comprise an area of transient erythema that appears within 1 hour of the incident and gradually fades in 24 hours. Death resulting from lighting strike is caused by cardiopulmonary arrest or electrothermal injury caused by the high-voltage current.

Stun Gun Electrocution

A stun gun can deliver 50,000 volts of electricity to the body through two contact points. The distance between the contact points is unique to the individual stun gun. These guns can cause burns on the skin from the two contact points. The distance between the two burns should be measured for comparison to a recovered gun.

Fires: Thermal Injury and Smoke Inhalation

Overview

Fires can cause injuries related to burns and smoke inhalation. Burns resulting from fires occur when there is contact with the body and the flame. The severity of the injury depends on the amount of contact time and area of the body that is burned. The damage may range from first- to fourth-degree burns. Flame burns may produce scorching of the skin and can progress to charring. Flash burns are caused by ignition from flash fires. These flash fires are caused by the sudden ignition or explosion of fuels, fine particulate matter, or gases. The initial flash ignition is usually short, burning the contacting surfaces uniformly. The hair is singed and there are partial-thickness burns. The burn may be superficial if the flash is very short (Di Maio and Di Maio 2001).

Additional burns may be seen because of thermal injury from the heat of the flame. These burns may be external or along the oral and respiratory tract. Depending on the circumstances, most fire victims suffer from smoke inhalation in addition to burn injuries.

Examination of Fire Victims

General

When examining fire victims it is important to consider the circumstances found at the crime scene. In fire-related deaths, it is important for the body to be photographed and examined *in situ* to establish the context of the body in relation to the fire scene. Evidence of the cause of the fire may be on the bodies of all fire victims. There may be an odor on the body from the accelerant used. All potential evidence should be collected from the body (see Collection of Evidence). Swabs should be taken of the burn and surrounding tissue for testing. Samples of fur and skin surrounding the injuries should be collected. Full-body radiographs should be taken of all fire victims to look for any evidence of antemortem trauma, such as projectiles or fractures. It should be noted that extreme heat from fires may cause characteristic fracturing of the bone (see below).

Live Victims

Surviving victims of fire usually have the smell of smoke on their fur. In addition to external burns, there may be burns around the face, inside the oral cavity, and along the upper and lower airways. Laryngospasm may be present. Findings in the airways may include mucosal erythema, ulceration, hemorrhage, edema, and carbonaceous particle accumulation. The animal may have carbonaceous sputum. If there is carbon monoxide poisoning, the skin and mucous membranes may be cherry red in color, which also may be result from burns or heat from the fire. Conjunctivitis or corneal abrasions may be found. In moderate to severe cases cytological exam of transtracheal aspirates may reveal burned ciliated cells, strands of mucus, and soot particles (Carson 1986).

Deceased Victims

Some bodies may not be charred or disfigured. Some may be seared and some may show little to no external evidence of injury except for the odor of smoke. Bodies that have minimal external injury have usually died from smoke inhalation (see below). With searing damage, the skin may be light brown in color and have a stiff, leathery consistency. There may be blisters on the skin with an erythematous rim but they are not indicative of antemortem injury. Blisters with this rim can be produced postmortem by heat causing contraction of the dermal capillaries, which forces blood to the periphery of the blister or burn (Di Maio and Di Maio 2001).

The body may be partially charred and swollen from the heat. If the body is severely burned, there may be splitting of the skin. The skin may be completely burned away exposing the underlying muscle, which may be ruptured by the heat. The skin that is not burned may have a seared, leathery texture. There may be areas of undamaged skin where the body was laying on a flat surface. The internal body walls may be burned away exposing the viscera, which may be seared or charred (Di Maio and Di Maio 2001).

It is usually impossible to determine antemortem burns from postmortem on gross examination. There may be microscopic evidence if the victim survived long enough to develop an inflammatory response, although the lack of this response does not indicate the burns were postmortem. Heat thrombosis of the dermal vessels can delay inflammatory cells from reaching the area of the burn (Di Maio and Di Maio 2001).

With fire victims, it is possible to see a postmortem epidural hematoma with charring of the head. They are usually large and thick overlying the frontal, parietal, and temporal areas with possible extension to the occipital area. They are chocolate brown in color with a crumbly or honeycomb appearance and are easy to distinguish from antemortem epidural hematomas (Di Maio and Di Maio 2001).

Burning of the body causes heat coagulation of the muscle tissue and contraction of the muscle fibers. This causes flexion of the limbs producing a pugilistic posture (pugilistic attitude). This pugilistic posture does not indicate whether the victim was alive or deceased before the fire (Di Maio and Di Maio 2001).

Burning of bones causes color changes and possible heat fractures. Burned bone may have a gray-white color. There may be a fine network of superficial fractures caused by the heat that can crumble with handling. The outer table of the skull can fragment and be completely absent. The feet may not be attached to the body if they were burned so severely they fragmented and were unrecognized at the scene (Di Maio and Di Maio 2001).

Entomology

There may be live or dead entomology evidence on burn victims either externally or internally. After the fire insects may feed on the body postmortem, which can determine the time the fire occurred. There also may be evidence that myiasis occurred prior to the fire. Dead insects may be found internally, especially inside the skull, which protects the insects from being consumed in the fire. The presence of blow fly larvae, and possibly other insects, indicates the animal was dead for a period of time prior to the fire, with enough for colonization and hatching. This entomology evidence can help determine the time of death of the victim. They also may provide clues to the location of death based on the species of blow fly. Maggots also may be assayed for toxicology testing, which may help determine the cause of death (see Chapter 14).

Smoke Inhalation and Thermal Injury

Overview

The cause of death in fire victims is most commonly caused by carbon monoxide poisoning, smoke toxicity, thermal damage to the airways or the body, or any combination of these. Immediate deaths may result from smoke inhalation or direct thermal injury to the body. The mouth, nostrils, and other airways usually contain soot with smoke inhalation victims. The absence of soot is not indicative of death prior to the fire. The leading cause of death in human victims of smoke inhalation is respiratory failure (Saxon and Kirby 1992). Damage to the respiratory tract usually results from both thermal and chemical causes.

Thermal Injury

Thermal damage may be seen if the animal breathes in hot gases resulting in edema and/or burns. This can cause damage to the oral mucosa, nasopharynx, pharynx, and possibly the lower respiratory tract. Thermal injuries can cause edema of the larynx, which may or may not be obstructive. It also can cause severe laryngospasm resulting in suffocation (Saxon and Kirby 1992). At any point in the first 24 hours the injury to the upper airway may cause upper airway obstruction (Tams 1989). The heat-damaged mucosa lining the airways sloughs into the lumen causing further airway obstruction in the first 2–6 days after the insult (Saxon and Kirby 1992) and impair surfactant production (Jutkowitz 2005). Furthermore, systemic inflammation from the burn wounds or from sepsis may indirectly cause acute lung injury or acute respiratory distress syndrome (ARDS) (Jutkowitz 2005).

Smoke Toxicity

Smoke toxicity refers to direct injury from the inhalation of smoke and poisoning resulting from the inhalation of toxic chemicals. These noxious chemicals are the byproducts of incomplete combustion of natural and synthetic material in the fire. Chemical injury is caused by the inhalation of toxic gases attached to carbon particles that are deposited in the deep lower airway. These poisonous gases include carbon monoxide, nitrous oxide, chlorine, sulfur dioxide, aldehydes, hydrogen cyanide, hydrogen chloride, and acrolein from the burning of room furnishings, clothing, plastics, and other materials. The combustion of some plastics may produce benzene whose anesthetic effects may allow easier passage of noxious particles into the lungs (Tams 1989).

All of these chemicals cause injury to the lungs producing pulmonary edema. The chemicals cause injury at the endothelial–epithelial interface, bronchociliary damage, inactivation of ciliary movement, and decreased production of surfactant causing alveolar collapse (Saxon and Kirby 1992; Di Maio and Di Maio 2001). In addition, macrophage function is impaired because of smoke poisons. In animals that survive the initial insult, pneumonia is the biggest life-threatening risk in the first week because of the denuded mucosal surfaces, impaired macrophage function, loss of ciliary function, and surfactant protection.

Carbon Monoxide Poisoning

Carbon monoxide (CO) is a colorless, odorless, poisonous gas weighing lighter than air that is a result of the incomplete combustion of hydrocarbon fuels (Carson 1986). It acts by competing with oxygen for binding sites, primarily on hemoglobin. Carbon monoxide has an affinity for hemoglobin that is 240 times higher than that of oxygen (Tams 1989). When CO binds with hemoglobin it forms carboxyhemoglobin, which inhibits its ability to carry oxygen. Furthermore, it causes the oxygen dissociation curve to shift to the left, which decreases oxygen release into the tissues. The ultimate result is hypoxia to the tissues of the body. The brain and the heart are the most sensitive tissues to hypoxia. There is a bright, cherry red or bright pink coloring to the skin or in areas of lividity.

The symptoms of CO poisoning are based on the percentage of carboxyhemoglobin in the body. The symptoms may be gradual as the CO in the air increases. At 10 to 20 percent carboxyhemoglobin levels, clinical signs of mild dyspnea, shortness of breath, and confusion appear. The animal becomes more disoriented and loses the will and capability to escape as CO levels increase. With higher levels increased irritability, nausea, vomiting, lack of coordination and convulsions may be seen. Respiratory failure and death may occur at levels greater than 50 to 60 percent (Tams 1989). Death may occur quickly with sudden high levels. This is thought to result from cardiac arrest because cardiac dysfunction usually occurs prior to central nervous system effects.

In CO poisoning the postmortem exam findings may include dilated bronchi and distention of the major blood vessels. The ventricles of the heart may be dilated, especially the right ventricle, which may result from the sudden increase in central venous pressure sometimes seen in CO toxicity. The cherry red color of the blood may or may not be present (Carson 1986). Brain changes may be seen related to anoxia, including necrosis in the cortex and white matter of the cerebral hemispheres, globus pallidus, and brainstem. Edema, demyelination, and hemorrhage in the brain and necrosis in the Ammon's horn of the hippocampus may occur (Carson 1986).

Tests for carboxyhemoglobin may be run at a human hospital. Venous blood should be used and transported on ice. The results are reported as the percentage of saturation of hemoglobin in the carboxyhemoglobin state (Tams 1989). The timing of sample collection is important and should be done as soon as possible. Once the animal is no longer exposed to CO, the carboxyhemoglobin level may return to normal levels within 3–4 hours when the animal breathes fresh air (Carson 1986). If the animal breathes 100 percent oxygen the levels drop more rapidly. This improves tissue oxygenation, especially for the brain and myocardium, and accelerates the elimination of the COHb. The half-life of carboxyhemoglobin is 4 hours at room air and 30 minutes at 100 percent oxygen (Tams 1989).

Cyanide Gas Poisoning in Fires

Cyanide gas is produced in a fire by the burning of many common synthetic substances. It is also produced when hydrogen cyanide salts come into contact with an acid. It is rare to be a contributory cause of death in human fire victims. The amount of gas produced in a fire is relatively low.

Cyanide binds to and inhibits the cellular respiratory enzyme mitochondrial cytochrome oxidase disrupting the ability of cells to use oxygen. It most severely affects the brain and heart. In most cases, death rapidly follows the onset of symptoms. The body may appear pink or cherry red, similar to carbon monoxide poison. The difference is the pink color in cyanide poison is caused by fully oxygenated blood because the tissues could not extract oxygen from the blood. It is possible for the victim to be cyanotic. The victims of cyanide gas poisoning may have a distinctive aroma of "bitter almonds" or "musty." The ability to smell the aroma is a genetic trait and a significant portion of the human population cannot detect the aroma (Dix et al. 2000).

Diagnostic testing for cyanide gas poisoning can be difficult. Decomposition causes the production of cyanide in the blood whether in the body or in a test tube. The testing for cyanide is also problematic in that other substances in the blood (sulfides) can react like cyanide, which causes falsely elevated cyanide levels (Di Maio and Di Maio 2001).

References

Carson, T.L. 1986. Toxic Gases. In *Current Veterinary Therapy IX Small Animal Practice*, ed. R.W. Kirk, pp. 203–205. Philadelphia: W.B. Saunders.

Di Maio, V.J., and D. Di Maio. 2001. *Forensic Pathology*, 2nd ed. Boca Raton, FL: CRC Press.

Dix, J., M. Graham, and R. Hanzlick. 2000. *Asphyxia and Drowning: An Atlas*. Boca Raton, FL: CRC Press.

Hedlund, C.S. 2002. Surgery of the Integumentary System. In *Small Animal Surgery*, 2nd ed., ed. T.W. Fossum, pp. 134–228. St. Louis: Mosby.

Jutkowitz, L.A. 2005. Care of the Burned Patient. In *Proceedings of the Eleventh International Veterinary Emergency and Critical Care Symposium*. Atlanta, GA, September 7–11, 2005. pp. 243–249.

Munro, H.M., and M.V. Thrusfield. 2001. 'Battered Pets': Non-accidental Physical Injuries Found in Dogs and Cats. *Journal of Small Animal Practice* 42:279–290.

Saxon, W.D., and R. Kirby. 1992. Treatment of Acute Burn Injury and Smoke Inhalation. In *Kirk's Current Veterinary Therapy XI Small Animal Practice*, ed. R.W. Kirk, and J.D. Bonagura, pp. 146–154. Philadelphia: W.B. Saunders.
Sinclair, L., and R. Lockwood. 2006. Cruelty toward Cats. In *Consultations in Feline Internal Medicine*, ed. J.R. August, pp. 693–699. St. Louis: Elsevier Saunders.
Smith, M.M. 1995. Oral and Salivary Gland Disorders. In *Textbook of Veterinary Internal Medicine: Diseases of the Dog and Cat*, Volume 2, 4th ed., ed. S.J. Ettinger, and E.C. Feldman, pp. 1084–1097. Philadelphia: W.B. Saunders.
Tams, T.R. 1989. Pneumonia. In *Kirk's Current Veterinary Therapy XI Small Animal Practice*, ed. R.W. Kirk, and J.D. Bonagura, pp. 376–384. Philadelphia: W.B. Saunders.

Chapter 8
Patterns of Non-accidental Injury: Gunshot Wounds

Introduction

Most animal gunshot victims have a common history of being outside and unattended. A gunshot study of animals revealed that most gunshot wounds involved animals that were allowed to wander outdoors unsupervised. In urban areas, dogs were more likely to be shot in the evening and early morning hours. Handguns were the most common firearm documented in urban areas. High-velocity rifles and shotguns were most common in rural areas. Air-powered firearms, including BB and pellet guns, were more prevalent in suburban areas (Pavletic 1985). In the study by Munro and Thrusfield, the veterinarians surveyed reported airgun injuries in a disproportionately higher number of cats than dogs. In fact, all firearm injuries were reported in a higher number of cats than in dogs (Munro and Thrusfield 2001).

Gunshot injuries may easily be mistaken for puncture wounds, bite wounds, or lacerations. Any animal with unexplained wounds should have full body radiographs taken. Additional clues of a gunshot injury include pneumothorax, pneumomediastinum, cardiac tamponade, dyspnea, lethargy, limping, fractures, peritonitis, hemoabdomen, and hemothorax. The animal also may present with symptoms of lead poisoning from a retained projectile in the body. This is commonly seen when a projectile is inside the joint, where there is slow dissolving of the bullet and slow absorption.

Overview of Firearms

A basic knowledge of firearms is necessary to properly interpret gunshot wounds. There are five categories of small arms: handguns, rifles, shotguns, submachine guns, and machine guns. Military firearms and ammunition are not covered in this chapter. Firearms also can be classified by their velocity, which has a direct impact on the amount of damage inflicted to the victim. High-velocity firearms include high-powered handguns and rifles. They fire a projectile at the speed of 2,500 ft/sec or higher which creates tremendous kinetic energy. Low-velocity firearms include handguns and air-powered pellet and BB guns. They fire a projectile at the speed of <1,000 ft/sec. Animals are often the target of the air-powered gun. Even these low velocity firearms can cause severe and even fatal damage.

Handguns

The four most common types of handguns are single-shot pistols, derringers, revolvers, and auto-loading pistols (automatics). Handguns have rifled barrels (see Rifling). The most common handgun in the United States is the revolver. These have a revolving cylinder that contains several chambers, which hold a single bullet cartridge. This cylinder rotates to align each chamber successively with the barrel and firing pin. The auto-loading pistol is also referred to as automatic pistol, automatic, or pistol. The automatic term comes from the auto-loader, which requires the trigger to be pulled for every shot fired. Each time the gun is fired, the pistol uses the forces from the fired cartridge to extract and eject the empty case, load a fresh cartridge, and then return the mechanism to the ready position to fire the new cartridge (Di Maio 1999). These cartridges usually are stored in a removable magazine, also called the clip, that is stored in the grip of the pistol.

Rifles

A rifle is a firearm with a rifled barrel that is made to be fired from the shoulder. The minimum barrel length requirement in the United States is 16 inches (Di Maio 1999).

Shotguns

A shotgun is a firearm with a smooth barrel that is made to be fired from the shoulder. The smooth bore is designed to fire multiple pellets. Most have a degree of *choke,* which refers to the partial constriction of the bore at the muzzle to control shot patterns. The minimum required barrel length in the United States is 18 inches (Di Maio 1999).

Caliber Nomenclature

The caliber of the weapon is supposed to refer to the inside diameter of the barrel before any rifling is cut into the metal. This would also match the caliber of cartridge used for that particular gun. However, this does not apply to all firearms; their munitions and caliber designations vary greatly (Di Maio 1999).

Rifling

Rifled barrels are found in handguns, rifles, submachine guns, and machine guns. This rifling is comprised of spiral grooves cut along the length of the interior (bore) of the barrel. The rifling marks are the grooves and the metal between the grooves called the *lands*. These marks are unique "fingerprints" to that individual gun. No two barrels are exactly alike, even when cut with the same tools. These rifling marks are imparted to the bullet as it travels down the barrel, allowing the bullet to be conclusively matched to the weapon from which it was fired. Each model of gun has a specific type of rifling, so the model of the gun may be determined by examining the bullet.

Rifling causes a rotational spin to the bullet along its longitudinal axis, which stabilizes the bullets flight through the air. The term *twist* refers to the number of inches or centimeters for one complete spiral (Di Maio 1999). When the twist is clockwise, it is referred to as a *right twist;* when counterclockwise it is called a *left twist*. Another type of rifling, introduced by Heckler and Koch, is when the bore has a rounded rectangular profile called polygonal boring. This type of rifling makes ballistic comparison of bullets very difficult (Di Maio 1999).

Ammunition

The small arms cartridge consists of a cartridge case, primer, propellant (gunpowder), and the bullet or other projectile. The cartridge case is usually made of copper and zinc. Shotgun shells are made of brass, plastic, and paper. The cartridge case is designed to expand and seal the chamber to prevent the gases from escaping to the rear when fired. The base of the cartridge cases have a head stamp containing letters, symbols, numbers, and/or trade name for identification (Di Maio 1999).

Small arms cartridges contain a primer at the base that explodes through the flash hole and ignites the gunpowder. The cartridge is classified as center-fire if the primer is located in the center, or rim-fire if the primer is located around the rim. In the United States, the primer is composed of chemical ingredients: lead stryphnate, barium nitrate, and antimony sulfide. Most primers contain all three chemicals, although some primers contain only two of the components. Gunpowder residue tests detect these compounds (Di Maio 1999).

The weapon used to fire the cartridge may impart unique class characteristics to the cartridge case or primer. These can be used to forensically match the cartridge from which the individual weapon was fired. These markings may be caused by the magazine, firing pin, extractor, ejector, and breach face of the weapon.

Propellants used in cartridges may be smokeless powder, Pyrodex (a synthetic black powder), or a combination of both. Smokeless powder may have chemical or graphite coating, which may be lost after discharge from a weapon. Uncoated powder grains are pale green or beige and may be found on the skin or wounds of the victim (Di Maio 1999).

The bullet is the located at the tip of the cartridge and leaves the muzzle of the firearm when the cartridge is discharged. There are two types of bullets, lead and metal-jacketed. Jacketed ammunition has a lead or steel core covered by jacket of gilding metal (copper and zinc), gilding metal-clad steel, cupro-nickel (copper and nickel), or aluminum. The bullets may be full metal–jacketed or partial metal–jacketed. Center-fire rifle ammunition used for hunting is partial metal–jacketed. Ammunition for revolvers and automatics may by full or partial metal–jacketed. The two most common forms of partial metal–jacketed bullets are semi-jacketed soft point and hollow point (Di Maio 1999). Both of these forms of ammunition are designed for greater *mushrooming* of the bullet when it strikes the target.

A rifled barrel creates certain class characteristics on the bullet when fired because of the rifling. The marks can indicate the make and model of the gun, and can be matched to the exact gun from which the bullet was fired. The class characteristics found on the bullet are the number, diameter, and width of the lands and grooves; depth of grooves; and direction and degree of twist. If someone tries to modify the rifling by physically altering the muzzle end of the bore, forensic scientist can still retrieve the interior markings. Mikrosil is a rubber casting compound that may be used in the barrel, creating a cast of the entire length of the bore. Then the marred end is cut off and the remaining rifling marks are used for comparison ballistic matching.

Bullets that are severely distorted or fragmented still may be analyzed to link it with other bullets fired from a specific gun or recovered at the scene. Quantitative compositional analysis may be conducted using scanning electron microscopy with energy dispersive x-ray (SEM-EDX) (Di Maio 1999). The bullet distortion may happen when the bullet is fired from a weapon not appropriate for that caliber of ammunition. Decomposition can affect the rifling marks on the bullet, depending on the composition of the bullet and location in the body.

The bullet that exits the body may contain tissue related to the place where the bullet penetrated the body. This is especially useful when multiple bullets are found at the scene to determine which bullet perforated the body. Tissue may be too small to be seen and may be retrieved through a washing process of the bullet. A low-velocity bullet usually has more tissue adherent to the bullet and typically is better preserved (Di Maio 1999). The bullet may be swabbed for microscopic tissue and DNA testing.

Firing of a Weapon

The firing of a weapon starts with pulling the trigger, which releases the firing pin. The firing pin strikes the primer, crushing it and igniting the primer composition, which produces an intense flame. The flame flows through the flash hole in the primer and ignites the powder in the cartridge, producing a large quantity of gas and heat. This heated gas increases the pressure on the base of the bullet and sides of the cartridge case. The pressure propels the bullet down the barrel with some of the gas leaking past and ahead of the bullet and the majority following after the bullet exits the muzzle. As the bullet emerges it is accompanied by a jet of flame, gas, powder, soot, primer residue, metallic particles stripped from the bullet, and vaporized metal from the bullet and cartridge case. The *flame* is from incandescent superheated gases, which can sear the skin in contact and near-contact wounds. A *ball of fire* accompanies the exit of the bullet as well, also called a *muzzle flash*. This is caused by superheated oxygen-deprived gases reacting to atmospheric oxygen. Revolvers have a cylinder-barrel gap in which soot and powder can exit, causing blackening and powder tattooing of the skin in close contact wounds. If the cylinder does not completely line up with the barrel, the bullet may be shaved and fragments cause stippling of the skin.

Examination of Gunshot Victims

It is important to have all the crime scene investigation information prior to examining a gunshot victim. This includes photographs, witness/suspect statements, and any recovered ammunition, casings, or weapon. All the wounds should be photographed before and after treatment. When examining a gunshot victim, it is important to consider that the animal may have suffered additional injuries, such as blunt force trauma. The skin of deceased animals should be reflected to look for subcutaneous bruising. All gunshot victims should have full-body radiographs to locate the projectile and injuries. The sequence of gunshot wounds often is hard to determine. The wound findings should be compared to witness and suspect statements.

To properly interpret gunshot injuries, the veterinarian needs to understand wound ballistics. Gunshot wounds can be very complex and a large amount of information must be analyzed and documented. The veterinarian must be able to classify the gunshot wounds as entrance or exit, recognize what can affect their appearance, and determine the gunshot range that caused them. The veterinarian also should recognize wound patterns associated with specific weapons and ammunition. It is important to properly retrieve gunshot residue and the projectile from the body, and cartridge casings at the scene without damaging the evidence. The trajectory of the projectile through the body must be determined and compared with investigation findings. Finally, the veterinarian must properly record the injuries and prepare the examination report. Most of the following information on gunshot wounds comes from human gunshot victims. The same principles and guidelines should apply to animals.

Wound Ballistics

The amount of damage caused by the gunshot is directly related to the amount of kinetic energy from the projectile that is absorbed by the tissues. The greater the energy transferred to the tissues, the greater the tissue damage. Kinetic energy refers to the energy possessed by a moving object. The kinetic energy is measured by the following equation:

$$\text{Kinetic Energy} = \text{Mass} \times \text{Velocity}^2/2$$

This equation shows that if the mass of the projectile is doubled, the kinetic energy is doubled; but if the velocity is doubled, the kinetic energy is quadrupled (Kraus 1992).

In gunshots, the projectile causes tissue to balloon outward, stretching and tearing in a process known as cavitation. Cavitation also creates a vacuum affect as it passes through the target, pulling debris and hair deeper into the wound track (Pavletic 2006). This shearing, compression, and contraction continues as it travels through the body, causing injury to the surrounding tissue, sometimes distant from the bullet's path. Depending on the kinetic energy of the projectile, this may cause rib fractures without a direct impact from the bullet.

In addition to the kinetic energy of the projectile, the degree of injury depends on the characteristics of the tissue through which it travels. If a high-velocity bullet passes through a leg without impact to the bone, the amount of damage depends on the kinetic energy transferred to the surrounding tissue. The thicker and denser the tissue, the more energy is absorbed. The lung and muscle are more resilient and elastic, which results in less damage because of the ability to absorb a portion of the cavitation process (Pavletic 2006).

A bullet can penetrate or perforate bone depending on the velocity, construction, angle of impact, type of bone, its thickness, and its surface configuration. Fracture patterns depend on the type of bone and angle of impact. Cancellous bone is softer and tends to absorb more of the energy, causing less fragmentation. Cortical bone tends to fracture and shatter. The angle of the bullet impact (such as 90 degrees versus tangential) and the weight and position of long bones also can affect the fracture pattern.

Tests were conducted by Vincent Di Maio using fresh human bone and 9-mm Parabellum ammunition loaded with 125 g round nose lead bullets. Using flat bone (4–6 mm thick) bullet penetration with depressed fractures started at 250 ft/sec with perforation at 290–300 ft/sec. Using bone 7–9 mm thick perforation started at 350 ft/sec. Using bone 10 mm thick, there was no perforation at velocities up to 460 ft/sec. Using human femurs, there was no perforation until 552 and 559 ft/sec (Di Maio 1999).

When a bullet penetrates bone, it causes fragmentation and a temporary cavity. This propels the bone fragments lateral and forward, causing additional injury. With the undulation of the cavity some of the fragments return to the center. The direction of the bullet can be determined by the appearance of the wound in the bone. The bone bevels out toward the direction of travel. The entrance tends to be round to oval, clean edges, and have a "punched-out" appearance. Superficial chips of bone may flake off the edges of an entrance hole. The exit wound is excavated out and appears funnel shaped. Entrance and exit wounds in thin bone can be difficult to determine (Di Maio 1999). There may be lead deposits on the edges of the entrance hole.

Gunshot wounds, tissue damage, and the bullet path are affected by the characteristics of the ammunition. The caliber of the bullet, presence of an outer jacket, and design of the jacket directly affect the injuries. The design of the projectile may be for greater tissue damage, such as for bullet fragmentation (frangibility) and partial or complete flattening upon impact (mushrooming).

Backspatter is the ejection of blood and tissue from an entrance gunshot wound. This may be found on the shooter, the weapon, and nearby objects. Backspatter is more likely to occur with contact wounds to the head than a distant wound to the body. A study was conducted of head gunshots using calves at the range of tight contact (5 cm) and loose contact (10 cm). The backspatter was categorized as macrospatter (stain diameter >0.5 mm) and microbackspatter (0.5 mm or less). Macrospatter was found with every shot with the stains' maximum traveling distance 72–119 cm, the majority 0–50 cm. Microbackspatter was found with every shot with the stains' maximum traveling distance of 69 cm; the majority were 0–40 cm. The microbackspatter stains were more numerous than the macrospatter. The micro-stains were circular or oval and the macro-stains were variable, from circular to exclamation marks. Both stains showed exiting direction of all angles, creating a 180-degree semi-circle spray, although the individual droplets were uneven and asymmetrical (Di Maio 1999).

Determining Entrance and Exit Wounds

General Characteristics

The type of bullet and the presence, separation, or fragmentation of the jacket affect the appearance of entrance wounds. Entrance wounds are typically smaller than exit wounds. The animal's hair may be pulled inward into the opening of entrance wounds. Dirt, debris, and hair may be dragged further into the wound track. Most entrance wounds have a zone of reddish to reddish-brown flattened, abraded skin called the abrasion ring. This occurs where the bullet rubbed raw the edges of the hole as it penetrated the skin. A fresh abrasion ring appears moist and fleshy but will eventually dry out. Some bullets do not cause abrasion rings such as centerfire rifle and jacketed/semi-jacketed handgun bullets (Di Maio 1999). The width of the abrasion ring varies depending on the caliber of the weapon, anatomical site of entrance, and angle of entrance. It may appear concentric (90-degree angle) or eccentric, from the bullet entering the skin at an oblique angle. The zone of abrasion is wider in the direction from which the bullet came if the skin surface is flat. Curves and depressions on the body can make this determination difficult. A gray coloration to the abrasion ring, called a bullet wipe, may be seen with entrance wounds. This gray area consists primarily of soot, and sometimes lubricant, from the surface of the bullet that is rubbed off as it penetrates the skin. This should not be confused with soot and searing found in contact wounds (Di Maio 1999).

Soot is produced by the combustion of gunpowder as it emerges from the muzzle. It contains carbon and vaporized metals from the primer, bullet, and cartridge case. The size, intensity, and appearance of the soot pattern around an entrance wound and the maximum range on which it can occur depend on several factors. These include the gunshot range, propellant, barrel length, angle of the muzzle, weapon caliber, type of weapon, target material, and whether or not the target is bloody (Di Maio 1999). If the muzzle is at a 90-degree angle to the body, the soot pattern is concentric around the entrance hole. At other angles, the soot pattern is eccentric. Soot may be removed by wiping or washing the wound. To prevent this, the wound should be sprayed with hot water, which eventually washes away only the blood. Hydrogen peroxide may be used to dissolve the blood and blood clots. Whenever there is doubt about whether or not the wound is an entrance injury with soot and searing of the skin, it should be excised and submitted for scanning electron microscopy with SEM-EDX analysis (Di Maio 1999).

The muscle around the entrance may have a cherry red color because of carboxyhemoglobin and carboxymyoglobin formed from the carbon monoxide in the muzzle gas. These levels may be detected on chemical analysis of the muscle. A control sample of muscle should be taken from another area of the body (Di Maio 1999).

High-velocity projectile entrance wounds may lack abrasion rings and cause micro-tears at the edges. These are small splits or tears that radiate outward from the perforation edges and may involve the partial or complete circumference (Di Maio 1999). Entrance wounds without abrasion rings have a round to oval punched-out appearance with clean margins. Rarely, an associated exit wound can appear the same on through-and-through gunshot wounds, making determination of entrance and exit difficult without other findings to indicate direction, such as bone fractures.

A distant gunshot wound to the head may have a stellate or irregular appearance. This is most often seen over a bony prominence and may be confused with a contact or exit wound. Large amounts of black soot may be found around the entrance wound and in the wound track in contact and near-contact wounds. Small amounts may be seen, along with occasional powder grains, in distant wounds. Grains of powder may be embedded in the adjacent skin with intermediate-range wounds (powder tattooing). This may be ball or flake (disk) powder.

The tumbling of the bullet, flattening, fragmentation, and kinetic energy absorbed by the body affect the appearance of the exit wounds. Exit wounds are usually larger and more irregular than entrance wounds. They may appear stellate, slit-like, circular, crescent-shaped, or completely irregular. Exits through tight skin usually cause larger irregular, often stellate, wounds. Exits in loose skin can be small and slit-like. Shored exit wounds have abraded margins because the skin was next to a firm surface when the bullet exited, abrading the everted wound margins. The pattern of the surface may be imprinted on the skin. They may have wide, abrasion collars that may resemble entrance wounds when dry. It is possible for exit wounds to be smaller than the entrance wound and smaller than the diameter of the bullet because of the elastic nature of skin. The shape of the exit wound does not correlate with the type of bullet used (Di Maio 1999).

It is possible for a bullet to have enough velocity to create an exit hole but not exit the body because of the elastic nature of the skin or an object next to the wound, causing shored margins. The bullet may be found partially protruding from the exit hole or it may have rebounded back into the wound track. With the use of semi-jacketed ammunition, the lead core may exit the body while the jacket remains in the body. It is the jacket that has ballistic importance, not the lead core. The jacket may be found adjacent to the exit site and only be visible on radiographs. It is important to note that the bullet path of an exiting bullet is not necessarily a straight line. The bullet may be tumbling or deformed and aerodynamically unstable. It can go off in any direction and veer from its projected trajectory. The shorter the path traveled through the body, the more stable the bullet may be upon exiting.

A graze wound is an abrasion created when a bullet strikes the skin at a shallow angle without perforating or tearing the skin. If the injury extends to the subcutaneous tissue, it is called a tangential wound. The entrance end has a partially abraded margin and the exit end is split. Any tears along the margin point in the direction of travel. There may be a piling up of tissue at the end of both graze and tangential wounds (Di Maio 1999).

Shallow through-and-through wounds in which the entrance and exit are close together are called superficial perforating wounds. The entrance usually has an abrasion ring and the exit usually has only a partial abrasion, which indicates the direction of travel. When a bullet passes through one part of the body (intermediary target) then re-enters another, it is called a re-entry wound. This wound usually is large and irregular with ragged edges and a wide irregular abrasion ring (Di Maio 1999).

Intermediary Targets

When a bullet passes through an intermediary object before hitting the body, it can cause significant changes in the wound appearance or number of wounds. For shotgun pellets, the intermediary object may cause wider dispersal of the pellets, making gunshot range determination more difficult. The object may fragment, and these fragments embed in the victim, causing pseudo-powder tattoo marks (stippling).

These fragments may be found embedded in the tip of the bullet. The bullet may become unstable and deformed after passing through the object, creating a larger and more irregular entrance wound with a wider and irregular abrasion ring. A semi-jacketed bullet passing through an intermediary object may become separated from the jacket and both may strike the body. Because of its light weight, the jacket may or may not penetrate the body or may not even hit the victim. The lead from the core can be deposited on the entrance wound of the body, simulating soot. This can cause the wound to be misinterpreted as a contact or similar close-range wound (Di Maio 1999).

Caliber Determination

The caliber of the bullet that caused the entrance wound cannot be determined by the size of the skin wound. In addition to the diameter of the bullet, the size of the wound is caused by the elasticity of the skin and location of the wound. An entrance in bone cannot be used to determine the caliber, but it can exclude certain calibers. Typically a bullet larger than the diameter of the entrance hole could not have been used. However, bone does have some elasticity and a 9-mm bullet can produce an 8.5-mm hole. The type of bullet can affect the caliber determination in bone. Lead bullets tend to expand on impact, creating larger entrance holes (Di Maio 1999).

Ricochet Bullets

Depending on the construction of the bullet, a bullet may strike an object at an angle and ricochet rather than penetrate. A round nose bullet, full metal–jacketed, or low-velocity bullet is more likely to ricochet than flat-nosed, lead, or high-velocity bullets. The bullet may fragment on impact, causing the fragments to spray out in a fan paralleling the plane of the ricochet surface. The surface may fragment with the impact of the bullet, which then strikes the body, causing secondary missile wounds. These may be confused initially with powder tattoo marks but they are larger and more irregular.

The ricocheting bullet usually tumbles and has an unpredictable trajectory. This causes larger, irregular entrance wounds with ragged edges and large, irregular abrasions surrounding the hole. These bullets tend to be penetrating and not perforating because of the loss of energy from the ricochet. Sometimes a lead bullet may have a flattened surface on one side that may appear like a ricocheted bullet. This flattening can actually be caused when the bullet strikes a heavy bone such as a femur or humerus. This usually involves a small-caliber low-velocity lead bullet such as the .22 rimfire (Di Maio 1999).

Bullet Wounds of the Skull

Gunshot wounds to the head in which the bullet does not enter the cranial cavity can cause severe cerebral injury, usually contusions, resulting in death. Tangential gunshot wounds to the skull (gutter wounds) may be first degree when only the outer table of the skull is grooved by the bullet and small bone fragments are carried away. In second-degree gutter wounds, pressure waves created by the bullet fracture the inner table. In third-degree wounds, the bullet perforates the skull in the center of the tangential wound. The outer table of the skull is fragmented and there are depressed fragments of the internal table. There may be comminution and pulverization of both tables in the wound track and fragments of bone may penetrate the brain. The next classification after third degree is superficial perforating wounds, in which there are separate entrance and exit holes in the skull (Di Maio 1999).

A keyhole wound can be produced when a bullet strikes the skull at a shallow angle. The bullet begins to penetrate, causing an entrance hole; then part of the bullet shears off and travels under the scalp, and the remaining bulk of the bullet enters the skull. At one end of this wound there is a typical entrance wound into the bone; the other end has external beveling associated with exit (Di Maio 1999).

Secondary fractures of the skull occur because of intracranial pressure waves generated by the gunshot. These most commonly occur in the thinner bone areas. In contact wounds the gas produced from the weapon discharge enters the cranial cavity and expands. The more gas produced, the more likely there will be secondary fractures. Distant wounds cause secondary fractures by the increased pressure produced by the temporary cavity formation. This is directly related to the kinetic energy lost by the bullet as it passes through the skull (Di Maio 1999).

Stippling

Stippling refers to multiple punctate abrasions of the skin caused by the impact of small fragments of foreign material. Powder tattooing is stippling caused by gunpowder. These abrasions cannot be wiped away. The powder may be identified by the shape such as ball, cylinder, or flake (thick disks). If the powder is partially burned or lacks shape, it can be analyzed to identify the material as gunpowder (Di Maio 1999).

Powder tattooing is truly an antemortem phenomenon. Their appearance depends on the form of the powder. Flake and cylindrical powder cause irregular-shaped marks of variable size and are reddish-brown in color. They are usually sparse compared with ball powder. Flake powder also can cause slit-like marks when striking on their side. If they penetrate the dermis there may be hemorrhage from the sites. Spherical (true) ball powder causes more dense, numerous fine, circular, and bright red marks. Initial impression is that of an area of petechiae. Flattened ball powder is similar to true ball powder but is fewer in number (Di Maio 1999). Postmortem tattooing can appear gray or yellow.

The pattern of powder tattooing depends on the type of powder, range, barrel length, caliber, and intermediary objects. The greater the gunshot range, the less dense the pattern. A shorter barrel has more unburned particles of powder than a long barrel. The hair coat of an animal may reduce or prevent this stippling or the grains may be on the surface of the hair. Ball powder readily perforates hair at close and medium range. Flake powder may penetrate at close range (Di Maio 1999).

Pseudo-powder tattooing is caused by non-gunpowder fragments and can be differentiated from powder tattooing easily. When a bullet passes through an intermediary target, it can cause the object to fragment, sending small particles to impact the skin. This also can occur for a bullet ricochet. These markings usually are larger, more irregular, and sparse compared with powder tattoo marks. Larger pieces of the object may be found embedded in the skin.

Insect feeding can resemble powder stippling. They often have a linear pattern indicating the feeding path of the insects. They may appear dry, red, or yellow, or have dark brown or black crusts. In humans, gunshot wounds located in hairy areas can produce hemorrhage in the surrounding hair follicles that can resemble stippling.

Determining Gunshot Range

General Characteristics

Gunshot range is defined as the range from the muzzle to the target. There are four categories of gunshot range: contact, near-contact, intermediate, and distant. Characteristic findings of gunshot wounds help define the distance from which the animal was shot. All contact wounds are defined by a tight zone of soot and/or searing of the skin. Subcutaneous hemorrhage around the entrance wound may appear purple to black and be mistaken for soot initially. The dried edges of a gunshot entrance wound may appear blackened, similar to soot. In addition to soot, all contact wounds have powder, carbon monoxide, and vaporized metals from the bullet, primer, and cartridge case deposited in the injury and along its tract (Di Maio 1999). In contact wounds, the explosive gases entering the body can propel the skin or body toward the muzzle, leaving an imprint of the muzzle and sometimes the sight of the barrel on the skin.

Contact wounds may be further characterized as hard contact, loose, angled, and incomplete. In hard contact wounds, the muzzle is pressed firmly to the skin, indenting the skin to envelop the muzzle. The edges of the wound are blackened by the soot and seared by the hot gases of combustion. This soot is embedded in the skin and cannot be removed by wiping or washing the wound. In loose contact wounds, the muzzle is placed lightly against the skin and is in complete contact. The gas indents the skin, creating a temporary gap through which it can escape. This soot can be wiped away easily. A few unburned powder grains may be found deposited in the zone of soot.

Angled contact wounds are caused by the barrel being held at an acute angle to the skin. The muzzle has incomplete contact with the skin allowing gas and soot to radiate outward creating an eccentric pattern of soot. A few powder grains may be found deposited in the zone of soot. The eccentric zone points to the direction in which the gun was directed. If the angle decreases, this allows more material to escape, producing powder tattooing. Incomplete contact wounds are caused by the curvature of the body. The muzzle is held against the skin, but there is a gap that allows escape of the gas. This produces an elongated zone of soot and searing. Powder tattooing may be seen.

In near-contact wounds the muzzle of the gun is held a short distance away from the skin but close enough to prevent powder tattooing. The zone of soot is wider and overlying the seared and blackened skin. The soot in the seared zone is embedded and cannot be wiped away. There may be a few clumps of unburned powder grains in the seared area. In near-contact angled wounds, two zones are created by the soot: a blackened seared zone on the same side as the muzzle and a light gray fan-shaped zone. This is the opposite of angled contact wounds. To differentiate the two, the bullet path must be correlated to the soot pattern. If both the bullet and soot zone point in the same direction, then it is an angled contact wound. If the bullet points one way and the zone another, it is an angled near-contact wound. As the angle increases, the entrance hole moves toward the center, making it difficult to differentiate between the two types of wounds.

Intermediate-range gunshot wounds are caused when the gun is fired from further away but close enough to produce powder tattooing of the skin. The transition between near-contact and intermediate-range is determined by the presence of distinct, individual tattoo marks. When the muzzle is at an angle, the area on the same size of the muzzle shows denser tattooing than on the opposite side. With revolvers, soot and powder may escape from the cylinder gap, producing tattooing of the skin. This pattern is usually sparse and may include fragments from shearing of the bullet.

Distant gunshot wounds have only the mark of the bullet perforation.

Wounds from Handguns

Handguns are low-velocity, low-energy weapons with muzzle velocity below 1,400 ft/sec. Hard contact wounds to the head from .22 Short or .32 Smith & Wesson Short cartridges can be difficult to interpret because of the small amount of powder in these cartridges. They may appear to be distant wounds because of the apparent lack of soot or unburned powder grains. A dissecting microscope is needed to examine the wound. The maximum distance for soot deposition of most handguns is 20–30 cm (Di Maio 1999).

A contact wound to skin over bone tends to be stellate or cruciform in appearance. This rarely occurs in contact wounds to the trunk. This is caused by the gas of discharge, which expands the subcutaneous tissue, lifting and ballooning the skin, and often causing tears radiating from the entrance hole. This tearing and its extent depend on the caliber of the weapon, amount of gas produced, firmness with which the muzzle was held to the skin, and elasticity of the skin. The margins can be re-approximated to reveal the original entrance hole. Less powerful calibers may cause very large, circular wounds with blackened, seared margins. Occasionally this is seen with more powerful cartridges (Di Maio 1999).

Contact wounds of the head tend to have soot deposited on the outer table of the skull located at the entrance wound. It also may be found on the inner table and dura. A wound caused by either a .22 Short or .32 Smith & Wesson Short cartridge usually does not have soot on the bone (Di Maio 1999).

Muzzle imprints with contact wounds from handguns can occur in the chest and abdomen and in places where there is a thin layer of skin overlying the bone. These imprints may be larger than the actual dimensions of the muzzle. A zone of abraded skin may be seen from the skin rubbing against the muzzle and flaring back to envelop the muzzle. This may be confused as a zone of searing from the hot gases, which have soot, whereas this zone of abraded skin does not (Di Maio 1999).

Contact wounds to the head, chest, or abdomen from handguns do not cause the massive injuries seen with rifles or shotguns because of the smaller gas explosion from the barrel. The exceptions seen are Magnum-caliber, or high-velocity, high-energy cartridge loadings of medium-caliber weapons.

Near-contact wounds may have small clumps of unburned powder piled up on the edges of the entrance injury and the seared zone of skin. This is most evident in wounds created by .22 Magnum handguns with cartridges containing ball powder. Near-contact wounds from handguns usually occur at ranges less than 10 mm (Di Maio 1999). The searing or burning of hair is rarely seen in humans. This is thought to result from the gas emerging and blowing the hair away.

Intermediate or distant range gunshots can cause irregular, cruciform, or stellate entrance wounds. This occurs in areas in which the skin is over a bony prominence or in places where the bone is curved with a thin, tightly stretched layer of skin. Intermediate-range wounds may have blackening of the skin in addition to powder tattooing. This soot is absent beyond 30 cm. The pattern of powder tattooing may indicate the range, depending on the weapon. From experiments on animals, the .38 Special revolver with a 4-in. barrel and cartridges with flake powder produce powder tattooing out to 18–24 inches; with flattened ball out to 30–36 inches; with true or spherical powder out to 36–42 inches. A .22 caliber rimfire revolver with a 2-in. barrel, firing .22 Long rifle cartridges with flake powder produces powder tattooing out to 18–24 inches; with ball powder out to 12–18 inches (Di Maio 1999). These maximum ranges should be used as a rough guide. Powder tattooing extends further out with ball powder than with flake in centerfire cartridges because of the aerodynamic form of the ball powder. However, in .22 rimfire the flake powder extends further than the ball powder because the balls are so light and small (Di Maio 1999).

Distant gunshot wounds from handguns begin beyond 24 inches for cartridges with flake powder and beyond 42 inches for ball powder. Further range determination is not possible.

Wounds from .22 Caliber Rimfire Weapons

The .22 rimfire cartridge is the most commonly fired cartridge in the United States. The four types of ammunition are the .22 Short, .22 Long, .22 Long Rifle, and .22 Winchester Magnum rimfire.

Contact wounds from the .22 Short have a no tears, little deposition of soot or powder, and some blackening and searing of the edges. There may be a muzzle imprint with hard contact wounds. Head contact wounds usually have no skull fractures. The bullet ricochets within the cranial vault and does not exit (Di Maio 1999).

Hard contact wounds to the head from .22 Long Rifle can range in appearance from a circular perforation with a narrow band of blackened seared skin to a larger, circular wound with ragged, blackened, seared edges. Soot, powder, and searing are evident and muzzle imprints are common. The bullet may perforate the body. Secondary fractures of the skull are seen with the bullet exiting (Di Maio 1999).

Contact wounds with the .22 Magnum cartridge are more destructive, causing stellate wounds. Ball powder can be found at the exit wounds. Extensive secondary fractures of the skull may be seen and the bullet usually exits. Muzzle imprints are common and the bullet may perforate the body (Di Maio 1999).

In intermediate-range wounds, the powder tattoo pattern depends on the powder and barrel length. Animal tests show a .22 handgun with a 2-inch barrel with Long Rifle cartridges loaded with ball powder extend out to 18 inches and is absent at 24 inches. Flake powder extend out to 18–24 inches and is absent at 30 inches (Di Maio 1999).

Distant gunshot wounds are circular usually and can measure 5 mm in diameter, including the abrasion ring. They may be 3 mm where the skin is very elastic and be misinterpreted as puncture wounds. The .22 hollow-point bullets do not usually mushroom on impact when fired from a handgun. They may mushroom when fired from a rifle because of greater velocity. The .22 Long Rifle bullets can produce linear fractures of the skull in distant-range wounds.

Wounds from Centerfire Rifles

Wounds from centerfire rifles are significantly different than those from handguns or .22 rimfire rifles. The muzzle velocity of centerfire rifles ranges between 2,400–4,000 ft/sec. The muzzle kinetic energy ranges from 1,000–5,000 ft-lb. A centerfire rifle can cause injuries to structures without actually contacting them (Di Maio 1999).

The bullets for centerfire rifles have either full or partial metal-jacketing. The full metal-jacketed bullet is used by the military. Soft-point rifle bullets have a partial metal-jacketing with the lead core exposed to facilitate expansion when the bullet strikes. Hollow-point rifle bullets are partial metal-jacketed hunting bullets with a lead core and cavity at the tip to facilitate expansion when it strikes. The last category of bullets is a miscellaneous group of controlled expansion projectiles (Di Maio 1999).

Contact wounds of the head produce a bursting rupture of the head. The entrance wounds have large irregular tears radiating from the site. There is usually soot and searing at the entrance. The entrance may be difficult to identify because of the destruction. The large quantities of gas produced emerge from the muzzle, delivering an explosive effect. If the rifle is discharged in the mouth, there are massive wounds to the mouth and face (Di Maio 1999).

Contact wounds to the chest and abdomen usually have a circular and large injury. There is usually no tearing of the skin. Soot is found in and around the wound, although there is usually less than that found in handgun wounds. The imprint of the muzzle is common. In addition, the front sight or the end of the magazine (in lever-action weapons) may be imprinted. The internal injuries produced usually are massive, with destruction of the organs. The musculature around the entrance and exit may have cherry red coloration from the large amount of carbon monoxide gas (Di Maio 1999).

Powder tattooing is present in intermediate-range wounds. The range for tattooing depends on the type of powder. Ball and cylindrical powder are used in centerfire bullets. Tests were conducted on rabbits. With the .30-30 rifle and cartridges located with cylindrical powder there was heavy powder tattooing with soot deposition at 6 inches; by 12 inches there were only a few scattered tattoo marks; by 18–24 inches there were none. With ball powder, tattooing extended out to 30 inches with moderate density; at 36 inches there were no tattoo marks. With the .223 rifle and cartridges loaded with cylindrical powder, there was rare tattooing out to 12 inches; at 18 inches there were no marks. With ball powder there was heavy tattooing at 18 inches; scattered at 36 inches; and absent at 42 inches. The skin of the rabbit is thinner and more delicate than humans and most other animals, so these findings should serve as a guide to the maximum distances at which powder tattooing can occur (Di Maio 1999).

The severity of the wound with intermediate and distant head wounds depend on the style of bullet and entrance site. Bullets entering through thicker bone cause greater injuries. Expanding bullets can cause as much destruction as contact wounds. The location of the entrance and exit wounds can require skull reconstruction. Distant and intermediate-range entrance wounds over bone can appear stellate because of temporary cavity formation and tearing of the skin (Di Maio 1999).

Distant wounds to the trunk may appear as round punched-out holes with microtears and no abrasion ring. The internal injuries are massive with pulpifaction of the organs. The chest or abdominal wall may be propelled outward and have an imprint of an overlying object (Di Maio 1999).

Exit wounds for all ranges are larger and more irregular than entrance wounds. They are usually 25 mm or less in diameter but can be as large as 40 mm (Di Maio 1999).

Radiographs of victims shot with hunting ammunition show a typical pattern called a *lead snowstorm*. Fragments of lead break off the lead core and are propelled into the surrounding tissues. The x-ray shows hundreds of small radiopaque fragments along the wound track. They can vary from dust-like to large irregular pieces. Pieces of the jacket may be seen. This phenomenon does not require the bullet to hit bone. The absence of the lead snowstorm does not rule out centerfire hunting ammunition. The bullet may be traveling at low velocity because of an extreme range or from passing through an intermediary target. A similar finding can be seen with head wounds from a .357 Magnum. The breakup of the bullet requires perforation of the bone and the fragments usually are larger and fewer in number with no lead dust (Di Maio 1999).

Hunting bullets or medium and large caliber exit the body. The .222 or .22-250 varmint cartridges tend to stay in the body. With other ammunition, the ability to perforate the body depends on the weight of the bullet, body area struck, and length of the wound path (Di Maio 1999).

Wounds from Shotguns

Shotguns have a smooth bore and can fire a single projectile, although often they are used to fire multiple pellets. Rifled shotgun barrels are used to fire slugs. The term *gauge* for a shotgun is used to describe its caliber, and refers to the number of lead balls of a bore diameter that can make up a pound. A 12-gauge would take 12 lead balls to make up a pound. The exception is the .410, which refers to the bore diameter of 0.410 inches (Di Maio 1999).

The ammunition for shotguns is comprised of a tube (paper or plastic); a thin brass or brass-coated steel head; a primer; powder; paper, cardboard, or composition wads; and lead shot. Some may have plastic or felt wads. Buckshot and birdshot shells have granular white polyethylene or polypropylene filler. This filler can cause pseudo-tattoo marks that extend out a greater distance than the powder tattooing. Birdshot is used for birds or small game and buckshot is used for large game. The smaller the shot size number, the larger the pellet diameter. Buckshot is labeled by the number of pellets per shell (Di Maio 1999).

Shotgun slugs are used for deer and bear hunting in heavily populated areas. The slug rapidly loses velocity, providing protection from shooting accidents. The Brenneke slug is solid lead with a pointed nose and felt and cardboard wads screwed to the base. There are 12 angled ribs on the surface. The Foster slug by Winchester is made of soft lead with a roundnose, deep concave base, and 12–15 angled, helical grooves on the surface. It has a cup wad and cardboard filler wads. It can be made with a hollow point as well. The Remington Foster slug may have a plastic insert on the tip and uses a combination of plastic and cardboard wads. The Federal Foster slugs have a one-piece plastic wad (Di Maio 1999).

The Sabot slug has an hourglass configuration with a hollow base with a plastic insert. This slug is enclosed in a sabot made of two haves of high-density polyethylene plastic. Once the unit exits the muzzle, the sabot falls away. Depending on the manufacturer, the slug may have a hollow point, a cup wad, and cardboard filler wad, and a nose section that separates on impact, producing four additional wound tracks (Di Maio 1999).

Shotguns are the most destructive of all small arms. The severity and lethality of birdshot and buckshot loads depends on the number of pellets that enter the body, organs struck, and amount of tissue destruction. There is no temporary cavity injury. Rifle slugs produce direct wounds as well as injury from temporary cavity formation. As the range increases, there is a decrease in the number of pellets that strike the victim. There is a rapid decline in velocity of the pellets as the range increases. The larger shot retains its velocity better than small shot. The maximum effective hunting range for birdshot is 45–65 yards. The maximum traveling range for lead birdshot is 110 yards for #12 shot and 396 yards for BB shot. The maximum range for buckshot is 528 yards for #4 Buck and 726 yards for #00 Buck. The effective range is much less because of the velocity needed to penetrate skin (Di Maio 1999).

The entrance wound of a shotgun slug is circular with a diameter measuring that of the slug, although the gauge cannot be determined. The wound edge is abraded (Fig. 8.1). The wads may enter through the entrance or strike adjacent skin, causing circular to oval imprints (Figs. 8.2, 8.3). With the Sabot slug, the two halves of the sabot may enter the body or impact the skin. With the Brenneke slug, the wadding enters the wound because it is screwed into the base. Slugs produce massive internal injuries similar to centerfire rifle hunting bullets. They tend to flatten and remain in the body. Comma-like pieces may break off of the disk (Di Maio 1999).

Wounds from buckshot depend on the gunshot range. A contact wound is circular and the diameter the same as the bore of the gun. The wound edges are abraded and seared. Soot may be deposited in loose contact wounds. Powder tattooing ap-

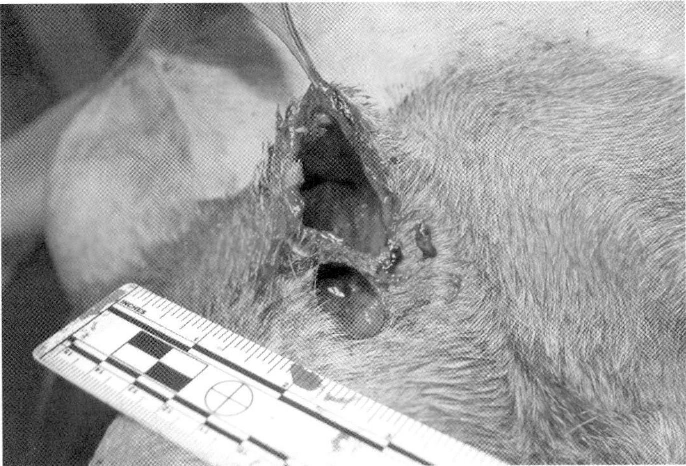

Fig. 8.1 Gunshot entrance wound caused by a slug. The slug entered over a fold of skin, causing the first wound, which is circular; then the slug expanded, causing the larger irregular second wound. For color detail, please see color plate section.

pears when the range increases beyond a few centimeters. In 12-gauge shotguns, this extends out to a maximum of 90–125 cm for ball powder and 60–75 cm for flake. The diameter of the entrance wound increases as the range increases. At 3 feet, the edges have a scalloped shape. At 4 feet the buckshot pellets separate to produce a large gaping wound with a few satellite holes. By 9 feet there are individual pellet holes. The wad follows the buckshot into the wound at close range. As this range increases, the wad impacts the skin, causing a circular or oval abrasion. This may be found among or adjacent to the pellet holes. Cork filler wads may fragment on firing, causing irregular abrasions on the skin (Di Maio 1999).

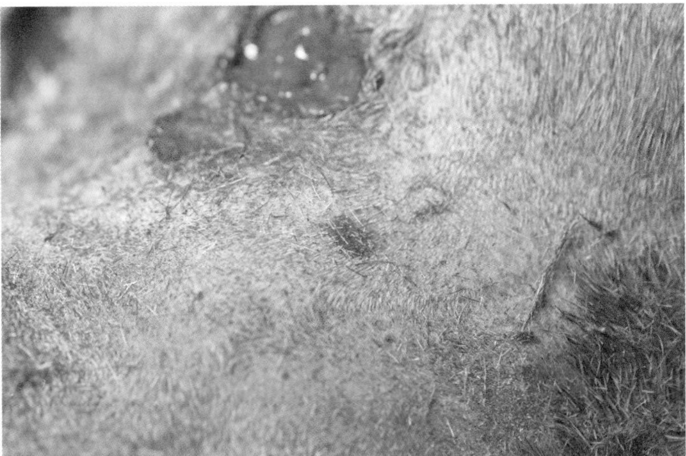

Fig. 8.2 Circular and linear abrasion adjacent to the gunshot wound (see Figure 8.1) from the impact of wadding. For color detail, please see color plate section.

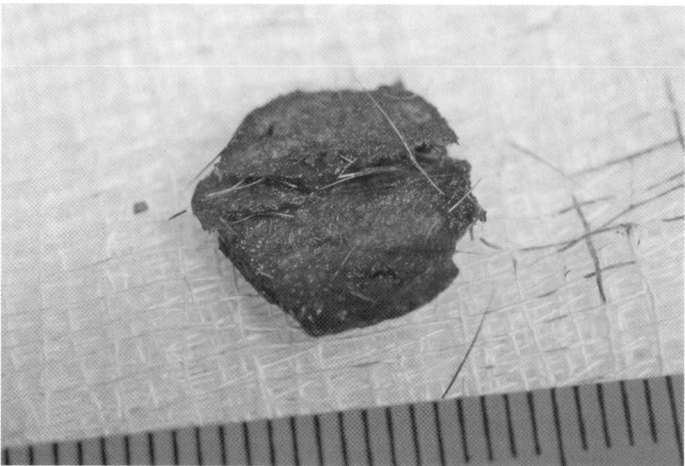

Fig. 8.3 Paper wadding found inside the second entrance wound (see Figure 8.1). For color detail, please see color plate section.

In general, contact shotgun wounds cause massive, mutilating damage. Large fragments of the skull and brain may be ejected from the head. This is caused by the charge of the shot, which directly fractures the skull, shreds the brain, and produces pressure waves. The gas expands, adding to the pressure waves, which shatters the skull. The entrance wound has large quantities of soot and the edges are seared and blackened. The pellet exit site may be difficult to determine because of the large amount of missing tissue and bone (Di Maio 1999).

Intermediate and close range wounds to the head cause similar mutilation of contact wounds. This is because the pellets travel in a single mass. There are large gaping tears at the entrance, which when re-approximated have an abrasion ring. The pellet exit site is difficult to determine (Di Maio 1999).

Contact wounds to the trunk have a circular entrance and a diameter measuring approximately that of the bore of the gun. The edges are seared and blackened without soot in hard-contact wounds. A muzzle imprint is common, including the front sight. The wound may be surrounded by a wide zone of abraded skin from the skin flaring against the muzzle. In loose-contact or near-contact wounds there is a circular area of soot that increases in diameter but reduces in density as the distance increases. Soot deposition continues out to approximately 30 cm. The muscle at the entrance may be cherry red from the carbon monoxide gas. This can spread 15 cm or greater from the entrance. It also may follow the path of the shot through the body (Di Maio 1999).

Powder tattooing occurs at ranges beyond 1–2 cm. This tattooing is less dense than that found with handguns. Testing on rabbits, conducted using a 12-gauge shotgun with a 28-in. barrel and flake powder in the shells showed powder tattooing out to 24 inches and absent by 30 inches; with ball powder the tattooing was present at 30 inches, few marks at 36 inches, and absent by 40 inches (Di Maio 1999). In addition to powder tattooing, petal marks may be seen from plastic shot cups 1–3 feet with 12-, 16-, and 20-gauge shotguns. In .410 shotguns, the petal marks appear at 3–5 inches and are absent at 2 feet.

Wadding may be found inside the wound. It may impact the edge of the entrance wound, causing an irregular abraded margin on one side. If the shell contains an over-the-shot wad and a plastic cup, there may be two sets of wad markings. As the distance increase, the wad loses energy and fails to mark the skin. With filler wads, marks may be seen out to 15 feet and plastic wads out to 20 feet (Di Maio 1999).

With distant wounds, the circular wound diameter increases until the pellet mass separates, producing individual pellet wounds. At 2 feet, birdshot (regardless of gauge) produced a 0.75- to 1-inch hole; at 3 feet the hole had scalloped margins and measured 7/8 inch for modified choke and 1.25 inches for a cylinder bore; at 4 feet, the hole was 1 inch for modified choke and 1.75 inches for cylinder bore with scattered satellite pellet holes; at 6–7 feet there was a cuff of satellite pellet holes around an irregular wound for a modified choke; the wound was ragged with a prominent cuff of pellet holes; at greater distances there was large variation in the size of the pellet pattern depending on the ammunition, choke of the gun, and range (Di Maio 1999). Range determination can only be made using the actual weapon and same brand of ammunition to conduct a series of test shots. Photographs should be taken and the pattern measured for comparison of test shots. Pellets should be measured.

Air Weapons

Air-powered guns range from toy BB guns to expensive and highly sophisticated air rifles. A BB gun can cause serious injury if it strikes the eye. Corneal penetration and globe disruption occur at 246–269 ft/sec. A steel BB has a muzzle velocity of 275–350 ft/sec. The air rifle has a rifled barrel and uses compressed air or gas to propel the projectile. In pneumatic type guns, the air is pumped into a storage chamber and can produce a maximum velocity of 770 ft/sec. The spring-air compression system uses a powerful spring compressed by manual action that produces velocities of 1,000 ft/sec. Carbon dioxide is used for gas-compression systems, which have the same muzzle velocity of spring rifles.

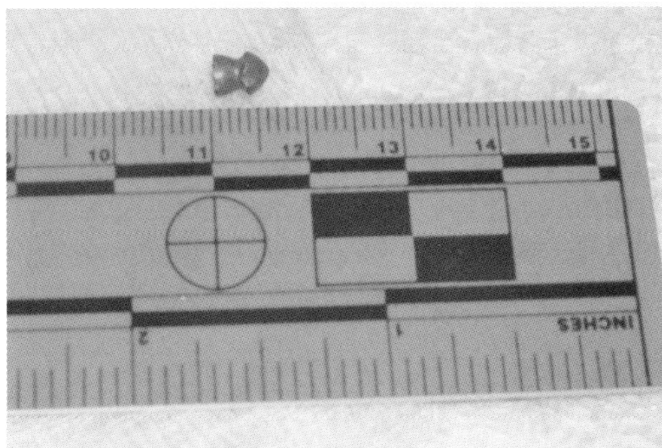

Fig. 8.4 Conical pellet from an air rifle that was fired into the neck of a dog and recovered from the opposite right shoulder (see Figure 8.5). For color detail, please see color plate section.

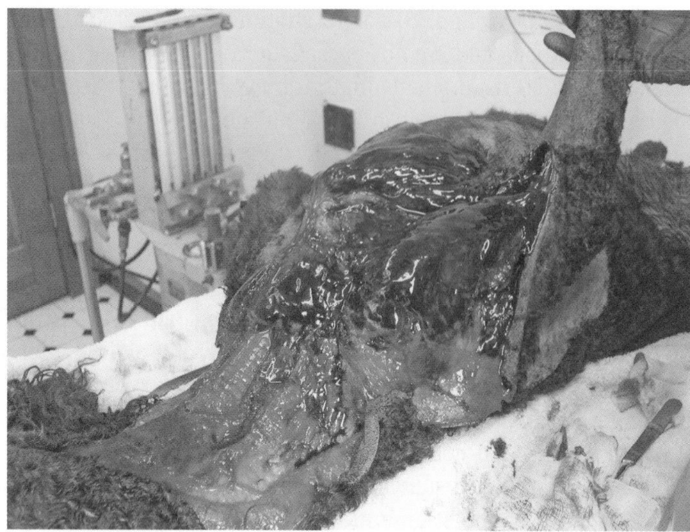

Fig. 8.5 This dog was shot with an air rifle. The pellet entered the left neck, perforated the trachea, punctured the right carotid artery, punctured the right jugular vein, and lodged in the subcutaneous tissue over the right shoulder. The dog died from massive exsanguination into the surrounding tissue and mediastinum. For color detail, please see color plate section.

The calibers used are 0.177, 0.20, and 0.22 inches. The most common ammunition for air-powered guns is the Diabolo pellet, an hourglass shaped, soft-lead missile (Fig. 8.4). The rifling of the barrel is on the front edge. These pellets lose velocity rapidly and are harmless at less than 100 yards. Pointed conical bullets are made for air rifles. Air rifles can cause significant, even fatal, injury if fired at close enough range (Fig. 8.5).

Retrieving Gunshot Residue

Gunshot wounds should be examined for evidence of soot and powder, and samples collected prior to cleaning the wound. Blood may hide the presence of soot and powder. The area should be sprayed with hot water or hydrogen peroxide to dissolve the blood. Soot and powder grains may be found around the entrance wound, inside the wound, and in the wound track. These areas should be swabbed or scraped to collect the residue. Any gunpowder grains should be collected and described (flake, ball, or cylinder). The animal may have licked at the wound, removing soot and gunpowder grains.

Retrieving Projectile and Wadding

To retrieve the projectile, the location of all bullets and fragments must be determined. Full-body radiographs should be taken to identify the presence of projectiles and injuries related to the gunshot. The presence of an exit wound does not necessarily mean the bullet exited (see Determining Entrance and Exit Wounds). The presence of BB or pellets without any entrance wounds is indicative of previous gunshot wound and is not significant. Bullet emboli are possible, causing the projectile to travel far away from the wound track through the bloodstream. Projectiles that enter the airway system may be coughed up and swallowed; therefore, the stomach contents should be inspected.

The bullet and all the fragments must be removed carefully to avoid causing any marks on the surface. The rifling marks on surface of the bullet are crucial for ballistics matching. It is best to use gloved fingers if possible to remove the bullet. Cotton, tape, or plastic IV tubing may be used to cover the ends of forceps or tweezers to prevent the instruments from causing any surface artifacts. If there are multiple projectiles, the bullet should be identified with a number or letter on the base or tip using a soft marking pencil. For shotgun wounds caused by pellets, a representative sample of the projectiles should be collected. All projectiles should be placed on cotton or tissue in a protective container.

The entrance wound should be examined for the presence of the wadding associated with shotgun wounds. The wadding may be composed of plastic, cork, or cardboard. Forensic examination of the wad can determine the gauge of the shotgun and make of the ammunition. Plastic wads and sabots may retain scratch marks to match to the weapon.

Manufacturers of ammunition make up a large batch of molten lead to make thousands of bullets to which they add a certain amount of trace elements that are unique to that batch. When there is no intact bullet and only bullet fragments are recovered, the lab can run an elemental analysis to determine the trace element contained in the bullet. This can be used to match other bullets found in the suspect's possession.

Retrieving the Cartridge Cases

At the scene, all unfired and fired ejected cartridge cases should be collected, taking care not to smudge any potential fingerprints. The end of the shell casing may have marks caused by the firearm. The firing pin has unique characteristics that are transferred to the bullet casing when the bullet is fired. These markings can be used to match the bullet casing to the gun from which it was fired. After the bullet is fired, the shell casing goes backward and contacts the breech face of the gun. This marking has unique and distinctive marks from the manufacturer of the gun. When a shotgun is fired the firing pin leaves a distinctive mark on the shell that is considered the fingerprint of the firearm.

Determining Trajectory

In order to evaluate trajectory it is important to determine what injuries and tissue destruction the gunshot caused. It is important to consider that the animal may have been in motion when shot. If the animal was shot more than once, the animal's response to the first impact must be considered to properly evaluate all the wounds.

An attempt should be made to re-create the incident using the exam findings, crime scene results, and witness interviews.

There are clues as to the bullet path. Blood clots indicate hemorrhage from laceration of a major vessel, several vessels, or severe tissue injury. In bone fractures, the bone bevels outward, indicating direction of travel. Lead may be deposited on the bone from the bullet. A bullet does not usually veer off the trajectory path after striking or perforating bone unless it has lost all of its forward velocity. In this case, the bullet may be found within 1–2 inches of the impact site.

In deceased victims, the bullet track should be carefully probed, taking care not to dislodge the missile or create false tracks. Special trajectory rods or metal or plastic rods from a craft store may be used. It is best if the rods have slight elasticity to allow easier manipulation. Sometimes the track is not obvious and both the entrance and exit wounds must be probed to get an idea of the path before proceeding with the necropsy. To visualize the bullet path, care should be taken to preserve the evidence of injury. This may require lifting out the chest or abdomen wall. In certain areas it may require reflecting the skin and dissecting the tissue layer by layer in a large area over the estimated wound track. This allows documentation of the injuries and prevents creating artificial tracks.

Recording the Injuries

All the wounds need to be photographed and recorded with written and diagram documentation. In the report, it is best to document the injuries under the "Evidence of Injury" section. A number should be assigned to each entrance wound and a letter to each exit wound. Describe the wound's location using measurements from a physical landmark, such as a nipple; from the ventral or dorsal midline; and from the head or rear as a cranial or caudal reference. General measurements should be taken of the animal's body (height at head, shoulders, pelvis, to ventral chest and abdomen; length from chest to rear, muzzle to rear). Describe the appearance of the wound (what features make it an entrance vs. exit) and the estimated range it was inflicted. Measurements of the wound and wound patterns should be documented. When there are dozens of gunshot wounds, as seen with shotgun pellets, they may be handled best in groups. For powder tattoo patterns, abrasion rings, burns, or muzzle imprints, measurements should be taken using a clock reference, making the midline of the body 12 o'clock. The path of the bullet through the body should be described. The injuries caused by the bullet should be described as well, including all organs penetrated or perforated. All recovered bullets, bullet fragments, pellets, and wadding should be documented by their location. A description of the bullet and wadding should be given with as much information as can be determined from examination. Lastly, an overall description of the bullet path through the body in relation to the planes of the body should be given (right to left, dorsal to ventral, sharply downward, etc.).

References

Di Maio, V.J.M. 1999. *Gunshot Wounds: Practical Aspects of Firearms, Ballistics, and Forensic Techniques*. Boca Raton, FL: CRC Press.

Kraus, K.H. 1992. Acute Management of Open Fractures, Including Gunshot, Shearing, and Degloving Wounds. In *Kirk's Current Veterinary Therapy XI Small Animal Practice*, ed. R.W. Kirk, and J.D. Bonagura, pp. 154–158. Philadelphia: W.B. Saunders.

Munro, H.M., and M.V. Thrusfield. 2001. 'Battered Pets': Features that Raise Suspicion of Non-accidental Injury. *Journal of Small Animal Practice* 42:218–226.

Pavletic, M.M. 1985. A Review of 121 Gunshot Wounds in the Dog and Cat. *Veterinary Surgery* 14:61–62.

Pavletic, M.M. 2006. Managing Gunshot Wounds in Small Animals. *Veterinary Technician* 27(1):36–44.

Chapter 9
Patterns of Non-accidental Injury: Asphyxia and Drowning

Overview of Asphyxia

Death resulting from asphyxia is defined as the failure of cells to receive or use oxygen (Di Maio and Di Maio 2001). This can result from partial oxygen deprivation (hypoxia) or total oxygen deprivation (anoxia). Asphyxia can be categorized into suffocation, strangulation, and chemical asphyxia. Chemical asphyxia is dealt with in Chapter 7 under Smoke Inhalation. In each of these categories there are subcategories that define the anatomical site and the nature of the force used to cause the asphyxia. In addition, drowning is considered a form of asphyxia and is dealt with later in this chapter.

Asphyxiation, specifically strangulation, is the most common cause of death in human sexual assaults. Any animal victim of asphyxia should be examined for possible sexual assault. Several forms of asphyxia require the assailant to be in close proximity to the victim. It is possible that the victim inflicted injury to the assailant during the struggle or there was a transfer of evidence from the assailant to the victim. Consideration should be given in all cases of abuse to these scenarios and appropriate measures taken to identify this evidence.

General Findings

The findings that are considered classic signs of asphyxia in humans are visceral congestion, petechiae, cyanosis, and fluidity of the blood (Di Maio and Di Maio 2001). Unfortunately, these signs are non-specific and can be associated with other causes of death. Other findings associated with each category of asphyxia may aid the determination of asphyxia as the cause of death. In some cases, the diagnosis of asphyxia may be a diagnosis of exclusion by the elimination of other causes of death and supported by the circumstances surrounding death. A full history should be obtained on the animal, including any emergency treatment that was rendered. Resuscitative injuries to the pharynx and larynx caused by intubation can be seen. These can mimic similar injuries produced by strangulation or neck holds, leading to misinterpretation of examination findings.

Visceral congestion is caused by obstructed venous return and capillovenous congestion, which are more susceptible to hypoxia. This produces dilation of the vessels and blood stasis (Di Maio and Di Maio 2001). Congestion also may be seen in the face. Petechiae seen are resulting from the sudden over-distention and rupture of small vessels, primarily the venules. They are commonly seen in the epicardium and visceral pleura (Di Maio and Di Maio 2001). Petechial hemorrhages on the surface of the lung are caused by small ruptures of blood vessels resulting from pressure changes in the lungs when air flow is obstructed through the nose and mouth.

The location of the petechiae also may depend on the mechanism of asphyxia. It should be noted that petechiae are nonspecific findings and may be seen in other conditions, such as bleeding disorders and septicemia. In humans, they may be found in the reflected scalp or the epiglottis and are considered unremarkable (Di Maio and Di Maio 2001). Petechiae also can develop postmortem in dependent areas in which the pooling of the blood overwhelms the vessels, causing mechanical rupture. These areas can enlarge to areas of ecchymoses. Cyanosis is also a nonspecific finding. The fluidity of the blood postmortem is caused by an increased rate of fibrinolysis that is seen in rapid deaths and is thought to result from high agonal catecholamine levels. This is considered a nonspecific finding and may be seen with other causes of rapid death (Di Maio and Di Maio 2001).

Microscopic Pathology Findings

Asphyxiation is a name given to different kinds of lesions that can produce similar histological findings. Thus, a complete history and necropsy would support the microscopic findings suggestive of suffocation, drowning, or strangulation. Areas of over-insufflation of the alveoli and alveolar collapse can be seen in cases of suffocation. Intra-alveolar hemorrhage in addition to the above lesions can be seen in strangulation. In the lungs of an animal that may have been drowned there is often proteinic reddish to light pink material in the lumen of alveoli.

Suffocation

Suffocation refers to death caused by failure of oxygen to reach the blood. The five categories of suffocation are vitiated atmosphere, smothering, choking, airway swelling, and/or obstruction, and compression of the chest or abdomen.

Vitiated Atmosphere (Entrapment Suffocation)

A vitiated atmosphere is one in which there is inadequate oxygen. This most commonly occurs when an animal becomes entrapped in a small space, such as a refrigerator or other similar closed spaces. With entrapment, initially there may be sufficient oxygen but as the animal continues to breathe, the oxygen supply is exhausted and they asphyxiate. The necropsy may reveal nonspecific acute visceral congestion (Di Maio and Di Maio 2001). Diagnosis of entrapment suffocation is made with exclusions of all other causes of death and analysis of the circumstances leading up to and surrounding death.

Smothering

Smothering is caused by the mechanical obstruction or occlusions of the external airways (Di Maio and Di Maio 2001). This may be done by placing a plastic bag over the animal's head and securing it or by placing the animal inside a plastic bag. It may be accomplished by placing a conforming object, such as a pillow, on top of the face and pressing down. It also may be the cause of death when an animal is buried alive.

The physical findings may indicate a struggle with abrasions and/or contusions on the external and internal surfaces of the face and mouth, including torn frenula. There may be trace evidence inside the mouth from the animal biting at the covering object. If a bag is secured around the neck, there may be scratches on the neck where the animal struggled to get it off. The animal may not be found with the offending object still attached or in proximity to the body. If the animal clawed at the object, the animal's nails may have retained embedded material. In humans, petechiae may be found on the face, sclerae, conjunctivae, or gingiva, but they are usually absent. There may be petechiae on the epicardium and pleural surface of the lungs, but these are nonspecific. Diagnosis usually is made by exclusion of other causes of death and the circumstances surrounding death.

Any recovered object is evidence that may be linked to the perpetrator(s) and victim. Plastic bags can be identified as to brand and manufacturer and the bottom edge can be linked to the roll from which they were torn. DNA from the animal's saliva, blood, or urine may be found on the inside of the bag or from the surface of the pillow. There may be fingerprints on the bag from the perpetrator. Nose prints on the bag may be linked to a specific dog victim because nose prints are unique to the individual dog.

When an animal is buried alive more than one type of asphyxia may cause death. Depending on the depth and weight of the fill on the body, compression of the chest can contribute to the suffocation. If the animal was buried alive, findings may include soil in the sinuses, deep airways, and stomach. It is possible for dirt to enter the airways passively, but one should not find a substantial amount of soil in the stomach. The soil also may lodge in the airway, causing an obstruction. Other evidence may be found in the grave (see Chapter 2).

Choking

Choking is caused by an obstruction in the internal airway by foreign material. This can occur in the posterior pharynx, larynx, trachea, or the bronchi. Most choking deaths are accidental ingestion or aspiration of foreign material, but they may caused by someone forcing an object into the mouth or the back of the pharynx. Findings of blockage of the airway by foreign material are diagnostic of choking. If the object was removed during resuscitative efforts, the diagnosis can be made only through the history. There are no other specific findings on necropsy.

Airway Swelling/Obstruction

Asphyxia may occur by severe airway swelling that obstructs the passage of air. It may involve the larynx and surrounding tissues, bronchi, or bronchioles. The swelling may result from a number of causes. Anaphylaxis can cause swelling in the larynx and surrounding tissues, leading to obstruction. The inhalation of steam can cause similar swelling, producing markedly edematous, beefy red mucosa in the larynx. Infection and neoplasia either within or adjacent to the airways can lead to obstruction. Chemical agents and irritating substances such as pepper can cause the lining of the airway to swell; obstruction is further complicated by the accumulation of mucus, inflammatory debris, and airway spasm. A blow to the neck can cause severe swelling of the larynx and surrounding tissue. This can take minutes to hours to develop and occlude the airway.

Compression of the Chest/Abdomen

Compression of the chest or upper abdomen can prevent breathing resulting in asphyxia, also called compression asphyxia. When extreme pressure is exerted on the chest, there is a sudden increase in intrathoracic pressure. This affects the cardiac hemodynamics, causing an increase in venous pressure. In humans, findings include marked dusky congestion of the head, neck, and upper trunk. Petechiae are found in face, sclerae, conjunctivae, periorbital skin, neck, and upper trunk. There may be external marks on the torso from the compressing agent or there may be no evidence of trauma. In animals, these marks may be seen when the skin is reflected back. Internally, there may be small hemorrhages in the neck and chest muscle attachments, rib fractures, and internal organ damage.

Strangulation

Overview

Strangulation is caused by the constriction of the jugular and carotid vessels with or without airway compression. The causes include manual strangulation (throttling), yoking, ligature strangulation (garroting), and hanging.

The cause of death in strangulation is cerebral hypoxia caused by the compression and occlusion of the arteries supplying the brain. These arteries include the carotids and vertebrals. Venous drainage is primarily through the jugular veins. The carotid arteries are easily compressed in contrast with the vertebral arteries, which are resistant to direct pressure. The vertebral arteries can be occluded by severe lateral flexion or rotation of the neck, as is seen in hanging (Di Maio and Di Maio 2001). When there is compression of the carotid and jugular vessels, the vertebral arteries continue to supply blood to the head. This increases the pressure in the capillovenules, causing them to rupture and producing petechiae. Petechiae associated with strangulation are indicative of local venous congestion (Di Maio and Di Maio 2001). If there are compression and release or partial compression of the vessels, the pressure may be altered and petechiae may be absent or reduced. If the compression of the neck vessels is sudden and complete, as with hanging, no petechiae may be found. The presence of petechiae is not diagnostic of strangulation because it is seen in other conditions.

General Findings

There are few descriptions of the features of strangulation in animals. The findings in these cases parallel those found in humans, so it seems appropriate that they apply to animals. There were two reported cases of attempted strangulation with detailed descriptions of their findings in the study by Munro and Thrusfield. In one case a dog, less than 2 years old, presented with evidence of a crushing injury to the trachea, severe laryngeal edema, lingual swelling, and fractures of the hyoid bone seen on radiographs. There was also edema of the lips and eyelids, subconjunctival hemorrhages and small internal eye hemorrhages. In the second case a dog, over 2 years of age, presented with swelling and edema of the neck, breathing difficulties, edema around the eyes, and bruising around the head and lips (Munro and Thrusfield 2001). These findings are similar to those in human victims of strangulation. Hyoid fractures may be difficult to see on radiographs and easily missed. This fracture caused by strangulation is more common after enough calcification of the bone occurs. In dogs, this occurs by 10–12 months of age.

Examination of the interior of the neck in all strangulation deaths should be done so as to minimize hemorrhage artifact. The best way is to remove all the viscera from the chest, abdominal cavities, and brain. The blood should be allowed to drain into the skull and body cavities. Then the neck can be dissected with less chance of causing artifactual hemorrhage. Antemortem fractures of the hyoid bone, thyroid, or cricoid cartilage can be determined only if there is visible hemorrhage at the fracture site. The neck should be dissected layer by layer to visualize injuries. The tongue and connected neck structures should be removed together by making an incision along the medial aspect of the mandible to free the oral tissues.

Manual Strangulation (Throttling)

Manual strangulation is caused by the pressure of the hand, forearm, or other limb against the neck. This compression of the internal structures causes occlusion of the blood vessels to the brain. There is usually compression of the carotids and jugulars, but the vertebral arteries continue to supply blood to the head. The face is usually congested and may appear cyanotic (Di Maio and Di Maio 2001). Petechiae may be seen on the face, conjunctivae, sclerae, or gingiva. Petechiae found on the mucosa of the larynx or epiglottis are not diagnostic of strangulation or asphyxia. Pulmonary edema may be seen, with foamy edema fluid found in the nostrils (Di Maio and Di Maio 2001). There may be evidence of sphincter incontinence at the scene of the assault.

There is usually injury to the external and internal structures of the neck with manual strangulation, although it is possible to see no injury at all. There may be abrasions, contusions, finger contusions, and fingernail marks on the skin. Fingernail marks are usually from the fingers and not the thumb because the thumb pad is used to apply pressure. These marks can appear as linear, semi-linear, scratches, or scrapes. Fingertips can cause erythematous impression marks or contusions. They appear curved, oval, triangular, dashed, rectangular, or exclamation mark–like (Di Maio and Di Maio 2001).

The animal may struggle and claw at the assailant's hand, arm, or limbs, retaining evidence on its feet and nails. There is often significant hemorrhage of the strap muscles of the neck and the surrounding soft tissue caused by the large amount of force used and the movement between the victim and assailant. Mild or absent hemorrhage may be seen if there is a large disparity of size between the assailant and victim, and movement is minimal between the two (Dix et al. 2000).

Fractures of the thyroid and cricoid cartilage may occur. Depending on the age of the animal and calcification of the hyoid, fractures of the hyoid bone may be found. The U-shape of the hyoid makes it susceptible to compression fractures and is usually only seen with manual strangulation (Di Maio and Di Maio 2001). Cartilaginous separations of the hyoid must not be mistaken for fractures. All antemortem fractures have visible hemorrhage at the fracture site. Microscopic hemorrhage is not indicative of antemortem fracture and can be a postmortem artifact (Di Maio and Di Maio 2001).

Hemorrhage within the tongue may be seen. On necropsy exam, multiple crosswise slices into the tongue should be made to look for internal hemorrhage within the tissue.

Yoking

Yoking refers to the compression of the neck by the forearm, usually from behind the victim. Because the forearm is a broad soft object, there may little to no external injury to the neck. If a large amount of force is applied and there is a lot of movement between the victim and assailant, there may be contusions on the neck. The damage to internal neck structures is variable and may include fractures of the larynx or hyoid. The presence of petechiae on the face, sclerae, conjunctivae, and gingiva may be found but is variable (Dix et al. 2000).

Ligature Strangulation (Garroting)

Ligature strangulation results from a constricting band that tightens, and is caused by a force other than the body weight. This ligature applies pressure to the neck, causing occlusion of the carotid arteries and depriving oxygen to the brain. A variety of ligatures may be used, including leashes, electrical cords, telephone cords, rope, plastic lock-ties, neckties, sheets, scarves, hose, and towels. The ligature mark appearance depends on the nature of the ligature, amount of force used by the assailant, and resistance of the victim. The mark may reflect the configuration of the ligature used, such as the weave of the rope or an imprinted pattern. Alternatively, the mark may be faint or absent, especially if the ligature was soft or removed immediately after death. The more narrow and firm the ligature, the more distinct the mark.

Typically, a ligature mark encircles the neck, creating a furrow, initially having a yellow parchment-like appearance in humans and turning dark brown over time (Di Maio and Di Maio 2001). There may be a break in the furrow where the assailant grasped the ends of the ligature and tightened. There are usually no abrasions or contusions unless the victim clawed at the neck. If two loops were wrapped around the neck, the skin that was pinched between the loops may be contused (Di Maio and Di Maio 2001). There may be multiple marks on the neck or atypical marks if the assailant repeatedly tried to get a grip with the ligature on the neck. Decomposition does not typically affect ligature marks. This is thought to be caused by the compression preventing access to the area by putrefying bacteria (Di Maio and Di Maio 2001).

The face and neck above the ligature are usually congested and edema fluid may be present in the nostrils. Scleral hemorrhage along with petechiae on the face, the periorbital region, conjunctivae, and gingiva may be seen. In ligature strangulation there is complete compression of the jugulars but incomplete compression of the arteries. The blood continues to go into the head through the vertebral arteries but cannot escape, causing increased intravascular pressure, congestion, and rupture of the vessels (Di Maio and Di Maio 2001). Injuries to the neck may or may not be present. Fractures of the thyroid cartilage may occur but hyoid bone fracture is rare. There may be minimal to severe soft tissue hemorrhage within the neck (Dix et al. 2000).

The ligature should be removed only by the veterinarian in a deceased animal and kept as evidence. The knot should be preserved, the ligature cut on the opposite side, and the ends taped together.

Hanging

General Findings

In hanging, the neck structures are compressed by some sort of ligature that is tightened by the weight of the body, resulting in asphyxia. There may be complete suspension of the body or partial suspension, with part of the body touching the ground or floor. Hanging can cause compression or constriction of the blood vessels. Obstruction of the airway may or may not occur. The airway obstruction may be caused by compression of the trachea, or through the elevation and posterior displacement of the tongue and floor of the mouth when the noose is above the larynx (Di Maio and Di Maio 2001). Cervical neck fractures are not seen with non-judicial hangings. In partial suspension hangings, the weight of the head can be enough to cause occlusion of the neck vessels.

The noose used in hangings may be constructed from anything that is handy and available. It may be comprised of rope, electrical cords, leashes, belts, phone cords, or from something softer such as strips of cloth. The point of suspension varies in location around the neck and is usually from the knot. The ligature causes a furrow on the neck but does not completely encircle the neck, producing an inverted V pattern. These marks can be misinterpreted as manual strangulation.

Initially the furrow may be light, with a congested rim and then change to darker brown as it dries out. The furrow is deeper and darker in color opposite the point of suspension and becomes lighter where it angles upward toward the point of suspension. The furrow may reflect the configuration of the ligature such as the weave of the rope, design on a belt, or configuration of the electrical wiring. With a thin, firm ligature, the groove is more distinct and well demarcated. There may be abrasions from the surface of the material or contusions. Nooses from softer material tend to cause a poorly defined groove or no marks at all. The upper margin may be red caused by postmortem congestion of the vessels and the lower margin may be pale (Di Maio and Di Maio 2001). There may be two furrows if the noose was composed of two loops. These furrows may be parallel, overlap, or have two different paths. They may pinch the skin between them, causing tissue hemorrhage. If a belt is used it may produce two parallel marks on the neck from where each edge dug into the skin. The longer the body is suspended, the more prominent the mark will be because of vessel congestion (Di Maio and Di Maio 2001).

Occasionally, the ligature marks are horizontal, depending on the position of the body. It is possible that an animal was first killed by ligature strangulation then strung up. In that case, the markings on the neck would be more horizontal and not the inverted V pattern seen in hanging. However, it is possible to have noose marks if the victim was deceased when hanged. In humans, these marks could be seen if the victim was hanged within 2 hours after death (Di Maio and Di Maio 2001).

Judicial Hanging

Judicial hangings involve a sudden drop of the body with complete suspension. In humans, death is caused by the fracture and dislocation of the upper cervical vertebrae and transaction of the spinal cord. If the body falls an insufficient distance, death is caused by strangulation. If the body falls too far, the victim may be decapitated. The classic hangman's fracture in humans, which is associated with cord injury at C2-C3, is caused by hyperextension and distraction. The fracture is through the pedicles of C2, where the caudal aspect remains fixed with C3 and the cranial aspect remains fixed with C1 (Di Maio and Di Maio 2001).

Other injuries to the cervical vertebrae may occur instead of the hangman's fracture. There may be fractures of the transverse processes of C1-C3 and C5, the cervical body of C2, the occipital bones, or the styloid processes. There may be separation of C2 and C3 with complete transection of the cord, fractures of the thyroid cartilage, the hyoid bone, and hemorrhage into the cervical muscle. There may be bilateral vertebral artery lacerations with basilar subarachnoid hemorrhage or bilateral internal carotid tears with subdural hematomas (Di Maio and Di Maio 2001). In animals, these injuries may or may not be seen caused by the thicker neck muscle in certain breeds.

Examination of Hanging Victims

The body should be photographed prior to being cut down. All knots should be preserved. The ligature should be removed only by the veterinarian. The nature, composition, width, location, type of knot, and mode of application should be documented prior to removal of the noose. The ligature should be slipped over the head or cut on the side opposite of the knot and the ends taped together. The ligature marks should be photographed with a ruler adjacent to the mark. The furrow should be described in detail, including the direction, depth, width, color, ligature patterns, area of neck involved, and its relation to local landmarks (Di Maio and Di Maio 2001).

The neck and body should be examined for other marks and injuries. The animal may have clawed at the noose, leaving abrasions on the neck and face. The animal may have been beaten, dragged, or otherwise assaulted either prior to or after it was hanged. In non-judicial hangings, there are often no internal neck injuries. Occasionally, fractures of the thyroid cartilage, hyoid bone, and cervical spine may be seen. Findings may include hemorrhage of the strap muscles of the neck and blood-tinged fluid in the nostrils (Di Maio and Di Maio 2001).

The victims of hanging often have protrusion of the tongue caused by the noose pushing the larynx upward, forcing the tongue out of the mouth. The tongue may be red, red-black, or black caused by drying (Dix et al. 2000). If the jugular veins were compressed for a period of time prior to compression of the carotid arteries, the face may appear congested. Petechiae may be found on the conjunctivae, periorbital regions, and gingiva. In most cases of hanging the compression of the neck occludes both the jugular and carotid vessels and petechiae are absent. The face is usually pale except for lividity (Dix et al. 2000). In hangings, the blood pools to the dependent portion of the body. The large amount of blood can overwhelm the vessels, causing them to rupture producing areas of pseudo hemorrhage called Tardieu spots.

One variation of hanging is the suspension of an animal upside down. Death can result if the animal is suspended for a sufficient period of time. The mechanism of death in upside down suspension is thought to be acute respiratory or cardiac failure or both. In humans, the length of time depends on the health of the victim, ranging from a few hours to a day or longer (Di Maio and Di Maio 2000). Expected injuries are related to the apparatus of suspension and its attachment to the body. Congestion of the head and petechiae on the face may be seen caused by postmortem lividity. There may be other injuries to the body if additional physical trauma was inflicted while the victim was suspended.

Drowning

Overview

Drowning is defined as death caused by submersion in a liquid, usually water. Submersion can be total or just enough to cover the mouth and nose. Although there are several physiological responses in the process of drowning, such as cardiac changes, the most important consequence is asphyxia.

Drowning of animals as a form of cruelty may be under-reported. These cases are not likely to be brought to the veterinarian for examination for a variety of reasons. There may be a witness to the abuse who is reluctant to come forward or the person who finds the animal tries to cover up the act and/or refuses to report the incident. In the study by Munro and Thrusfield, there were three reported cases of drowning or attempted drowning. It is interesting to note that two of the three cases happened inside the home (Munro and Thrusfield, 2001).

When an animal is submersed under water, there may be a period of panic and hyperventilation. The animal may attempt to hold its breath but the carbon dioxide concentrations build up in the bloodstream, which causes the animal to take an involuntary breath. This in turn causes aspiration of the water into the lungs, which may be small or large in volume. A large volume of water may be swallowed, which can be found in the stomach. This can cause the animal to vomit and possibly aspirate the gastric contents. Fresh water dilutes the surfactant, which causes collapse of the alveoli and reduced lung compliance. The hypertonicity of salt water actually draws water from the interstitial space into the alveoli, which increases alveolar filling known as secondary drowning (Hawkins 1995). The amount of water aspirated is more significant than the type of water (Dix et al. 2000). In humans, consciousness is lost within 3 minutes of submersion (Rohn and Frade 2006). Once consciousness is lost, water can enter the airways passively. After consciousness is lost, cerebral hypoxia continues until death occurs. In humans this happens usually within 10 minutes (Rohn and Frade 2006).

The term *dry drowning* has been used to describe victims of drowning, in which the lungs do not have the typical heavy, boggy, and edematous appearance seen in drowning lungs. The theory is that in some cases of drowning there is sudden laryngospasm through a vagal reflex when water enters the larynx or trachea. There may be the development of thick mucous, foam, and froth that forms a physical plug, preventing water aspiration. The animal still expires from cerebral hypoxia. The problem some human pathologists have with this theory is that the physical plug has not been seen and laryngospasm cannot be demonstrated after death because of the relaxation of the musculature. They believe instead that these lung findings are just one of a spectrum of the changes seen in drowning with the opposite end being wet drowning with the heavy, boggy lungs that contains massive amounts of edema fluid (Di Maio and Di Maio).

In near-drowning incidents the animal survives submersion in water. Depending on the circumstances, these also may be classified as *attempted drowning* or *inflicted submersion injury*. The injuries seen usually are caused by hypoxemia and the aspiration of the water. The water aspirated is usually small in quantity but enough to cause pulmonary damage. The amount of damage depends on several factors, including whether fresh or salt water, and the presence of debris, sand, or chemicals in the water. Any water purged by the animal should be saved for analysis. Aspiration pneumonia may result from the debris and chemicals in the water, or the aspiration of the animal's own vomit. The bacteria present in the water can cause secondary bacterial pneumonia. Hypoxemia injuries can include cerebral edema, herniation, and death. Adult respiratory distress syndrome can occur as a result of near-drowning, so all patients should be hospitalized and monitored for worsening symptoms (Hawkins 1995).

Effect of Submersion on Deceased Victims

Prolonged submersion in water causes the skin to wrinkle and this may be most evident on the animal's foot pads. When a body is placed in water, the remains are subject to several actions, depending on the type of and characteristics of the water. The temperature, depth of water, salinity, oxygenation, current, shores, bottoms, and life forms present within the water all affect what happens to the body (Haglund and Sorg 2002). The body may be subjected to abrasions or buried in sediment. The floating limbs are more subject to abrasions and disarticulation caused by their movement. The mandible may disarticulate before or after the limbs (Haglund and Sorg 2002). Aquatic and marine life may consume the internal viscera. Bones may be subject to modifications, such as encrustation by marine life and dissolution (see Chapter 3).

The body may initially float or sink, depending on the fat content and the density and viscosity of the water. In animals, the fur or feathers increases the body's buoyancy. The finding of heavy weights attached to the body may be indicative of body dumping or cruelty. The body may sink over time, and as decomposition progresses, the gaseous build-up within body cavities and interstitial spaces may overcome external water pressure, causing the body to resurface. If the body has sunk to sufficient depth, the decomposition gas will not cause the body to resurface (Haglund and Sorg 2002). In cold water, the decomposition is delayed; it may be months before the body resurfaces. When the body is floating, the exposed surface area is subject to insect infestation and bird scavenging. The submerged portion of the body is subject to water life scavenging.

The onset of rigor is variable, caused by antemortem struggling, which can deplete ATP (adenosine triphosphate) and water temperature. The pattern of lividity reflects the position of the body when it was submerged. Lividity may be pink in cold water drowning. Decomposition in the water is affected by a variety of factors, including the temperature, salinity, pH, and bacterial content of the water (Haglund and Sorg 2002). It is generally slower in water than on land. Decomposition also is slower in cold water than in warm. It is faster in bacteria-laden, stagnant water than in fresh, flowing water (Dix et al. 2000). Decomposition accelerates once the body is out of the water resulting from the proliferation of bacteria in the body. Because of this, a necropsy should be performed as soon as possible.

The formation of adipocere may occur in bodies that are submerged in cold water (see Chapter 14). Adipocere is a grayish-white to brown, firm, wax-like material found primarily in the subcutaneous tissue and other fatty deposit areas. Adipocere formation hinders decomposition and also may interfere with postmortem estimates (Haglund and Sorg 2002).

Gross Examination Findings

There are no pathognomonic necropsy findings to diagnose drowning. It is a diagnosis of exclusion based on the circumstances of death and nonspecific necropsy findings. In wet drowning, as opposed to the findings in dry drowning, there is white or hemorrhagic edema fluid in the nostrils, mouth, and airways. Compression of the chest can cause the fluid to flow out. This pulmonary edema fluid is nonspecific and can result from other causes. Foam may be found coming out of the nose or mouth and may be found in the trachea and deeper airways. This foam can continue to form when wiped away. It may be white, off-white, or blood tinged and is caused by admixing of moving air with water. This *foam cone* is the most suggestive indicator that a victim was alive when in the water (Dix et al. 2000). The absence of foam does not rule out drowning or that the victim was deceased when submerged. Studies of pediatric drowning in humans found that attempted resuscitation can decrease the incidence of frothy exudates. In addition, as the time interval between the drowning and autopsy increases, the incidence of frothy exudates decreases significantly. This increased time interval also decreases the incidence of pleural effusion findings (Somers et al. 2006).

The lungs are large and bulky, and may bulge from the open thoracic cavity caused by the presence of water and entrapped air. They are heavy because of pulmonary edema and the aspirated liquid within the lungs. On cut section, the lungs usually are brick-red in appearance and large quantities of edema fluid flow out (Di Maio and Di Maio 2001). The right ventricle may be dilated. The brain is swollen, with flattening of the gyri, but this is also nonspecific (Di Maio and Di Maio 2001). The presence of water, vomitus, sand/silt, or flora from the water in the mouth, airways, lungs, stomach, or sinuses are nonspecific because they can enter these areas passively when the body is submerged. However, if these findings are found in a body that was not in found water they are indicative that the body was submerged at some time. Samples of all water and debris found should be taken for testing. The water can also help identify the location of drowning (see Diatoms).

The body should be examined for evidence of antemortem injury and other contributing factors or causes of death. Radiographs should be taken of the entire body. If the body has been immersed in water for a prolonged period of time, the blood from the wounds can be leached out by the water. This can give the wound the appearance that it was postmortem versus antemortem.

Diatoms

Overview

Diatoms are microscopic unicellular algae with a uniquely extracellular coat composed of silica. There are over 10,000 morphologically distinct varieties of diatoms that range in size from 5 to greater than 500 μm. They are present in every naturally occurring body of water, from a puddle to the ocean. They may be found also in moist soil and the atmosphere. The type of diatoms found in a certain location is unique and specific to that area. The season also affects what type is found. The diatom populations have monthly fluctuations in their concentrations in a particular body of water (Pollanen 1998). In one body of water, several types of diatoms may be found, but all are located in a separate and specific area. These characteristics can help identify the location and even season of death. Because of the presence of diatoms in all types of water, the analysis for diatoms has been developed as a conclusive test for drowning.

Diatoms can enter the body in three different ways: through inhalation of airborne diatoms, ingestion of material containing diatoms, and aspiration of water containing diatoms. This last route is the foundation for forensic diatom testing, which in conjunction with other findings provides a diagnosis of drowning. When water enters the lungs, either through aspiration if the victim was alive or by postmortem submersion, diatoms may enter the lung tissue passively. They stay in the lungs and do not disseminate unless the heart is beating. When the diatoms perforate the alveolar-capillary barrier they enter the bloodstream and are disseminated to various organs, including the femoral bone marrow. The detection of diatoms in the bone marrow is then compared with the water that was aspirated into the airways or stomach, or from the site at which the body was recovered. A positive match indicates that drowning was the cause of death and the victim was breathing upon entry into the water (Pollanen 1998). A negative test may be seen with dry lung drowning, i.e., when there is no aspiration of water. However, a negative test does not rule out drowning.

The testing of soil for diatoms has been used also to determine cause of death or site of death in severely decomposed or skeletonized bodies found on land. If a body was submerged, presumably drowned, and then pulled from the water and then dumped on land or buried, the diatoms from the outside of the body and within the lungs are deposited in the soil underneath the body. Because diatoms may be found in moist soil, samples from underneath and adjacent to the body are tested and compared to soil samples further away but near the body. These samples also may be compared to water diatoms from nearby bodies of water to determine the site of submersion. A higher concentration of diatoms in the soil associated with the body than the surrounding soil is indicative that the victim died by drowning.

Diatom Testing

The acceptance of diatom testing has been questioned because of the ubiquitous nature of diatoms in the environment. The validity of this test is supported by the *criterion of concordance,* which demands that the diatoms recovered from tissue be comparable to the diatoms in the putative drowning medium (Pollanen 1998). The concentration of diatoms in bone marrow and other tissues is directly proportional to the concentration found in the drowning medium. Aquatic diatoms are diagnostically different that those living in other environments. Any contamination is detected by the investigator when comparison is made with the putative drowning medium. This removes the ambiguity of the origin of the diatoms and proves the diatoms were introduced during the drowning process. New testing modalities may further increase the sensitivity and reliability of the diatom test (Rohn and Frade 2006). A recent study using a quantitative diatom-based reconstruction technique was able to confirm drowning as the cause of death and the site of drowning (Horton et al. 2006).

The diatom test may be conducted on bone marrow or from other tissue in the body. It has been found that the sternum may be the best source for diatoms because the depositional interval for diatoms is shorter than for the femur (Rohn and Frade 2006). The testing of other tissue may provide additional confirmation to bone marrow findings; however, caution must be used when testing other tissues to prevent contamination. The body must not be decomposed and the chest cavity must not have been damaged while submerged.

When collecting and preparing samples for diatom testing, certain precautions should be taken to prevent contamination from other water supplies. This includes changing gloves when touching or handling a single area and limiting contact of samples to only triple-distilled water (Di Maio and Di Maio 2001). A sample of the drowning medium should be collected from the scene at the site where the body was recovered for comparison testing. Approximately 500–1000 ml should be collected in a clean container. Additional samples should be taken of the water in the stomach, sinus, or airways. All water samples should be kept separate from the body and stored in separate containers to prevent contamination. Water samples should be refrigerated to prevent microbe growth. The tissue test for diatoms is conducted on the femoral bone marrow. Tests may be performed also on other tissue from closed organ systems such as an encapsulated kidney from a non-decomposed body.

The body and leg should be cleaned prior to the removal of the femur to prevent contamination with exogenous diatoms. Before removing the bone from the body, it is important to change gloves to prevent contamination of the surface of the bone. The femur should be washed in distilled water. The femur should be placed in a sealed plastic bag and frozen prior to submission to the laboratory for testing (Pollanen 1998).

Strontium Testing

Strontium is a trace metal found in the crust of the earth and is widely present in sea water. It is found in smaller quantities in fresh and domestic water. Blood strontium quantification has been used as a supportive test for the diagnosis of drowning and can be performed at most medical laboratories. The foundation for the use of this test is that strontium has a naturally low level in plasma. Elevated levels in the blood are supportive of drowning. The water content of strontium affects blood levels, with salt water containing higher levels than fresh water. Decomposition in the water also reduces the detectable blood levels of strontium (Pollanen 1998).

References

Di Maio, V.J., and D. Di Maio. 2001. *Forensic Pathology,* 2nd ed. Boca Raton, FL: CRC Press.

Dix, J., M. Graham, and R. Hanzlick. 2000. *Asphyxia and Drowning: An Atlas*. Boca Raton, FL: CRC Press.

Haglund, W.D., and M.H. Sorg. 2002. Human Remains in Water Environments. In *Advances in Forensic Taphonomy*, ed. W.D. Haglund, and M.H. Sorg, pp. 201–218. Boca Raton, FL: CRC Press.

Hawkins, E.C. 1995. Diseases of the Lower Respiratory System. In *Textbook of Veterinary Internal Medicine: Diseases of the Dog and Cat*, vol. 1, 4th ed., ed. S.J. Ettinger, and E.C. Feldman, pp. 767–811. Philadelphia: W.B. Saunders.

Horton, B.P., S. Breham, and C. Hillier. 2006. The Development and Application of a Diatom-Based Quantitative Reconstruction Technique in Forensic Science. *The American Journal of Forensic Medicine and Pathology* 51(3):643–650.

Munro, H.M., and M.V. Thrusfield. 2001. 'Battered Pets': Non-accidental Physical Injuries Found in Dogs and Cats. *Journal of Small Animal Practice* 42:279–290.

Pollanen, M.S. 1998. *Forensic Diatomology and Drowning*. Amsterdam: Elsevier Science.

Rohn, E.J., and P.D. Frade. 2006. The Role of Diatoms in Medicolegal Investigations I: The History, Contemporary Science, and Application of the Diatom Test for Drowning. *The Forensic Examiner* 15(3):11–15.

Somers, G.R., D.A. Chiasson, and C.R. Smith. 2006. Pediatric Drowning: A 20-Year Review of Autopsied Cases: II. Pathologic Features. *The American Journal of Forensic Medicine and Pathology* 27(1):20–24.

Venker-van Haagen, A.J. 1995. Diseases of the Throat. In *Textbook of Veterinary Internal Medicine: Diseases of the Dog and Cat,* vol. 1, 4th ed., ed. S.J. Ettinger, and E.C. Feldman, pp. 567–575. Philadelphia: W.B. Saunders.

Chapter 10
Patterns of Non-accidental Injury: Poisoning

Sharon M. Gwaltney-Brant

Overview of Intentional Poisonings

Incidence

For a variety of reasons the actual incidence of intentional animal poisonings cannot be accurately determined. Perhaps most importantly, many intentional poisonings are never actually witnessed by animal owners, which may result in a poisoning case being mistaken for an infectious, metabolic, or other condition. It may be mistakenly assumed that an intentional poisoning has occurred when animals are accidentally exposed to toxic agents in their environment. Many toxicoses manifest as non-specific signs (e.g. vomiting and depression) that can make the diagnosis of an unwitnessed poisoning challenging. Additionally, a nationwide means of reporting animal poisonings does not exist. Animal and (some) human poison control centers do maintain databases on the animal poisoning cases they receive, but there is no central reporting agency to which animal poisonings can be compiled that accurate accounting of intentional poisonings can be made. In most cases, animal poisonings reported to poison control centers are done so for real-time treatment recommendations, so if an animal has died there is little incentive to report to a poison control center. Even if a central reporting center did exist, animal owners or veterinarians might be reluctant to report suspected intentional poisonings because of lack of sufficient evidence or, in the case of veterinarians, time.

Intentional poisonings include abuse or misuse of products and malicious intent. Abuse may include intentional intoxication of an animal as a "joke" (e.g. intentionally blowing marijuana smoke into a pet's face), whereas in cases of misuse of an agent, the actual intent generally was not to cause harm to the animal (e.g. giving acetaminophen to an ill cat). Malicious poisonings may be aimed at destroying animals that the poisoner considers pests, occasionally with unfortunate consequences for non-target animals that also may be exposed, or the poisoning may be done in retaliation against the animal or its owners. Rarely, malicious poisoning is done strictly for the sadistic pleasure it brings the poisoner.

Because of these limitations, one can assume that the incidence of intentional animal poisonings reported to poison control centers (animal and human) very likely greatly underestimates the actual incidence. In spite of this, poison control data can show some trends that may be of interest in evaluating intentional animal poisonings. Based on information from human and animal poison control centers, intentional exposures comprise less than 1 percent of all exposures of animals to potentially toxic agents, and malicious poisonings account for less than 0.5 percent of all poisonings reported (Hansen et al. 2001). Of intentional exposures, abuse/misuse of agents accounts for approximately one-half of feline exposures, with the majority of these being off-label use of dog flea control products on cats (ASPCA 2006). Malicious exposures in cats account for approximately one-third of intentional exposures, whereas in dogs over one-half of intentional exposures to potentially toxic agents are reported as malicious in nature (Hornfeldt 1997; ASPCA 2006).

Demographics

Although intentional poisonings can occur in any species, such poisonings are most commonly reported in dogs and cats. Dogs account for more than 75 percent of malicious poisoning cases; cats account for approximately 15 percent; and other species, including wildlife, comprise the remainder of reported malicious poisonings. Of the malicious canine poisonings reported to the ASPCA Animal Poison Control Center between 2002 and 2005 (ASPCA 2006), 22 percent involved either Labrador retrievers or German shepherds (Table 10.1). German shepherds and their mixes appear to be over-represented in malicious poisonings, as they account for just 4.2 percent of all toxicoses (Gwaltney-Brant 2006), although they were involved in 11 percent of malicious poisonings. Conversely, pure- and mixed-breed Labrador retrievers appear to be under-represented in malicious intent (11 percent) compared with overall poisonings (17.6 percent) and their relative popularity (15.0 percent). These trends are similar to those found in an earlier study of malicious poisonings in dogs during 1999 and 2000, with the exception that in the previous study Rottweilers and their mixes accounted for 6 percent of malicious poisonings compared with 3 percent in the more recent study (Hansen et al. 2001). No specific breed trends have been reported in feline malicious poisonings.

Table 10.1. Top ten dog breeds involved in malicious poisonings (ASPCA 2006).

Breed	Percent
German shepherd	11%
Labrador retriever	11%
Mixed breed, Unspecified	8%
Chihuahua	6%
American pit bull terrier	5%
Great Dane	5%
Golden retriever	3%
Great Pyrenees	3%
Jack Russell/Parson Russell	3%
Rottweiler	3%

Index of Suspicion

In the majority of poisoning cases, whether intentional or accidental, it is usually the acute onset of significant clinical signs that appear to have no obvious cause that triggers suspicion of poisoning. Less commonly, insidious illness resulting from chronic exposure to a toxicant may occur. In all cases, it is important to consider all potential differentials before settling on a diagnosis of poisoning and, lacking direct evidence of exposure to a potential toxicant, poisoning should be considered a diagnosis of exclusion.

Evidence and History

Occasionally, an animal owner may witness the exposure of the pet to a potential toxicant, may find evidence of the toxicant on the animal's coat or fur, or the animal may quickly vomit up the agent, making it evident that an ingestion has occurred. More frequently, animal poisonings are not witnessed, and diagnosis of poisoning relies on other observations.

Historical information is essential to determine as much as possible the events leading up to the poisoning of the patient. Whether the animal was indoors or outdoors prior to development of clinical signs, the number and status of other animals in the same environment, the rapidity of onset and progression of clinical signs, and the presence of children or adolescents in the environment all are factors that may provide clues to the source and intent of a poisoning.

The patient's prior health history, including any current medications, should be obtained to determine if any pre-existing conditions are present that may alter the patient's response to therapy or exacerbate signs of toxicosis.

Clinical Findings

There are few toxicants that produce definitively diagnostic clinical signs, although in many cases the clinical signs provide valuable clues as to the potential agent involved. As with any emergent patient, the potential poisoning patient should be examined thoroughly, and abnormalities in vital signs and cardiovascular, hematological, neurological, musculoskeletal, and gastrointestinal (GI) function should be noted in detail. Examination of skin, eyes, and oral mucosa for ulceration or inflammation should be performed. Blood should be drawn for baseline clinical chemistry and hematological analysis; at this time, evaluation for defects in hemostasis may be performed. Ancillary clinical procedures that may aid in narrowing down the potential agent involved in a poisoning include radiography, ultrasonography, and endoscopy.

Olfactory clues to poisonings include the garlicky odor associated with toxicants such as arsenic, thallium, and zinc phosphide or the bitter almond odor of cyanide. Many pesticides, especially insecticides, have a hydrocarbon odor. Bleaches, alcohols, and ammonia-based products leave their distinctive odors on the coat or breath of the animal.

Animals found dead should be examined externally for evidence of antemortem clinical signs. Vomit or diarrhea staining of the hair coat indicates antemortem GI dysfunction, whereas rapid onset of rigor mortis can be suggestive of antemortem seizures or hyperthermia. Samples of residues on the hair coat should be taken, and any vomitus or diarrhea should be collected, carefully labeled and sealed, and saved for future analysis. Once external examination and sample collection is complete, a necropsy should be performed.

Environmental and Physical Evidence

Evaluation of the environment in which the animal lives may aid in detecting potential sources of poisonings. This is especially important when malicious poisoning is suspected, as potential sources of accidental poisoning need to be identified and eliminated to add weight to the case for intentional poisoning. Indoor environments should be evaluated for potential exposure to items such as plants, pharmaceuticals, illicit drugs, cleaning and other household products, lead-containing items, pesticides, and potentially toxic foods. Outdoor habitats should be similarly evaluated for the above-mentioned items as well as mushrooms, lawn care and pool products, poisonous and venomous animals, water-borne toxicants (e.g. blue-green algae), compost piles, mulches, automotive materials, and garbage containers.

Environmental clues to intentional poisonings might include the unexpected presence of scattered food products, product containers, or granular or pelleted materials in the animal's habitat. Open gates or doors to areas where potential toxicants are stored may indicate the recent presence of an uninvited person to the animal's environment.

Diagnostics

Investigation of intentional animal poisonings requires close attention to detail in evaluation of history and clinical findings, accurate and appropriate sample collection, maintenance of chain of custody of evidence, and judicious use of analytical testing. The veterinarian's role in evaluating a suspected malicious poisoning encompasses all of these requirements, as well as appropriate contact with the necessary public authorities (animal control and/or law enforcement) to ensure that adequate evidence is collected to provide for successful prosecution should the perpetrator be found.

Necropsy Considerations

Forensic necropsy of suspected malicious poisoning victims ideally should be performed by a board-certified pathologist at a veterinary diagnostic laboratory; this is especially important if the case is expected to be pursued by the legal system. Although most veterinary practitioners have been trained to perform a basic necropsy, cases of malicious poisoning may have few or subtle lesions that may be overlooked. Additionally, forensic necropsies require detailed record keeping so that accurate testimony can be given, often years after the necropsy was performed.

If referral of a body to a diagnostic laboratory is not possible, the veterinary practitioner should perform a thorough and complete necropsy, maintaining numerous records. A tape recorder may be used to dictate findings, which later can be transcribed into a written report. Initial examination should include photographs of the body and any external abnormalities. Foreign material on the hair coat or in the oral cavity should be swabbed and saved for possible future analysis.

Once the external examination is complete, a thorough examination of internal organs should be performed. It is important that the prosector not jump to conclusions or make assumptions during the necropsy. Each organ system should be examined thoroughly and samples collected methodically. Epidermis and subcutaneous tissues around any identified injection sites should be excised and saved. For exclusionary purposes, samples may be submitted for non-toxicology–related tests (e.g. microbiology) based on lesions found at necropsy. Stomach contents should be examined closely for evidence of foreign objects, such as granules and pellets, plant material, foods, pill casings, tablet fragments, or illicit drugs. Samples of all major organs should be taken and preserved in fixative for histopathological examination; for large organs, such as liver, sections should be taken from multiple areas rather than a single site.

Toxicology Testing

Sample Collection and Submission

When investigating potential malicious poisonings, sample collection is essential for confirmatory tests to be performed. When collecting samples, it is always best to err on the side of taking too many samples, because one can always throw away unneeded samples but it is not possible to resurrect material that has been discarded. Live animal samples include stomach contents from lavage and/or vomitus, urine, feces, whole blood, serum or plasma, and hair. The patient's oral cavity should be inspected for agents lodged in the teeth or trapped in mucosal folds; these items should be collected and saved for future analysis. Because some analytes may be damaged by contact with red blood cells, it is best to collect both whole blood and serum or plasma. In general, glass containers are preferred over plastic because plastic can leach contaminants into samples over time. If plastic containers must be used, harder plastics pose less risk of sample contamination. Never store samples in syringes, as leakage may occur and syringes with needles are hazardous to receiving personnel. Serum and plasma may be frozen prior to shipping, whereas whole blood should be refrigerated, never frozen. Urine may be either refrigerated or frozen. Vomitus, gastric contents, and feces should be stored in glass or hard plastic and may be frozen prior to shipping. Hair samples are most useful for topical exposures and they may be stored in hard plastic or glass vials.

For necropsy specimens, samples of liver, kidney, urine, stomach/intestinal contents, and feces should be saved for toxicological analysis. If exposure to anticholinesterase agents (organophosphates or carbamates) is suspected, samples of brain and retina (submit entire eyeball) may be evaluated for cholinesterase activity.

It is important to remember that there is no single toxicology screen that can detect all known toxic agents, and testing at random can prove to be expensive and futile. Determining which toxicant to look for in a chemical analysis is based on the clinical, historical, and environmental findings in the case, which will hopefully provide the clinician with a list of potential rule outs to consider. In a 2003 outbreak of suspected malicious poisonings of dogs in a public park in Portland, Oregon, the clinical signs shown by the affected dogs (oral ulcerations, GI signs, progressive respiratory distress) allowed veterinarians to suspect paraquat and request the appropriate analysis; paraquat poisoning was confirmed in several of the dogs (Cope 2004). Some laboratories offer specific screening tests based on clinical findings. For instance, Michigan State University's diagnostic laboratory (see Appendix 25) offers a convulsant screen that analyzes for toxicants frequently associated with seizures or convulsions, including bromethalin, metaldehyde, organophosphate insecticides, carbamates, strychnine, and tremorgenic mycotoxins. In general, however, one needs to have an idea of what toxicant is suspected to request the appropriate analysis.

An important aspect in the interpretation of toxicology results is to realize that exposure to a potential toxicant does not necessarily indicate that a toxicosis has occurred. With all toxic agents, a threshold below which signs will not develop exists (i.e. "The dose makes the poison"). This is especially important to remember as our ability to analyze and detect agents in samples improves, and our ability to measure the presence of agents at minute levels means we will at times detect the presence of agents at levels consistent with casual exposure but not toxicosis. Close attention should be paid to the normal background levels indicated by the testing laboratory that accurate interpretation of analytical results occurs.

Finally, once a diagnosis of toxicosis has been confirmed through evaluation of clinical findings and laboratory results, the determination of malicious intent still can be difficult to establish. This is especially true in cases of malicious animal poisonings, as the victims cannot testify that they saw the perpetrator expose them to the poison. Ancillary trace evidence should be collected and retained, including any potentially poisoned foods materials (e.g. cans of tuna or pet food mixed with rodenticides or ethylene glycol) along with their containers. The food materials can be analyzed for the presence of the toxic agent, and fingerprints or trace evidence on the containers may provide sufficient evidence that the suspected perpetrator was in possession of the tainted material at some time.

Chain of Custody

Maintaining chain of custody of collected evidence entails complete documentation of sample collection (date/time of collection, condition of sample, type of storage), witnesses to sample collection, and the name of parties responsible for sample during collection, storage, and transit (Galey 1995). Courier services with tracking capabilities should be used when transporting samples to maintain chain of custody (see Chapter 3).

Human Laboratories

Human hospital laboratories may be of assistance in determining exposure to agents commonly associated with toxicosis in humans. The current bench-top test for ethylene glycol in dogs is not sensitive enough for cats, as cats can develop ethylene glycol toxicosis at levels below the 50 mg/dl limit of that test. Human hospitals use a quantitative test that gives the actual serum level; therefore, human labs are a good resource to use when faced with potential ethylene glycol exposure in a cat. Other tests that can be performed by human hospitals include serum iron levels, total iron binding capacity, acetaminophen levels, and salicylate levels. Additionally, most hospitals use ToxiLab as a quick screening test for a variety of commonly abused human drugs, including opioids, marijuana, amphetamines, barbiturates, antidepressants, and cocaine. These tests also may be of benefit in determining exposure of animals to these agents, with the caveat that most of these tests have not been validated in species other than humans.

Over-the-Counter Testing Kits

Recently, over-the-counter home testing kits for a variety of illicit drugs (opioids, marijuana, amphetamines, barbiturates, cocaine, and benzodiazepines) have become readily available in many pharmacies. These kits are easy to use, affordable and, anecdotally, have been used with varying success in diagnosing cases of canine poisonings with these agents.

Agents Used in Animal Poisonings

Introduction

There are virtually an unlimited number of agents that might potentially be used to maliciously poison animals, making diagnosis of malicious poisonings challenging. However, in spite of the wide variety of agents available, most poisoners tend to use a narrow range of agents. An informal survey by the author of toxicologists at veterinary diagnostic laboratories across the country indicated that the primary poisons of choice in intentional poisonings are anticoagulant rodenticides and ethylene glycol. Other commonly reported poisons involved in malicious poisonings included organophosphate insecticides, carbamates, strychnine (particularly in the northwestern United States), caffeine, and methylxanthines.

Ethylene Glycol

Sources

Ethylene glycol (EG) is most commonly found in automotive antifreezes and windshield de-icers, but it is also present in brake fluids, inks, and some paints. Automotive antifreeze is 95 percent EG, although it is usually diluted to 50 percent in automobile radiators. EG is inexpensive, easily obtained, and palatable. It can be mixed readily with other foods to entice target animals to ingest it and is fairly well known for its toxicity to animals, all of which may contribute to the fact that it is often used in malicious poisonings.

Cats are very sensitive to EG; less than a tablespoon of undiluted EG is fatal to most cats. Dogs are about four times less susceptible than cats to EG.

Mechanism of Action

The toxicity of EG is primarily caused by its conversion to highly toxic metabolites (Thrall et al. 2006). Parent EG is an alcohol, which accounts for the initial inebriation that develops. As EG is converted to acidic metabolites, severe metabolic acidosis ensues. The metabolite oxalic acid binds with serum calcium to form calcium oxalate crystals, which collect in the renal tubules. The renal damage likely results from a combination of metabolic derangement of the tubular epithelium caused by the toxic metabolites as well as mechanical injury caused by the presence of calcium oxalate crystals in the kidney.

Clinical Signs and Clinical Laboratory Findings

EG toxicosis is characterized by three stages: inebriation, acidosis, and renal failure. The inebriation stage occurs within 30 minutes of exposure and may persist up to 12 hours. The primary signs are central nervous system (CNS) depression, ataxia, disorientation, tremors, muscle fasciculations, hypothermia, polyuria, and GI irritation. In dogs ingesting lower dosages of EG, signs may subside and apparent recovery may occur, whereas cats tend to remain markedly depressed. Acidosis develops within 12 to 24 hours after exposure and is characterized by deepening CNS depression, tachypnea, tachycardia, pulmonary edema, metabolic acidosis, high anion gap, and high osmolal gap. Hypocalcemia occurs in approximately one-half of EG intoxicated patients, although hypocalcemic tetany is uncommon. Calcium oxalate crystalluria can be seen as early as 3 hours postexposure in cats and 6 hours in dogs, but the absence of crystalluria does not rule out an ethylene glycol toxicosis. Elevations in blood urea nitrogen (BUN) and serum creatinine may occur as early as 12 hours in cats and 24 hours in dogs. Oliguric or anuric renal failure subsequently develops, accompanied by vomiting, depression, anorexia, renal pain, oral ulceration, and seizures.

Diagnostics

Diagnosis of ethylene glycol toxicosis can be challenging, as the signs of toxicosis vary depending on the stage in which the patient is presented. Early stages of inebriation can resemble intoxication by alcohol or marijuana. Because many automotive antifreezes contain fluorescent dye, examination of a suspected EG victim's fur, paws, face, mouth, vomitus, and urine with a Wood's lamp may reveal fluorescence, indicating exposure. Fluorescence may be detectable in urine up to 6 hours after ingestion, but the absence of fluorescence does not rule out the possibility of EG exposure.

An on-site ethylene glycol test kit (PRN Pharmacal, Pensacola, FL) is available to test for EG in dogs; the test measures blood levels of EG $>$50 mg/dl and is not sensitive enough for cats. False-positives may occur if the animal has been exposed to metaldehyde, glycerol, formaldehyde, or propylene glycol (which is present in some injectable medications and some commercially available activated charcoal formulations). False-positives do not occur after exposure to ethanol or methanol. The test is most accurate when performed at least 1 hour after suspected EG ingestion.

A newer immunohistochemical-based test, the Kacey test, recently has been introduced on the market for testing EG exposures in dogs and cats. The original version of this test measured blood levels of EG at 2 and 5 mg/dl and was too sensitive to be of practical use; many dogs with minor exposures who would have tested negative with the PRN test would have been positive with this test. Recent modification to the test results in the ability of this test to measure blood levels of EG at 20, 50, and 75 mg/dl. The 20 mg/dl is designed for cats because of their increased sensitivity. It is not yet known if this is sufficiently sensitive to trust a negative result, but a positive result in a cat warrants treatment. The 50 mg/dl is for testing dogs, and the results should be comparable to the PRN test. The 75 mg/dl level is superfluous, as treatment for dogs and cats should be started at lower levels. Unlike the PRN test, this test *does* give false-positives with ethanol and methanol; it is not known if the other agents that give false-positives (metaldehyde, propylene glycol, etc.) with the PRN test will do so with the Kacey test. The advantages to this test are its ability to measure lower levels of EG, making it useful for cats, and its speed and ease of use when compared with the PRN test. Disadvantages include false-positives with ethanol and methanol (common ingestions in dogs) and the fact that the test has not yet been fully validated.

Other confirmatory laboratory changes associated with EG exposure include increased osmolality with high osmolal gap, high anion gap, elevated BUN, elevated creatinine, and hyperglycemia. Hyperkalemia, hypocalcemia, hyperphosphatemia, and isosthenuria or hyposthenuria are present variably. Calcium oxalate crystalluria is strongly suggestive of exposure, but absence of crystalluria does not rule out EG intoxication.

Ultrasonography of kidneys in later stages of EG toxicosis may reveal a *halo* sign, with areas of higher echogenicity within the cortical and medullary regions surrounding an area of lower echogenicity at the corticomedullary junction and central cortical areas. The halo sign is most often associated with the onset of anuria (Thrall et al. 2006).

Trace mineral analysis of kidneys generally reveals renal calcium concentrations greater than 8,000 ppm and a calcium:phosphorus ratio of greater than 2.5 (Rumbeiha 2006).

Lesions

Gross lesions of EG toxicosis may be absent in animals that die of acidosis or hypothermia prior to the onset of renal injury. Animals dying of renal failure may have pale, soft, swollen kidneys that can be gritty on cutting. Other potential lesions in animals dying of renal failure include uremia-associated oral and gastric ulceration, mineralization of gastric mucosa (gritty on cutting), and ulcerative colitis (especially in cats). In uremic animals surviving several days, mineralization of the endocardium, lungs, and intercostal muscles may be evident as white, gritty plaques (Maxie 1985). Histopathological lesions in the kidney reveal the presence of birefringent crystals within the renal tubules associated with renal tubular degeneration and necrosis. Mineralization of the tubular basement membrane often is present. In cases that survive more than a few days, evidence of tubular regeneration may be evident. Calcium oxalate crystals may be found in other areas occasionally, including the liver and meninges. Evidence of metastatic mineralization may be found in the gastric mucosa, media of arteries and arterioles, pulmonary interstitium, epicardium, myocardium, and meninges.

Differential diagnoses for ethylene glycol are many and vary with the stage at presentation of the animal. The initial inebriation seen in EG toxicosis is similar to that seen with ingestion of other alcohols or glycols (e.g. methanol, propylene glycol) as well as marijuana and some medications affecting CNS function (e.g. baclofen). Other alcohols can produce acidosis, high serum osmolality and ethanol may cause transient hypocalcemia (Thrall et al. 2006). Differential diagnoses for acute renal failure include non-steroidal anti-inflammatory drug (NSAID) toxicosis, aminoglycoside ingestion, grape/raisin ingestion, *Lilium* or *Hemerocallis* ingestion (cats), and ingestion of vitamin D or its analogues (e.g. calcipotriene). Non-toxicologic rule outs to consider for renal failure include leptospirosis, borreliosis, hemolytic uremic syndrome hemoglobin/myoglobin nephropathy, renal dysplasia, and acute decompensation of chronic renal failure.

Anticoagulant Rodenticides

Sources

Anticoagulant rodenticides include a large number of different compounds, including warfarin, pindone, brodifacoum, bromadiolone, chlorphacinone, difethiolone, and diphacinone. First-generation anticoagulants include warfarin and pindone, whereas second-generation anticoagulants encompass most of the other agents. Second-generation anticoagulants were developed to poison warfarin-resistant rats and mice. Anticoagulant rodenticides are available as grain-based pellets, paraffin-based blocks, meal baits, tracking powders, grains, and dusts (Murphy and Talcott 2006). Rodenticides are not color coded, so identification of a particular rodenticide can be difficult if the packaging is not available.

Mechanism of Action

Anticoagulants are vitamin K antagonists as they inhibit the recycling of vitamin K epoxide hydroxylase, thereby inhibiting the recycling of vitamin K in the body. This ultimately results in decreased synthesis of vitamin K–dependent clotting factors II, VII, IX, and X. As these factors become depleted, a process that usually takes 3–5 days to become clinically evident, evidence of coagulopathy develops.

Clinical Signs and Clinical Laboratory Findings

The clinical signs seen with anticoagulant rodenticide toxicosis depend on the site of hemorrhage. Frank hemorrhage may occur from the oral cavity, nose, rectum, vulva, or prepuce, or from minor skin lesions that fail to stop bleeding. Internal hemorrhage into the lungs, mediastinum, thymus, or trachea may present as acute dyspnea, whereas hemorrhage into muscle or subcutis may present with large hematomas. Lameness may occur because of bleeding into joint cavities and neurological signs may develop if bleeding into the brain or spinal cord occurs. Hemorrhage into the abdomen may manifest as weakness, lethargy, anorexia, and pallor. Failure of blood to clot may be noted upon venipuncture for blood collection.

Laboratory abnormalities may include decreases in hematocrit and plasma protein levels secondary to hemorrhage as well as elevations in coagulation parameters. Prothrombin times tend to elevate first in all animals except horses, in which partial thromboplastin time (PTT) can elevate first within 24 hours of exposure to anticoagulants (McConnico et al. 1997).

Diagnostics

Elevations in coagulation parameters with associated hemorrhage are highly suspicious for exposure to anticoagulant rodenticides, especially in otherwise healthy animals. Reduction in coagulation parameters in response to vitamin K1 therapy within 12–24 hours of initiation of treatment is supportive of anticoagulant rodenticide toxicosis. Pre-existing liver disease may be a non-toxic cause of coagulopathy; therefore, a complete serum chemical profile should be obtained. These coagulopathies tend to be poorly responsive to vitamin K1.

Anticoagulant rodenticides can be detected in plasma, serum, liver, and other tissues. Many veterinary diagnostic laboratories perform a rodenticide screen to detect the major rodenticides, including all of the anticoagulants. Because of the varying half-life of anticoagulant rodenticides and the fact that the initial dose ingested is rarely known in an intentional poisoning, the concentrations of anticoagulant found in the liver or serum often do not correlate well with the severity of the clinical syndrome seen. However, detection of anticoagulant in tissues of an animal with a coagulopathy is highly supportive of anticoagulant toxicosis.

Lesions

Lesions are related to hemorrhage either externally or into a variety of bodily sites, including meninges, thymus, larynx, renal or perirenal, thoracic cavity, abdominal cavity, liver, pericardial sac, GI tract, nasal cavity, joints, muscles, and mediastinum. On necropsy, blood clots poorly, and usually there is a generalized pallor to tissues.

Differential diagnoses for anticoagulant rodenticide toxicosis include coagulopathies secondary to disseminated intravascular coagulopathy, congenital clotting factor deficiencies, von Willebrand's disease, paraneoplastic syndromes, liver disease, platelet defects, and infectious disease (e.g. ehrlichiosis).

Bromethalin

Sources

Bromethalin is a neurotoxic rodenticide that is occasionally mistaken for an anticoagulant because of similarity of its name with the anticoagulants bromadiolone and brodifacoum. Bromethalin is formulated in pellets or block forms for residential use and 2 to 10 percent solutions are available for use by licensed pest control operators (Dorman 2006).

Mechanism of Action

Bromethalin requires activation to desmethyl bromethalin to exert its toxic effect. Interestingly, as guinea pigs are deficient at desmethylation, they are highly resistant to the effects of bromethalin (Dunayer 2003). Desmethyl bromethalin is thought to uncouple oxidative phosphorylation in the CNS, resulting in decreased adenosine triphosphatase (ATP) production and failure of ATP-dependent ion pumps. Dissociation of fluid into myelinated areas of the brain and spinal cord results in edema of myelin sheaths and interference with nerve conduction. Some of the adverse effects of bromethalin within the CNS may also result from lipid peroxidation of cerebral membranes (Dorman 2006).

Clinical Signs and Clinical Laboratory Findings

Clinical signs associated with bromethalin are dose dependent in onset and severity. Very large ingestions result in onset of severe CNS signs within 24 hours of exposure characterized by muscle tremors, hyperexcitability, hyperesthesia, hyperthermia, and focal motor or generalized seizures. Death generally occurs within 24–36 hours after ingestion. Ingestion of lower doses results in a syndrome characterized by delayed onset (3–6 days) of neurological signs, including hind limb ataxia, paresis or paralysis, and depression. Cats may show abdominal distention secondary to enlarged bowel loops. Other potential signs include behavior changes, nystagmus, abnormal posturing, opisthotonos, muscle tremors, vomiting, and anorexia. Signs may progress over a 1- to 2-week period to end in death, or signs may stabilize with gradual improvement possible over days to weeks.

Clinical laboratory findings with bromethalin toxicosis are expected to be unremarkable. Alterations in electrolyte status secondary to dehydration and anorexia are possible.

Diagnostics

There is no specific antemortem test to confirm bromethalin exposure, so diagnosis is based on history and clinical findings. Postmortem evaluation of fat, liver, kidney, and brain can detect the presence of bromethalin.

Differential diagnoses for bromethalin toxicosis include head trauma, neoplasia, cerebral vascular disorders, infectious encephalitides (including rabies), and other toxic agents such as antifreeze, metaldehyde, zinc phosphide, and psychotropic drug ingestion.

Lesions

Gross necropsy findings usually are unremarkable. Histopathological evaluation of animals dying from bromethalin toxicosis reveals extensive vacuolation of the white matter within the CNS. The presence of typical lesions along with analytical evidence of bromethalin within tissues is confirmatory for bromethalin toxicosis.

Cholecalciferol Rodenticides

Sources

Cholecalciferol rodenticides, such as anticoagulant rodenticides and bromethalin, come in a variety of formulations and colors, making identification of unpackaged baits often impossible. Most cholecalciferol baits contain 0.075 percent of the active ingredient, which equates to 23.4 mg of cholecalciferol per ounce of bait.

Mechanism of Action

Cholecalciferol enhances absorption of phosphorus and calcium from the GI tract and distal tubules of the kidney and enhances the mobilization of calcium from bone. The end result is increased serum calcium and phosphorus levels, which can persist up to several weeks after exposure (Rumbeiha 2006). Sustained elevations in serum calcium and phosphorus result in soft-tissue mineralization, most notably within the kidney, but the CNS, myocardium, GI tract, and lung also may have extensive mineralization. Most animals that die from cholecalciferol die because of renal failure; however, death secondary to cardiac arrhythmia, seizure, or pulmonary hemorrhage is possible.

Clinical Signs and Clinical Laboratory Findings

Initial signs of toxicosis generally develop about 36–48 hours after ingestion and are characterized by depression, weakness, and anorexia. Vomiting, constipation, polyuria, polydipsia, and dehydration occur as renal injury develops. GI ulceration caused by uremia and gastric mucosal metastatic mineralization is possible and the presence of hematemesis is considered a grave prognostic indicator (Rumbeiha 2006).

Serum phosphorus tends to rise early within the first 12 hours of exposure, with serum calcium levels rapidly following suit. Elevations in BUN and serum creatinine occur as renal failure develops. Urine specific gravity is usually low (1.002 to 1.006), and calciuria may be noted early in toxicosis.

Diagnostics

Live animal testing may include serum intact parathyroid hormone, which is expected to be depressed in cholecalciferol toxicosis. Ionized calcium 25-hydroxycalciferol ($23(OH)D_3$) levels in serum are elevated over 15 times normal in cholecalciferol toxicosis.

In the dead animal, bile and kidney can have $25(OH)D_3$ levels measured. Alternatively, trace mineral analysis of the kidney may reveal renal calcium levels at 2,000 to 3,000 ppm with a calcium:phosphorus ratio of 0.4 to 0.7, which is strongly suggestive of cholecalciferol toxicosis (Rumbeiha 2006).

Differential diagnoses for cholecalciferol intoxication include ingestion of other vitamin D3 analogues (calcipotriene, calcitriol), paraneoplastic hypercalcemia syndromes (especially lymphoma and anal sac apocrine gland adenocarcinoma), acute or chronic renal failure, hypercalcemia of granulomatous diseases, and hyperadrenocorticism.

Lesions

Gross lesions in animals dying from cholecalciferol may be minimal, but may include gastric ulceration, oral uremic ulcers, and mineralization (gritty on cutting) in the kidney, lung, and heart. Histological examination confirms mineralization of multiple organs, but these lesions also are seen in other conditions, such as uremia and hypercalcemia of malignancy.

Strychnine

Sources

Strychnine is available for use as a rodenticide, and is frequently used to poison coyotes, particularly in the northwestern United States. Most baits are 0.5 percent to 1 percent strychnine sulfate and the baits are frequently formulated as red- or green-colored grains such as wheat, milo, corn, and oats.

Mechanism of Action

Strychnine exerts its toxic effect by inhibiting the release of the inhibitory neurotransmitter glycine from the Renshaw cells on the anterior horn of the spinal cord. Inhibition of inhibitory nerve transmission results in uncontrolled neuronal activity, producing exaggerated reflexes and marked muscle spasms. Extensor muscles are more severely affected, resulting in hyperextension that can progress to tetanic convulsions.

Clinical Signs and Clinical Laboratory Findings

Onset and severity of clinical signs are dose dependent, with severe signs developing within 10 minutes after large ingestions (Talcott 2006). Lower levels of exposure may result in delayed onset of mild ataxia and muscle stiffness within 2 hours of exposure. Initial signs may include anxiety, apprehension, tachypnea, and hypersalivation followed by ataxia, muscle spasms, and stiffness. Muscular signs generally begin in the face and progress to the neck and limb muscles. Violent generalized tonic-extensor convulsions may follow, accompanied by impairment of respiratory efforts. Animals may be hyperesthetic with convulsions worsening on exposure to sensory stimuli (light, sounds, touch). Convulsions can be continuous or intermittent with periods of depression between convulsive episodes. Death is caused by respiratory compromise.

Diagnostics

There are no consistent clinical pathological abnormalities associated with strychnine that would aid in diagnosis of the acutely ill patient.

Strychnine can be identified via analysis of vomitus, gastric contents, serum, or urine. Although strychnine may be found in liver, bile, or kidney, generally these samples are considered less likely to yield positive results than stomach contents (Talcott 2006).

Differential diagnoses for strychnine toxicosis includes other toxicants that can cause tremors and seizures such as metaldehyde, tremorgenic mycotoxins, 4-aminopyridine, methylxanthines, *Clostridium tetani* toxin, cocaine, amphetamine, organophosphorus and carbamate insecticides, organochlorines, and pyrethroids (especially in cats).

Lesions

Because strychnine toxicosis results in a biochemical lesion, no specific gross or histopathological lesions are associated with strychnine toxicosis.

Zinc Phosphide

Sources

Zinc phosphide (and similar compounds, aluminum and magnesium phosphides) is a metallophosphide rodenticide available as pastes, tracking powders, or grain-based pellets.

Mechanism of Action

Zinc phosphide is corrosive to the GI tract, and in the acidic environment of the stomach, zinc phosphide is converted to phosphine gas. Phosphine gas is also corrosive and it complexes with metal ions, interfering with cellular respiration and producing reactive oxygen species that damage cellular structures. The phosphine gas is eructated and inhaled, resulting in pulmonary injury. Systemic absorption of phosphine results in damage in tissues with high oxygen demand, such as heart, brain, kidney, and liver (Knight 2006).

Clinical Signs and Clinical Laboratory Findings

Initial signs after ingestion of zinc phosphide include emesis within the first hour of ingestion resulting from the strong emetic effect. Other signs may have a delay of up to 4–12 hours and include vomiting (± blood), depression, and anorexia. A garlicky or rotten fish odor may be noted in the vomitus or on the patient's breath. Care should be taken to avoid exposure of veterinary personnel to the odor, as phosphine gas poses a risk to humans if inhaled. Pain from the GI injury may result in behavior changes. As systemic absorption of phosphine occurs, anxiety, pacing, weakness, ataxia, dyspnea, convulsions, and collapse may take place. Other signs that might be seen include persistent retching, vocalization bruxism, urinary and bowel incontinence, fasciculations, disorientation, recumbency, and convulsions. Cardiac arrhythmias, hypotension, and shock may occur. Evidence of renal or liver injury may develop as late as 1–2 weeks after acute exposure.

Clinical chemistry abnormalities may include elevations of hepatic and renal values, metabolic acidosis, and a variety of electrolyte disorders. Hematological alterations may include methemoglobinemia, hemolysis, and coagulopathy.

Diagnostics

There is no specific diagnostic antemortem test to detect zinc phosphide exposure. Suspicion of exposure may be aroused by the garlicky or rotten fish odor that may be detected on the animal's breath or in vomitus. Samples taken for toxicological analysis should be placed in airtight containers and frozen promptly, as phosphine gas rapidly dissipates. Zinc phosphide toxicosis can be associated with elevated zinc levels in gastric contents, liver, and kidney.

Differential diagnoses for zinc phosphide toxicosis include strychnine, metaldehyde, tremorgenic mycotoxins, organophosphate and carbamate insecticides, 4-aminopyridine, sodium monofluoroacetate, and CNS stimulant medications.

Lesions

Gross lesions of zinc phosphide toxicosis may include generalized hyperemia of viscera and GI tract, and pulmonary edema. Histopathological lesions reported include generalized congestion, vacuolar degeneration and interstitial edema of the brain, and edema of the myocardium (Knight 2006). None of these findings is specific or, by itself, diagnostic of zinc phosphide toxicosis.

Sodium Monofluoroacetate (1080)

Sources

In the United States, sodium monofluoroacetate (1080) is currently registered only for the use of livestock protection collars for sheep and goats, but at one time it was used as a rodenticide; therefore, unlicensed persons still may have access to the agent for the intentional poisoning of other species (Parton 2006).

Mechanism of Action

The proposed mechanism of action of 1080 is related to its effects on the tricarboxylic (TCA; Kreb's) cycle of cellular respiration (Parton 2006). Fluoroacetate combines with acetyl coenzyme A, forming fluoroacetyl coenzyme A, which in turn combines with oxaloacetate to produce fluorocitrate. Fluorocitrate is converted to 4-hydroxy-*trans*-aconitate, which binds to and inhibits aconitase. This results in inhibition of the oxidation of citric acid, essentially shutting down the TCA cycle and resulting in energy depletion, an accumulation of lactic and citric acid, and acidosis. High citrate levels inhibit phosphofructokinase, further impairing cellular energy metabolism (Goh et al. 2005). Organs most susceptible to 1080 are those with high metabolic rates, such as brain, kidneys, and heart. Accumulated citric acid also binds to serum calcium, resulting in decrease in ionized calcium.

Clinical Signs and Clinical Laboratory Findings

Clinical signs occur 30 minutes to 2 hours after ingestion. Carnivores show CNS excitation characterized by agitation, hyperesthesia, frantic behavior, vocalization, and tonoclonic convulsions (Goh et al. 2005). GI signs include hypersalivation, vomiting, defecation, and tenesmus. Urinary incontinence and hyperthermia may also occur. Late signs include convulsions, collapse, dyspnea, and cardiorespiratory arrest. Death occurs from cardiopulmonary failure within 2–12 hours after the onset of clinical signs.

Clinical pathological abnormalities associated with 1080 toxicosis include hyperglycemia, acidosis, hypokalemia, and hypocalcemia. Cats may show decreases in ionized rather than total calcium (Goh et al. 2005).

Diagnostics

Gastric contents, bait, or vomitus may be evaluated for 1080 analysis; in most cases a minimum of 50 g of material is required for analysis. Very low levels of sodium monofluoroacetate may be found in urine, serum, plasma, and fat tissues using high power liquid chromatography (Goh et al. 2005).

Differential diagnoses for 1080 toxicosis include other agents capable of causing acute onset of CNS stimulation and convulsions, including amphetamines, strychnine, methylxanthines, organochlorines, hypocalcemic tetany, acute head trauma, and lead.

Lesions

No specific gross or histological lesions are expected with 1080 exposures.

Metaldehyde

Sources

Metaldehyde is a molluscicide commonly used to control snails and slugs on horticultural and home garden crops. Baits are available as powders, liquids, pellets, and granules. Many formulations contain bran or blackstrap molasses to attract the molluscs, making these products appealing to pets, especially dogs. The pelleted forms can resemble dry dog kibble. Most formulations of metaldehyde contain 1.5–5 percent metaldehyde and some are combination products containing insecticides such as carbaryl.

Mechanism of Action

The exact mechanism of action of metaldehyde is not fully elucidated. Metaldehyde may act by affecting γ-aminobutyric acid (GABA) neurotransmission in the CNS, resulting in decreased levels of GABA within the CNS. Reduced GABA levels result in decreased inhibitory neurotransmission leading to stimulation. Depletion of other neurotransmitters, such as serotonin and norepinephrine, also has been associated with the decreased seizure threshold seen in metaldehyde toxicosis (Puschner 2006).

Clinical Signs and Clinical Laboratory Findings

Signs of metaldehyde toxicosis occur within 3 hours of ingestion. Initial signs are related to CNS stimulation, including agitation, anxiety, diarrhea, hyperthermia, muscle rigidity, cyanosis, tremors, and seizures. Later signs may include profound CNS depression, narcosis, and respiratory depression. Evidence of liver injury may develop over 2–3 days after exposure. The syndrome in cats can be somewhat different; signs include dyspnea, ataxia, hyperthermia, muscle spasms, mydriasis, nystagmus, and opisthotonos; sensory stimuli may trigger seizures (Puschner 2006). A formaldehyde odor may be noticed in the vomitus or on the animal's breath.

Diagnostics

Laboratory abnormalities associated with metaldehyde include profound acidosis. Chemical analysis of stomach contents, serum, urine, and liver can detect metaldehyde. Samples should be kept frozen prior to analysis.

Differential diagnoses of metaldehyde toxicosis include other CNS stimulants such as strychnine, 1080, zinc phosphide, bromethalin, organophosphorus and carbamate insecticides, pyrethrins (cats), 4-aminoppyridine, and tremorgenic mycotoxins.

Lesions

No specific gross or histopathological lesions are found in metaldehyde-intoxicated animals. The stomach contents may have a distinct formaldehyde odor and rapid onset of rigor mortis may be noted.

Organophosphorus Insecticides

Sources

Organophosphates (OPs) are widely used insecticides, many of which are gradually declining in use with the availability of less toxic insecticides. OPs are available in a variety of forms, including powders, dusts, granules, emulsions, sprays, dips, shampoos, flea and tick collars, and foggers. As a class OPs include agents with very minimal potential for mammalian toxicity (e.g. tetrachlorvinphos) and those that are highly toxic to mammals (e.g. disulfoton).

Mechanism of Action

OPs act through the inhibition of acetylcholine esterase (AChE), an enzyme that breaks down the neurotransmitter acetylcholine within synapses of the autonomic nervous system, parasympathetic system, neuromuscular junctions, and cholinergic synapses within the CNS. Inhibition of AChE results in accumulation of acetylcholine at these synapses, resulting in overstimulation of the postsynaptic neurons and muscles. Some OPs have the ability to "age" on the AChE molecule, resulting in permanent disability of that molecule. This accounts for the prolonged effects that can be seen with OPs when compared with carbamates.

Clinical Signs and Clinical Laboratory Findings

Clinical signs of OP toxicosis are classically described as those resulting from overstimulation of nicotinic, muscarinic, and central receptors. Nicotinic signs include muscle tremors, tetany, and stiffness followed by weakness, paresis, and paralysis because of depolarizing neuromuscular blockade. Muscarinic signs include salivation, lacrimation, urination, defecation, miosis, increased bronchial secretions, dyspnea, bradycardia, abdominal pain, and emesis. Central signs are related to cholinergic overload and include anxiety, restlessness, depression, seizures, respiratory depression, and coma. Not all signs are present in an individual animal and signs vary with the toxicity, dose, and route of exposure to the OP, as well as the species involved and stage of toxicosis. In dyspneic animals, sympathetic effects (e.g. tachycardia, mydriasis) may override the expected parasympathetic effects (bradycardia, miosis).

Clinical laboratory findings generally are unremarkable, although animals that have had extended seizure activity may have acid-base, electrolyte, or fluid imbalances.

Diagnostics

Measurement of cholinesterase activity can aid in the diagnosis of OP toxicosis but laboratory turnaround times generally are too long to be of use in acute toxicosis. Heparinized whole blood samples should be kept refrigerated to maintain cholinesterase activity. For the emergent animal, an atropine test dose may be used in cases in which OP toxicosis is suspected but not confirmed. A dose of 0.02 mg/kg of atropine is administered intravenously and the animal monitored for resolution of hypersalivation or for an increase in heart rate. If hypersalivation resolves or the heart rate increases more than 5 beats per minute, the cause of the signs is not an OP, as it would require at least 10 times that dose of atropine to override the effects of an OP. Stomach contents, vomitus, hair, and suspected baits can be submitted to a veterinary diagnostic laboratory for an OP screen. Brain and retina may be submitted for cholinesterase levels. These are especially important in cases in which animals have died quickly after developing signs, as blood cholinesterase may not have had a chance to become depressed.

Differential diagnoses for OP toxicosis include carbamates, tremorgenic mycotoxins, ethylene glycol, organochlorines, metaldehyde, strychnine, and zinc phosphide.

Lesions

No specific gross lesions are expected in animals that have died from OP toxicosis. Hair or stomach contents may have a petroleum, sulfur, or garlicky odor. Histopathologically, pulmonary edema and pancreatitis may be seen.

Carbamate Insecticides

Sources

Carbamates are widely used insecticides, many of which are gradually declining in use with the availability of less toxic insecticides. Carbamates are available in a variety of forms, including powders, dusts, granules, emulsions, sprays, dips, shampoos, flea and tick collars, and foggers. As a class, carbamates include agents with very minimal potential for mammalian toxicity (e.g. carbaryl) and those that are highly toxic to mammals (e.g. methomyl).

Mechanism of Action

Carbamates act through the inhibition of AChE, an enzyme that breaks down the neurotransmitter acetylcholine within synapses of the autonomic nervous system, parasympathetic system, neuromuscular junctions, and cholinergic synapses within the CNS. Inhibition of AChE results in accumulation of acetylcholine at these synapses, resulting in overstimulation of the postsynaptic neurons and muscles. Unlike OPs, carbamates do not age and are rapidly broken down in the body. For this reason, signs generally are of shorter duration than those of OP toxicosis.

Clinical Signs and Clinical Laboratory Findings

Clinical signs of carbamate toxicosis are classically described as those resulting from overstimulation of nicotinic, muscarinic, and central receptors. Nicotinic signs include muscle tremors, tetany, and stiffness, followed by weakness, paresis, and paralysis caused by depolarizing neuromuscular blockade. Muscarinic signs include salivation, lacrimation, urination, defecation, miosis, increased bronchial secretions, dyspnea, bradycardia, abdominal pain, and emesis. Central signs are related to cholinergic overload and include anxiety, restlessness, depression, seizures, respiratory depression, and coma. Not all signs are present in an individual animal and signs vary with the toxicity, dose, and route of exposure, as well as the species involved and stage of toxicosis. In dyspneic animals, sympathetic effects (e.g. tachycardia, mydriasis) may override the expected parasympathetic effects (bradycardia, miosis).

Clinical laboratory findings generally are unremarkable, although animals that have had extended seizure activity may have acid-base, electrolyte, or fluid imbalances.

Diagnostics

Measurement of cholinesterase activity is less helpful in carbamate toxicosis, as carbamates tend to rapidly dissociate from the AChE molecule and depressed AChE levels may not be found. Heparinized whole blood samples should be kept refrigerated to maintain cholinesterase activity. For the emergent animal, an atropine test dose may be used in cases in which OP toxicosis is suspected but not confirmed. A dose of 0.02 mg/kg of atropine is administered intravenously and the animal monitored for resolution of hypersalivation or for an increase in heart rate. If hypersalivation resolves or the heart rate increases more than 5 beats per minute, the cause of the signs is not a carbamate, as it would require at least 10 times that dose of atropine to override the effects of a carbamate. Stomach contents, vomitus, hair, and suspected baits can be submitted to a veterinary diagnostic laboratory for a carbamate screen. Given the inconsistency of cholinesterase levels in carbamate toxicosis, this may be the best means of confirming exposure to carbamates. Brain and retina may be submitted for cholinesterase levels. These are especially important in cases in which animals have died quickly after developing signs, as blood cholinesterase may not have had a chance to become depressed.

Differential diagnoses for carbamate toxicosis include organophosphates, tremorgenic mycotoxins, ethylene glycol, organochlorines, metaldehyde, strychnine, and zinc phosphide.

Lesions

No specific gross lesions are expected in animals that have died from carbamate toxicosis. Hair or stomach contents may have a petroleum, sulfur, or garlicky odor. Histopathologically, pulmonary edema may be seen.

Paraquat

Sources

Paraquat is a restricted use pesticide that has been associated with outbreaks of suspected malicious poisonings of dogs in the Pacific Northwest in 2003 and 2004 (Cope 2004). Paraquat was once widely used for agricultural purposes and outdated stocks tend to be readily available.

Mechanism of Action

Concentrated paraquat is highly corrosive to tissues, and ingestion results in marked oral, esophageal, and GI ulceration. The systemic toxicity of paraquat stems from the extensive cyclic oxidation–reduction reactions it undergoes in tissues resulting in the formation of oxygen-derived free radicals that bind cellular macromolecules and cause tissue injury. Paraquat preferentially isolates to the lung, where progressive tissue injury develops, leading to respiratory compromise. Dermal exposures can result in localized dermal irritation and ulceration, whereas ocular exposure can result in severe corneal injury.

Clinical Signs and Clinical Laboratory Findings

The signs seen with paraquat toxicosis are dose dependent, with higher doses resulting in fulminant respiratory compromise, pulmonary edema, and multi-organ failure. Moderate doses result in slower onset of pulmonary, hepatic, and renal failure with death generally resulting from hepatic failure. Low doses result in progressive pulmonary fibrosis, with death occurring in days to weeks from pulmonary fibrosis. Initial signs in oral paraquat toxicosis are vomiting, anorexia, lethargy, oroesophageal ulceration, abdominal pain, and oral pain. Within 3 days after ingestion, evidence of renal failure and hepatocellular necrosis develop with vomiting, diarrhea, polyuria, and polydipsia becoming apparent. Within several days of ingestion, evidence of pulmonary injury becomes apparent. Animals are tachypneic, dyspneic, and cyanotic. Death is caused by respiratory compromise.

Clinical laboratory findings are not specific to paraquat. Elevation in hepatic enzymes and renal values may be seen in animals developing hepatic and renal insufficiency. Elevations in serum lipase can be seen after exposure to paraquat (Cope 2004).

Diagnostics

The development of acute GI upset followed within days by progressive respiratory compromise is highly suggestive of exposure to paraquat. Radiographic changes to the lungs include bilateral ground-glass pulmonary shadows, diffuse consolidation and pneumomediastinum; the latter change is considered one of the earliest changes in paraquat-poisoned dogs (Oehme and Mannala 2006). Paraquat can be measured from the stomach contents, vomitus, or bait from an acute exposure or from urine up to 48 hours after ingestion. Measurement of paraquat in tissues is best done using lung and kidney, but by the time pulmonary fibrosis has developed tissue levels of paraquat may be below the range of detection.

Lesions

Gross lesions of paraquat poisoning include ulcerative stomatitis and esophagitis. Pulmonary lesions include edema and hemorrhage in acute cases, and shrunken and fibrotic lungs in chronically affected animals. Histopathological changes in the lung include hyperplasia of type II pneumocytes with fibroplasia. Evidence of proximal renal tubular degeneration and midzonal hepatic degeneration also may be present.

Acetaminophen

Sources

Acetaminophen is an analgesic and antipyretic that is widely available in a wide variety of formulations, both as a single drug or in combination with other drugs, such as hydrocodone and pseudoephedrine. Cats may be at increased risk for malicious poisoning by acetaminophen because many lay people are aware that cats are highly sensitive to acetaminophen and it is readily available and inexpensive.

Mechanism of Action

The mechanism of toxicity of acetaminophen stems from the formation of toxic metabolites that deplete cellular glutathione, resulting in oxidative injury to cell components. Oxidative injury to red blood cells results in methemoglobinemia and possibly hemolysis. Cats are highly susceptible to methemoglobinemia because of deficiency in methemoglobin reductase and the fact that feline red blood cells have eight sulfhydryl groups to which the toxic metabolites can bind. Ferrets appear to be approximately as sensitive to acetaminophen as cats. In most other animals, the primary effect of acetaminophen is hepatotoxicity resulting from oxidative damage to hepatocytes. Methemoglobinemia can occur in these species but generally only at very high acetaminophen dosages.

Clinical Signs and Clinical Laboratory Findings

Methemoglobin formation can occur within a few hours of ingestion and is characterized by cyanotic to muddy mucous membranes, chocolate brown blood, respiratory distress, facial and/or paw edema, depression, hypothermia, and vomiting. Evidence of hepatic injury may take greater than 24 hours to develop. Animals may develop vomiting, anorexia, diarrhea, icterus, and depression.

Clinical laboratory abnormalities reported with methemoglobinemia include hemolysis, hemoglobinemia, and hemoglobinuria. Increases in hepatic enzymes, particularly serum alanine transaminase (ALT) generally are apparent within 24 hours in animals at risk of developing acute hepatic failure. As hepatic failure develops, BUN, cholesterol, and albumin levels drop, whereas serum bilirubin increases.

Diagnostics

In cats and dogs, the presence of methemoglobinemia should raise suspicion of acetaminophen exposure. The concomitant presence of facial and paw edema are highly suggestive of acetaminophen toxicosis. Most human hospitals can determine serum, urine, or plasma levels of acetaminophen in a timely manner and may be useful in diagnosing the acutely ill patient.

Differential diagnoses for methemoglobinemia include other agents, such as nitrites, naphthalene, phenols, and phenazopyridine. Differential diagnoses for acute hepatic insufficiency include leptospirosis or other infectious hepatitis, and hepatopathy induced by other toxic agents such as hepatotoxic mushrooms, aflatoxin, iron, blue-green algae, and *Cycad* palms.

Lesions

Gross lesions of acetaminophen toxicosis include generalized icterus, methemoglobinemia, and mottled or swollen liver. Histopathological lesions include centrilobular hepatocellular degeneration and necrosis with congestion. Degeneration of renal tubular epithelium has been described in dogs with acetaminophen toxicosis.

Ibuprofen

Sources

Ibuprofen is an NSAID available in a large number of OTC and prescription products in various formulations, both alone and in combination with other medications, such as pseudoephedrine or hydrocodone.

Mechanism of Action

Ibuprofen is thought to inhibit the conversion of arachidonic acid to prostaglandins by blocking the action of cyclooxygenase (COX) enzymes. The pharmacological effects of ibuprofen (analgesic, antipyretic, anti-inflammatory) result from inhibition of COX-2 enzymes, whereas the adverse effects of ibuprofen are largely caused by inhibition of COX-1 enzymes. COX-1 enzymes are responsible for producing prostaglandins that allow for the maintenance of normal gastric mucosal barriers, renal blood flow, and platelet aggregation. Adverse effects of COX-1 inhibition include GI ulceration and renal tubular injury. Sensitivity to adverse effects of ibuprofen is species- and individual-specific, and in general cats and ferrets are about twice as sensitive as dogs.

Clinical Signs and Clinical Laboratory Findings

Clinical effects from ibuprofen are dose dependent. At lower dosages, GI ulceration may develop 1–5 days after acute exposure characterized by vomiting, abdominal pain, hematemesis, melena, and diarrhea. Severe cases may manifest with acute hypovolemic shock, pallor, and anemia; perforation of GI ulcers may result in signs of peritonitis. As dosages increase (>175 mg/kg in dogs), renal injury develops manifested by vomiting, anorexia, depression, polyuria, and polydipsia. At very high doses (>400 mg/kg in dogs) acute CNS signs may be present, including depression, seizures, and coma. Ferrets are especially sensitive to the CNS effects of ibuprofen, and depression, ataxia, and coma are seen frequently.

Clinical laboratory abnormalities expected in animals with GI hemorrhage include decreased hematocrit and serum protein. Severe ulcers may be associated with elevations in white blood cell counts, whereas severe sepsis secondary to peritonitis may result in hypoglycemia and leukopenia secondary to sequestration of white blood cells. Animals developing renal failure secondary to ibuprofen toxicosis have elevations in BUN and serum creatinine, hyposthenuric urine, glucosuria, and proteinuria; and numerous cellular casts may be present in urinary sediment.

Diagnostics

There is no readily available screening test for ibuprofen. Although levels can be determined from blood collected during acute toxicosis, long turn around times generally preclude these tests as being useful for diagnosing the acute patient.

Differential diagnoses for ibuprofen overdosages resulting in GI signs include hemorrhagic gastroenteritis, hypoadrenocorticism, GI foreign body, inflammatory bowel disease, GI neoplasia, and anticoagulant rodenticides. Differentials for renal injury secondary to ibuprofen toxicosis include other leptospirosis, borreliosis, aminoglycoside antibiotic toxicosis, grape/raisin ingestion, *Lilium* or *Hemerocallis* ingestion (cats), and other NSAID intoxicants. Differentials for acute CNS effects include trauma, infectious encephalitides, CNS depressant or stimulant medication, alcohols, marijuana, ivermectin, and other macrolides, and ethylene glycol.

Lesions

GI lesions of ibuprofen toxicosis may include ulcers within the stomach, duodenum, or colon. Oral ulcers may develop in severely azotemic animals with renal insufficiency from ibuprofen toxicosis. Histopathological examination of affected kidneys reveals proximal renal tubular degeneration and necrosis with intraluminal casts. Papillar necrosis is a less common finding in animals with ibuprofen toxicosis. No specific CNS lesions have been described in animals with CNS signs from ibuprofen.

Amphetamine

Sources

The amphetamine family contains a large number of products, including amphetamine, dextroamphetamine, fenfluramine, methamphetamine, pemoline, and phentermine. These drugs have been used to manage human conditions such as obesity, attention deficit disorder, and narcolepsy, and some of these products are being used in veterinary medicine for various behavioral disorders. All members of this class of drugs are controlled substances and there is high potential for abuse. Illicit production of amphetamines, especially methamphetamine, occurs in clandestine laboratories.

Mechanism of Action

The exact mechanism for the effects of amphetamines on the CNS is not fully elucidated. It is known that amphetamines stimulate the cerebral cortex, reticular-activating system, and medullary respiratory center. Amphetamines also stimulate release of norepinephrine from adrenergic terminals as well as directly stimulate both α- and β-adrenergic receptors. Other actions of amphetamines include monoamine oxidase inhibition and dopamine excitatory receptor stimulation.

Clinical Signs and Clinical Laboratory Findings

Most formulations of amphetamines have the potential to cause rapid onset of clinical signs. Signs of amphetamine toxicosis include agitation, restlessness, anxiety, mydriasis, hypersalivation, vocalization, hyperthermia, tachypnea, ataxia, tachycardia and other arrhythmias, tremors, and seizures. Late in toxicosis animals may become depressed, weak, and bradycardic.

Clinical laboratory abnormalities may include acidosis, electrolyte abnormalities, and hypoglycemia, although none of these is specifically diagnostic for amphetamine toxicosis.

Diagnostics

Amphetamines can be detected in blood, urine, and saliva. OTC test kits can detect amphetamine metabolites in urine and anecdotally have been used to diagnose amphetamine toxicosis in dogs. Other sympathomimetics with similar metabolites (e.g. pseudoephedrine) cross react with these tests.

Differential diagnoses for amphetamines include other CNS stimulants such as pseudoephedrine, phenylpropanolamine, cocaine, methylxanthines, metaldehyde, concentrated permethrin (cats), organophosphorus and carbamate insecticides, organochlorines, tremorgenic mycotoxins, lead, and herbal supplements containing ma huang, ephedra, or guarana. Non-toxic differentials include head trauma, hepatic encephalopathy, and infectious encephalitides (e.g. rabies).

Lesions

No specific lesions would be expected in animals that succumb to amphetamine toxicosis. Rapid onset of rigor mortis and generalized congestion of major organs may be noted.

Marijuana

Sources

Marijuana is composed of the dried leaves, stems, seeds, and flowers of *Cannabis sativa*. The primary active component in marijuana is δ-9-tetrahydrocannabinol (THC), the concentration of which will vary depending on growing conditions such as temperature, light, moisture, soil pH, and trace elements. Recreational use of marijuana by humans is generally through inhalation of smoke, although ingestion is also popular.

Mechanism of Action

THC and other cannabinoids in marijuana bind to cannabinoid receptors within the nervous system (Volmer 2006). Two cannabinoid receptors, CB1 and CB2, have been identified. CB1 is widely distributed throughout the brain, especially in areas controlling memory, perception, and movement. Cannabinoids stimulate dopamine release, enhance GABA turnover, and may enhance the release of norepinephrine, dopamine, and serotonin (Donaldson 2002). CB2 is found in peripheral nerves where stimulation by THC may provide an analgesic effect.

Clinical Signs and Clinical Laboratory Findings

Signs of marijuana toxicosis include depression, ataxia, vomiting, mydriasis, weakness, disorientation, hypersalivation, hypothermia, bradycardia, and tremors. Other signs that may occur include nystagmus, stupor, apprehension, hyperesthesia, hyperexcitability, and tachycardia.

Clinical laboratory abnormalities are not expected with marijuana intoxication.

Diagnostics

Stomach contents and urine may be analyzed for the presence of cannabinoids and levels in urine can be elevated for several days after an acute exposure. OTC test kits include marijuana and could be considered but anecdotal evidence suggests that the use of these kits in dogs can yield inconsistent results.

Differential diagnoses of marijuana intoxication include alcohols, ethylene glycol, propylene glycol, CNS depressant drugs, centrally acting skeletal muscle relaxants, macrolide parasiticides, and hallucinogenic mushrooms. Non-toxic differentials include head trauma, hepatic encephalopathy, and infectious encephalitides (e.g. rabies).

Lesions

No specific lesions are expected in animals with marijuana toxicosis. Fortunately, deaths from marijuana exposures in animals are quite rare.

Cocaine

Sources

Cocaine is an alkaloid derived from the shrub *Erythroxylum coca* (Volmer 2006). Cocaine is a schedule II drug but is widely available as an illicit street drug. Cocaine comes as a powdered hydrochloride salt or *free base* form consisting of flakes, crystals, or rocks. The hydrochloride salt is readily dissolved in water and can be taken intravenously or intranasally. Free base cocaine may be smoked or taken orally.

Mechanism of Action

Cocaine has strong sympathomimetic properties and it blocks the reuptake of norepinephrine and serotonin at adrenergic nerve endings, resulting in excessive stimulation of adrenergic receptors (Volmer 2006). Cocaine also sensitizes sympathetic effector cells, resulting in exaggerated response to endogenous catecholamines. Cocaine also may have a direct cytotoxic effect on the myocardium.

Clinical Signs and Clinical Laboratory Findings

Clinical signs may occur within 10 to 15 minutes of exposure and include hyperactivity, ataxia, mydriasis, vomiting, hypersalivation, hyperthermia, tachycardia, tachypnea, tremors, and seizures.

No specific clinical laboratory abnormalities are expected with cocaine, although severely symptomatic animals may have alterations in fluid, electrolyte, and acid-base status. Additionally prolonged hyperthermia may predispose to disseminated intravascular coagulopathy, whereas prolonged seizure activity may result in rhabdomyolysis, myoglobinuria, and renal injury.

Diagnostics

Cocaine can be detected in serum, plasma, gastric contents, and urine. Many readily available and affordable OTC test kits are available on the market and may prove useful in diagnosis of cocaine toxicosis.

Differential diagnoses for cocaine toxicosis include other CNS stimulants such as amphetamines, pseudoephedrine, methylxanthines, metaldehyde, concentrated permethrin (cats), organophosphorus and carbamate insecticides, organochlorines, tremorgenic mycotoxins, lead, and herbal supplements containing ma huang, ephedra, or guarana. Non-toxic differentials include head trauma, hepatic encephalopathy, and infectious encephalitides (e.g. rabies).

Lesions

No specific gross or histopathological lesions are expected with cocaine toxicosis.

Phencyclidine

Sources

Phencyclidine (PCP) was originally developed as a human anesthetic but was withdrawn because of adverse side effects during use. Because of its emergence as a drug of abuse, PCP was later removed from the veterinary market as well (Volmer 2006). PCP is a schedule II drug, but it is easily and inexpensively synthesized in illicit laboratories and is a popular recreational drug. Ketamine is an analogue of PCP with about one 1/10 to 1/20 the potency of PCP.

Mechanism of Action

The exact mechanism of action of PCP is not known, but the overall effect is to dissociate the somatosensory cortex from higher cortical centers (Volmer 2006). The binding of PCP to *N*-methyl-D-aspartate (NMDA) receptors result in noncompetitive blockade of glutamate receptors, blocking excitatory neurotransmission within the cortex and limbic structures in the brain. PCP may block reuptake of norepinephrine and dopamine, inhibit GABA, and stimulate opiate receptors.

Clinical Signs and Clinical Laboratory Findings

Phencyclidine can result in rapid onset of behavior abnormalities in animals, including jaw snapping and blank staring. Muscular rigidity, hypersalivation, hyperthermia, and seizures also may be seen.

No specific clinical laboratory abnormalities are expected with phencyclidine toxicosis, although acidosis and electrolyte abnormalities resulting from muscle activity and/or dehydration may be seen in some case.

Diagnostics

Most veterinary diagnostic laboratories are not equipped to analyze for PCP, so samples may need to be sent to human laboratories if PCP exposure is expected. Veterinary clinicians should contact their veterinary diagnostic laboratory to verify whether the lab will be able to analyze the sample. PCP can be detected in urine, serum, and stomach contents. PCP may be detectable in urine up to 2 weeks after exposure.

Summary

Collecting evidence for suspected malicious animal poisonings requires attention to detail, meticulous record keeping, appropriate sample collection, maintaining chain of custody, selection of appropriate diagnostic tests, and accurate interpretation of test results in light of the patient's clinical syndrome.

References

ASPCA. 2006. AnTox™ Database 2002–2005. Urbana, IL: ASPCA Animal Poison Control Center.

Blodgett, D.J. 2006. Organophosphate and Carbamate Insecticides. In *Small Animal Toxicology,* 2nd ed., ed. M.E. Petersen, and P.A. Talcott, pp. 941–955. St. Louis: Saunders.

Carson, T.L. 2006. Methylxanthines. In *Small Animal Toxicology,* 2nd ed., ed. M.E. Petersen, and P.A. Talcott, pp. 845–852. St. Louis: Saunders.

Cope, R.B. 2004. Helping Animals Exposed to the Herbicide Paraquat. *Veterinary Medicine* 99(9):755–762.

Donaldson, C.W. 2002. Marijuana Exposure in Animals. *Veterinary Medicine* 97(6):437–439.

Dorman, D.C. 2006. Bromethalin. In *Small Animal Toxicology,* 2nd ed., ed. M.E. Petersen, and P.A. Talcott, pp. 609–618. St. Louis: Saunders.

Dunayer, E.K. 2003. Bromethalin: The Other Rodenticide. *Veterinary Medicine* 98(9);732–736.

Galey, F.D. 1995. Diagnostic and Forensic Toxicology. *Veterinary Clinics of North America: Equine Practice* 11(3):443–454.

Goh, C.S.S., D.R. Hodgson, S.M. Fearnside, J. Heller, and N. Malikides. 2005. Sodium Monofluoroacetate (Compound 1080) Poisoning in Dogs. *Australian Veterinary Journal* 83(8):474–479.

Gwaltney-Brant, S.M. 2006. Epidemiology of Animal Poisonings. In *Veterinary Toxicology: Basic & Clinical Principles*, ed. R.C. Gupta. San Diego: Elsevier Academic Press.

Hansen, S.R., L.A. Murphy, S.A. Khan, and C. Allen. 2001. *An Overview of Malicious Animal Poisonings*. North American Congress of Clinical Toxicology. October 4–9, 2001. Montreal, Quebec, Canada.

Hornfeldt, C.S., and M.J. Murphy. 1997. Poisonings in Animals: The 1993–1994 Report of the American Association of Poison Control Centers. *Veterinary and Human Toxicology* 39(6);361–365.

Knight, M.W. 2006. Zinc Phosphide. In *Small Animal Toxicology,* 2nd ed., ed. M.E. Petersen, and P.A. Talcott, pp. 1101–1118. St. Louis: Saunders.

Maxie, M.G. 1985. The Urinary System. In *Pathology of Domestic Animals,* vol. 2, 3rd ed., ed. K.V.F. Jubb, P.C. Kennedy, and N. Palmer, p. 375. San Diego: Academic Press.

McConnico, R.S., K. Copedge, and K.L. Bischoff. 1997. Brodifacoum Toxicosis in Two Horses. *Journal of the American Veterinary Medical Association* 211(7):882–886.

Murphy, M.M., and P.A. Talcott. 2006. Anticoagulant Rodenticides. In *Small Animal Toxicology,* 2nd ed., ed. M.E. Petersen, and P.A. Talcott, pp. 563–577. St. Louis: Saunders.

Oehme, F.W., and S. Mannala. 2006. Paraquat. In *Small Animal Toxicology,* 2nd ed., ed. M.E. Petersen, and P.A. Talcott, pp. 964–977. St. Louis: Saunders.

Parton, K. 2006. Sodium Monofluoroacetate (1080). In *Small Animal Toxicology,* 2nd ed., ed. M.E. Petersen, and P.A. Talcott, pp. 1055–1062. St. Louis: Saunders.

Puschner, B. 2006. Metaldehyde. In *Small Animal Toxicology,* 2nd ed., ed. M.E. Petersen, and P.A. Talcott, pp. 830–839. St. Louis: Saunders.

Rumbeiha, W.K. 2006. Cholecalciferol. In *Small Animal Toxicology,* 2nd ed., ed. M.E. Petersen, and P.A. Talcott, pp. 629–642. St. Louis: Saunders.

Talcott, P.A. 2006. Strychnine. In *Small Animal Toxicology,* 2nd ed., ed. M.E. Petersen, and P.A. Talcott, pp. 1076–1082. St. Louis: Saunders.

Thrall, M.A., H.E. Connally, G.F. Grauer, and D. Hamar. 2006. Ethylene Glycol. In *Small Animal Toxicology,* 2nd ed., ed. M.E. Petersen, and P.A. Talcott, pp. 702–726. St. Louis: Saunders.

Volmer, P.A. 2006. 'Recreational' Drugs. In *Small Animal Toxicology,* 2nd ed., ed. M.E. Petersen, and P.A. Talcott, pp. 273–311. St. Louis: Saunders.

Chapter 11
Patterns of Non-accidental Injury: Neglect

Introduction

Neglect is the most common form of animal abuse encountered. The term neglect is commonly used to refer to the failure to provide adequate food, water, and shelter. Neglect can be more generally defined as the failure to provide for an animal's needs. This includes proper medical care, adequate space, appropriate food, maintaining the animal's hair coat and nails, and providing sanitary conditions. Neglect can also apply to any situation that has a negative impact on the animal, such as embedded collars, short tie-outs, and heavy chains. Some state laws and local ordinances have vague definitions that are open for interpretation, whereas others have clear, detailed definitions of what constitutes neglect.

Neglect can be an act of omission or commission. In cases of neglect, it is important to note what would have been obvious to the owner, such as a foul odor from an embedded collar. In criminal cases, the issue of intent is a vital criterion in deciding on appropriate charges and sentences. Neglect is often a continuum of action or lack of action by the owner over a prolonged period of time. The issue becomes at what point in this continuum the owner had to have knowledge of the problem and still failed to take appropriate action. This can be defined as implied malice. In addition, it can help define the animal's suffering. The veterinarian's assessment of the animal's condition and environmental findings is the foundation for these legal issues.

Environment Examination

The animal's environment usually holds the most critical information in neglect cases. The veterinarian needs all this information, especially photographs, to analyze the physical findings in context with the environment and determine what tests to perform. Often multiple problems are found at the scene. Common findings include crowding, short tie-outs, lack of shelter, and exposure to the elements. Usually there is a lack of potable water, containers that the animal cannot access (i.e. 5-gal buckets with food or water only at the bottom), inappropriate food (dog food for puppies, large kibble for small-breed puppies), and food unfit for consumption. Neglect cases often have environments that are malodorous, filthy, and cluttered with hazardous material, with urine and feces covering most surfaces. The level of ammonia in the environment can contribute to eye and respiratory problems.

It is important to look for evidence of infectious diseases at the scene, such as vomiting and bloody diarrhea. The presence of infectious disease may be a primary or secondary problem. Severe environmental infestations of fleas can cause anemia in the live animals. Any deceased animals should have a necropsy performed to determine cause of death and rule out any infectious disease.

A time estimate should be given for the conditions to have been present. This may be evident by old, dried, moldy feces; debris covering the fronts of pen/cage doors; moldy food; and algae in the water container. There may be botanical evidence, such as vines growing over pens and the lack of grass around the place dog was tied-out. In cases in which there are deceased animals, entomological evidence may provide an estimate for the time of death (see Chapter 14).

Starvation

Overview

Starvation is the result of inadequate nutrition. This can be caused by complete withholding of food, poor quality food, inappropriate food, intermittent feeding, or a lack of appetite by the animal. In all cases of starvation, the environment must be investigated. Every attempt should be made to obtain the prior medical history on the animal to determine if there was any pre-existing medical condition and find the animal's healthy body weight. A body condition score should be given for the animal (see Chapter 3). The animal's initial weight should be recorded and then charted while hospitalized or with follow-up examinations. Dehydration is often found in starved animals, and the estimated percentage should be recorded. Blood work should be performed on all victims because starvation and dehydration can have severe detrimental effects on the body. Full-body radiographs should be taken of every victim because it is common to find evidence of other abuse in addition to starvation.

Process of Starvation and the Physical Ramifications

Starvation, also referred to as protein-calorie malnutrition, causes the gradual loss of lean body mass and adipose tissue because of the lack of intake of protein and calories, increased demand, or both (Table 11.1). Starvation causes weight loss, stunted growth in young growing animals, and loss of subcutaneous fat and muscle. Pregnant starving animals may give birth to weak neonates or dead fetuses. It is important to place the state of starvation in context with the animal's life stage. Young growing animals are more profoundly affected than adults. An animal can succumb to starvation prior to consuming all its own body fat and muscle for nourishment.

Starvation causes a progressive decrease in the metabolic rate. The energy needs of the animal are met primarily through the oxidation of fats, which reduces the body protein breakdown. In the liver there is a loss of amino acids for glucose production (Labato 1992). The stored lipid in the body is the primary source of energy

Table 11.1. Basal caloric requirements of dogs and cats.

Large-breed dog	40 kcal/kg/day
Medium-breed dog	50 kcal/kg/day
Small-breed dog	60 kcal/kg/day
Cat	70 kcal/kg/day

Source: Labato, M.A. 1992. Nutritional Management of the Critical Care Patient. In *Kirk's Current Veterinary Therapy XI Small Animal Practice*, ed. R.W. Kirk, and J.D. Bonagura, pp. 117–125. Philadelphia: W.B. Saunders.

and varies from animal to animal. Because amino acids are not stored in the body, the protein of the body must be maintained by intake. The protein content of a healthy animal is approximately 14–20 percent of the lean body weight. Of an animal's total body protein, only about one-third is available as a potential energy source (Labato 1992).

During periods of starvation the body uses fat as its preferential energy supply, saving protein as the final source. In the process of starvation, this protein source is broken down into amino acids, which can then be oxidized as a direct energy source, stripped of nitrogen, and converted to glucose, or the amino acid can be put back together as a protein to maintain crucial organs. Cats are unique (vs. dogs) because during starvation they are capable of down-regulating their energy requirements and increase the use of fat for energy, but their need for protein remains unchanged. Therefore, the protein in their body is not conserved.

When an animal has been subjected to trauma or is suffering from a severe illness or sepsis, the metabolic rate increases. When this increased metabolism is associated with starvation, the body rapidly uses up its fat stores, resulting in the subsequent use of the body protein (Labato 1992). When an animal is in a hypermetabolic state of starvation because of injury or illness, which is compounded by a lack of nutritional intake, the animal experiences certain deleterious effects, including immune dysfunction and decreased wound healing. The compromised immune system increases the animal's susceptibility to infection and sepsis and the lack of protein intake slows down wound healing.

Starvation affects the immune system in several different ways. The cell-mediated immunity becomes impaired, in as soon as 3–5 days of anorexia. There is often decreased lymphocyte activation. Other immune system effects are seen as well, including impaired antibody and interferon production, and decreased T lymphocytes, immunoglobulin A (IgA), and inflammatory response. There may be decreased leukocyte function because leukocyte products are proteins such as lymphokines, immunoglobulins, and bacteriocidal enzymes. Findings also may include atrophy of the thymus, spleen, and peripheral lymph nodes. There may be T-cell dysfunction, which can cause decreased immunoglobulin production. The total lymphocyte count may be decreased or normal, with the T-cell proportion decreased. Although total immunoglobulin levels may be normal or even increased, their binding affinity is decreased compared with normal animals. The IgA levels may be decreased in the lacrimal, salivary, and mucosal secretions. Lastly, the bacteriocidal activity of neutrophils and macrophages, in addition to the concentration of complement proteins, are reduced. The amount of this reduction is directly related to the severity of the starvation (Labato 1992).

Starvation has several adverse effects on the body and numerous organ systems. Reduced elasticity of the lungs may develop (Labato 1992). There is impairment of the respiratory defense system, thereby predisposing the animal to secondary pneumonia. Starvation and stress reduce the humoral and cellular immune responses and are thought to be the mechanisms behind the impairment. Dehydration is believed to increase mucus viscosity in the respiratory tract, which decreases or stops mucociliary movement (López 2001).

In starvation, there is a substantial decrease in the size of organs. In the heart, there is reduced cardiac contractility in addition to reduced mass of the ventricles (Miller and Bartges 2000). The cardiac muscle is less able to use lactic acid (Labato 1992). Starvation also results in reduced cardiac output, contractile force, and ventricular compliance (Allen and Toll 1995).

Under the conditions of starvation, the kidney functions as a gluconeogenic organ (Labato 1992). Acute starvation may increase uric acid production because of the increased catabolism of nucleic acids, purines, and amino acids. Increased uric acid levels in the urine may result because of hyperuricemia, which increases the risk of urate urolith formation (Allen and Toll 1995).

The gastrointestinal tract can have profound changes, such as prolonged gastric emptying and gastrointestinal transit times. Gastric erosions and ulcerations may be seen, especially if the animal has exhibited pica (see Pica). The intestinal villi flatten because of the lack of local trophic and nutritional factors, which reduces the absorptive area. With starvation, fat and carbohydrate digestion are impaired (Labato 1992). Hepatic lipidosis may or may not be seen in cats suffering from chronic starvation. In addition to the reduction of the basal metabolic rate, there is decreased insulin secretion. There is also increased fluid and sodium retention, which can cause hypertension, although the causes are unknown (Miller and Bartges 2000).

Animals suffering from starvation, especially if they are hypoproteinemic, may have ulceration of the lingual or buccal mucosa. This is because the oral cell turnover is the fastest in the entire body. The cause of the ulceration is possibly that the lack of protein for cell regeneration causes sloughing of the epithelial cells. In addition, decreased IgA secretion in stressed and debilitated animals allows bacterial and fungal growth in the mouth (Burrows, Batt, and Sherding 1995).

Dehydration

Dehydration is commonly seen in starvation cases. Dehydration can be simply due to the lack of access to water or potable water, or if the animal becomes too weak to drink. Water deprivation can lead to death within days, whereas animals may survive for weeks without food. Severe dehydration can cause profound electrolyte imbalances and result in death. Large water deficits of 15–20 percent of body weight can lead to death. A starving animal without access to water will die sooner than one that does have access to water.

Behavior: Pica, Cannibalism

Cannibalism

Cannibalism may be seen by the mothers of puppies or kittens. This behavior, usually brought on or exacerbated by a stressful environment, often involves a mother that is nervous or high strung. Situations in which there is a lack of adequate food, water, shelter, or there is a perceived threatening environment may cause the mother animal to commit cannibalism where they may not otherwise. Cannibalism also may be seen as a natural behavior and not one of maternal neglect when the puppy or kitten is very young and sickly.

Cannibalism is not just limited to maternal animals. This behavior may be seen between young or adult animals in neglect situations. In cases of starvation in which one of the animals has died, it is not uncommon for the surviving animals to eat the recently deceased animal when there is no other food source. The absence of puppies or kittens in situations in which there are a number of sexually intact adult animals living together of both sexes is usually the result of cannibalism. This is especially true when the adult animals are suffering from malnutrition or starvation and living in crowded conditions. In addition to cannibalism, other possible explanations must be investigated. The animals may be unable to successfully breed because of their age or disease or the owner could have disposed of the puppies or kittens either through selling them, giving them away, or killing them. Regardless, the investigator and prosecutor need to understand the significance of the lack of offspring.

The behavior of cannibalism may just involve the feet and lower extremities of the deceased animal (Fig. 11.1). It should be recognized that this is not a normal predatory feeding pattern, and in fact demonstrates a reluctance to feed on their own species. In other cases, it may involve eating the entire body except for the head and tail. Sometimes bones of intact or disarticulated carcasses are found at the

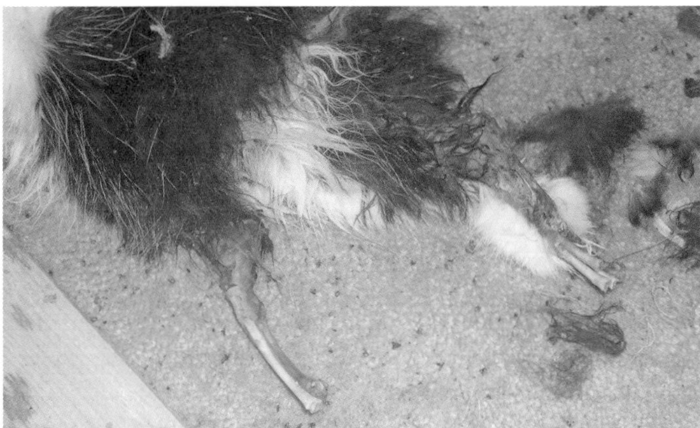

Fig. 11.1 Cat hoarding case with cannibalism of the hind feet of a cat. For color detail, please see color plate section.

scene of starved animals. It is not uncommon for an animal to take a piece of the body to another location to feed, leaving bones scattered around the scene. It is important to first identify the bones as coming from a domestic animal. Further bone examination may reveal marks that are consistent with predation. It must then be determined if the marks are from a domestic animal (the species at the scene) or a non-domestic animal. If the animals and bones are found in an enclosed structure where there is no access to other animals, then a reasonable deduction can be made regarding the source of the marks.

Pica

Pica refers to the indiscriminate craving and ingestion of non-food items, such as plastic, rocks, dirt, and wood. This behavior is commonly seen in animals suffering from starvation, most notably dogs. The items ingested may cause gastric mucosa or intestinal injury, resulting in ulceration, hemorrhage, or perforation (Fig. 11.2). Pica also may be seen with stress or boredom in animals. If the items pass through the gastrointestinal tract, the feces will show what the animal has been ingesting. Melena may be present if there is upper gastrointestinal bleeding. For starvation and neglect victims, it is very important to examine the feces of the animal for the first 24 hours.

Laboratory Findings

Underlying Disease Considerations

In starvation cases, it is important to test for underlying diseases. These may be a primary problem or one that is secondary to the animal's compromised immune system. They may also be a contributing cause to the animal's condition or death.

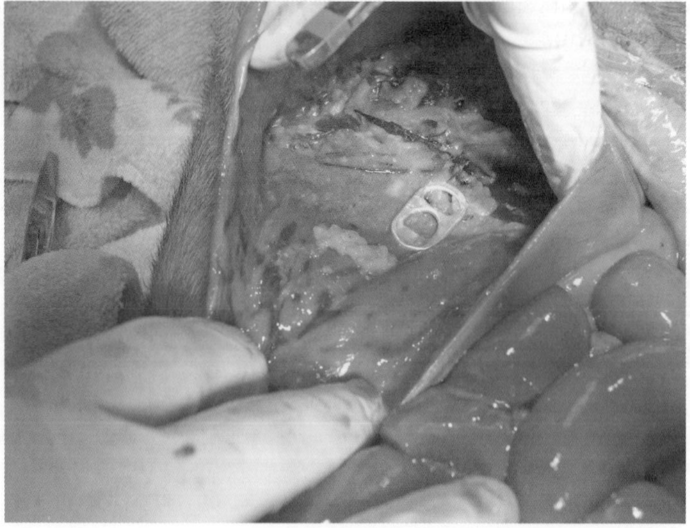

Fig. 11.2 Stomach contents of starving dog with evidence of pica: pieces of plastic, metal tab from soda can, and gastric ulceration. For color detail, please see color plate section.

Laboratory tests should include a full chemistry profile, electrolytes, complete blood cell count, thyroid function, urinalysis, and fecal exam. In addition, the animal should always be screened for infectious diseases such as parvovirus, panleukopenia, feline leukemia, and feline immunodeficiency virus. Postmortem, the bone marrow may be tested for feline leukemia; the spleen and small intestine may be used for parvovirus and panleukopenia testing.

Starvation

Starvation has a profound affect on the entire body affecting several laboratory results (see Chapter 3). The albumin level is a good indicator of prolonged starvation, reflecting a prolonged negative nitrogen balance. In early starvation, the levels are normal because the serum concentrations are slow to change. The albumin results must be interpreted in light of other conditions that may affect the levels, such as dehydration, over-hydration, blood loss, hemodilution, and liver disease. The half-life of albumin in dogs is 8.2 days (Labato 1992).

Transferrin is a glycoprotein that binds and transports iron. It has a smaller body pool and shorter half-life than albumin and more accurately reflects acute changes in body protein content. The level of serum transferrin should be measured using radioimmunodiffusion. However, an estimate can be reached through the total iron-binding capacity measurement (Labato 1992).

Hypoglycemia may not be present in a starving animal. The gluconeogenic mechanisms in animals can be very effective in maintaining normal blood glucose. Hypoglycemia is more likely to be seen in juvenile animals or adults that have decreased or depleted hepatic glycogen and fat stores (Leifer 1986).

In starvation, the body struggles to maintain serum electrolyte concentrations. As starvation persists, the total body potassium, magnesium, and phosphate are depleted. The serum concentrations actually may be normal and do not reflect the total body stores (Miller and Bartges 2000).

Creatine phosphokinase (CPK) is a skeletal muscle enzyme. Elevations of CPK may be related to skeletal muscle injury or starvation. In starvation, the CPK may be significantly elevated, in some cases greater than 8,000 U/L. This elevation is caused by the consumption of protein for energy. If the animal is severely emaciated, the CPK may be normal because of the depletion of available protein stores and subsequent lack of protein breakdown for energy use.

The urine specific gravity is usually low and the urine volume is increased in starvation. Polyuria and polydipsia have been noted in a study of dogs. This may be caused by the decrease in protein intake or serum urea nitrogen; therefore, less urea is filtered by the glomerulus and reabsorbed by the renal medulla (Allen and Toll 1995). The serum creatinine may be artificially increased when measured using the Jaffe method. Non-creatinine chromogens, such as acetoacetate, which is produced during starvation, interfere with the Jaffe method. Measurements of creatinine and serum urea nitrogen using the enzyme method are unaffected by the non-creatinine chromogens (Allen and Toll 1995).

Non-regenerative anemia is commonly seen in animals suffering from starvation. The anemia may be caused by blood-sucking parasites such as hookworms and fleas, certain diseases or toxins, or any chronic disease state, including starvation (anemia of chronic disease).

The animal's immune status may be evaluated by measuring the total lymphocyte count. In dogs and cats, a total lymphocyte count of less than 800/μl is indicative of immune suppression (Labato 1992).

Dehydration

Dehydration can cause several changes in laboratory values depending on the severity of dehydration. These include increased total protein, hematocrit, urine specific gravity, and blood urea nitrogen. It is important to factor in the effects of starvation, such as decreased total protein, albumin, hematocrit and blood urea nitrogen. Dehydration can cause falsely elevated levels. Once a starving and dehydrated animal is re-hydrated, the laboratory tests should be repeated for more accurate results.

Stress and Inflammation

In addition to starvation, the animal is often suffering from stress and inflammation caused by concurrent disease and the environmental conditions. Stress and inflammation can affect the laboratory results (see Chapter 3).

Bone Marrow Fat Analysis

During the process of starvation, the body consumes its own fat stores and muscle protein for nourishment, with fat being the primary source. The body uses the fat stores of the body in a sequential manner, using the most expendable fat stores first and the more vital areas last. The external fat stores are used first, then the internal thoracic and abdominal cavity fat, followed by the deep organ fat (heart and kidney). The very last place the body consumes body fat is the bone marrow.

A bone marrow fat analysis can be performed postmortem to determine if the animal was suffering from the final stages of starvation. The normal range is 60 percent or higher in dogs and cats. End-stage starvation cases can be as low as 0–10 percent. It is important to note that a normal bone marrow fat percentage does not rule out starvation. A low bone marrow fat percentage indicates the animal had depleted all its fat stores. An animal can succumb to starvation prior to the consumption of all the fat stores.

Because this is a percentage analysis, and not a quantitative analysis, it is possible for the test to be performed on animals that are moderately to significantly decomposed. The bone marrow fat can become rancid with time but freezing can preserve it for up to 1 year. With cool or cold environmental conditions, the bone marrow fat may be preserved for a longer period of time postmortem.

Some university laboratories perform bone marrow fat analysis (see Appendix 25). The test requires a minimum quantity of bone marrow to get an accurate percentage. If the amount of available bone marrow is in question or the animal is small, then several, if not all, of the long bones should be submitted for testing. The bones should be clean of most blood and tissue prior to submission. The bones should be frozen prior to transport to preserve the bone marrow and shipped on ice overnight to the lab.

Some situations of starvation in animals may be similar to anorexia nervosa in humans, in which there is intermittent nutritional intake. In animal cases, the perpetrator may intermittently feed the animal and the food may be inadequate in quantity or nutritional value. A study of bone marrow changes in human patients with anorexia nervosa was conducted. Bone marrow samples were obtained via aspiration and biopsy that found there was an excellent correlation between cytological and histological findings. There have been studies suggesting that examination with magnetic resonance imaging may be useful in people with anorexia nervosa. The main cytohistological changes were bone marrow focal or diffuse hypoplasia to aplasia, with partial or focal gelatinous degeneration, or atrophy of the bone marrow. Gelatinous degeneration of the bone marrow, identified histochemically as hyaluronic acid, is an extreme condition often associated with bone marrow necrosis. There was no consistent correlation of peripheral blood changes associated with bone marrow changes, making it a poor predictor of the degree of bone marrow involvement. Severity of bone marrow changes were correlated to the amount of weight loss, not the length of the condition of the anorexia nervosa. The study found that anorexia nervosa patients initially have an increased bone marrow fat tissue fraction because of a relative increase in the size and number of adipocytes as the hematopoietic tissue disappears. Eventually, the adipocytic tissue collapses as gelatinous degeneration of the bone marrow develops (Abella et al. 2002).

Gross and Microscopic Findings

The most common gross finding in starvation is the lack of fat. This may be external fat, omental fat, and/or deep organ fat. In some cases of starvation, the animal will still have an adequate amount of fat. The presence of fat on the body does not necessarily contradict other affirmative findings of starvation. It may not be known if the animal was originally overweight or obese prior to the starvation. An animal may succumb to starvation prior to the depletion of the body fat stores.

Serous atrophy of fat occurs rapidly in animals suffering from starvation. It has a gray gelatinous appearance compared with the normal white or yellow. Although this may be seen around any deep organ, such as the perirenal fat, it is most readily seen around the heart, especially in the coronary groove and around the auricles. Microscopically, the lipocytes are atrophied and there is edema in the interstitial tissues (Van Vleet and Ferrans 2001).

In starvation, there is a substantial decrease in organ sizes. In dogs, starvation causes gross cardiac edema, myofibrillar atrophy, and interstitial edema of the myocardium. There is reduced glycogen content, decreased protein synthesis, proteinase activation, and mitochondrial swelling (Allen and Toll 1995).

Muscle atrophy is seen in malnutrition and starvation because of the metabolism of protein for nutrients. Except for cachexia resulting from febrile disease, this atrophy occurs gradually (McGavin and Valentine 2001). The muscles of the entire body are affected to different degrees. The postural muscles are spared and in some cases the type I fibers may have hypertrophied. This is compensatory hypertrophy resulting from the increased workload. In atrophied muscles, as the volume of muscle decreases some of the muscle nuclei disappear (McGavin and Valentine 2001).

On gross examination, the muscles appear more flabby, thinner, smaller, and darker than normal muscle and devoid of fat. In muscles with lipofuscinosis, the muscle has brownish discoloration. The pigment, lipofuscin, is also referred to as the "wear and tear" pigment. It is a yellow-to-brown, granular, iron-negative lipid pigment found in skeletal muscle, myocardium, neurons, liver, kidney, and adrenal cortex. This pigment accumulates in secondary lysosomes and is later converted to small, dense aggregates known as residual bodies in electron microscopy. These tissues accumulate lipofuscin with age or past or present episodes of cachexia or starvation (McGavin and Valentine 2001).

The hair coat of starved animals may appear dull and thin because of the need for protein to produce the hair coat. The hair is unable to complete the normal hair cycle so it cannot shed. The epidermis and dermis may show atrophy with reduced muscle, subcutaneous fat, and hyperkeratosis. Peripheral edema is found if the animal is subjected to prolonged, severe protein deficiency (compared with calorie intake) because of low serum albumin (Hargis and Ginn 2001).

Small intestinal crypt ectasia is a common finding in animals with chronic anorexia or starvation. Villous atrophy may be seen. The stomach may contain gastric erosions or ulcers.

If the animal had severe anemia, the gums and tongue may appear very pale postmortem. Microscopically, extramedullary hematopoiesis is indicative of antemortem anemia. This may be found in the lung, liver, and kidney tissue. This indicates chronic blood loss anemia. With antemortem non-regenerative anemia, the bone marrow may show increased hemosiderin deposits because of an inadequate bone marrow response from a bone marrow disorder (Searcy 2001). If the animal also had a chronic suppurative infection, the bone marrow may show granulocytic hyperplasia (Searcy 2001). For histopathology of the bone marrow, the proximal femur should be submitted in formalin. The bone can be split to allow better fixation.

Gross changes that suggest dehydration include prolonged skin tenting (skin pinch test) of the upper eyelid or skin over the neck, sunken eyes, and dry or tacky mucus membranes. There are no specific microscopic lesions present in all species with dehydration. Papillary necrosis in the kidneys has been observed in racing greyhounds with dehydration.

Animal Hoarders

Overview

There has been a tremendous amount of research on the subject of animal hoarding. Several books and articles have been written on the topic. Animal hoarders are animal abusers whose actions are the result of a complex and poorly understood mental condition (Sinclair, Merck, and Lockwood 2006). In 1997, the Hoarding of Animals Research Consortium (HARC) was established to study and increase awareness of this issue. Updates are posted on their website: www.tufts.edu/vet/cfa/hoarding. An animal hoarder is defined as someone who has accumulated a large number of animals that overwhelm his or her ability to provide a minimum of care, including adequate nutrition, sanitary conditions, and veterinary care. Animal hoarding is about the need to accumulate and control animals, which supersedes the needs of the animals. In addition, animal hoarders usually hoard other items, such as newspapers, magazines, clothes, videos, and so on. Often, hoarding is precipitated by a personal loss or some other major negative event in the hoarder's life.

Hoarders have a tremendous impact on the animals, the people, and the community. Hoarding constitutes cruelty to animals and is often accompanied by elder or child abuse. One of the major problems with animal hoarders is they do not believe they are doing anything wrong. The hoarder fails to acknowledge the deteriorating conditions of the animals or environment. They also do not recognize the adverse effect on their own or other household members' health and well-being.

Hoarding is not a lifestyle choice, it is pathology. Because animal hoarders do not see the harm of their actions, they are not motivated to get treatment. Even in non-animal hoarders, of those who seek treatment only 15 percent show sustained improvement (Lockwood 2006). Animal hoarders have nearly a 100 percent recidivism rate. This becomes an issue that the courts must address by getting the right of inspection as part of sentencing. It is important to share this burden of monitoring with other agencies, including animal control, adult protective services, police, and the health department.

There are several warning signs of animal hoarding (Lockwood 2006), as follows:

- They will not let visitors see their facilities.
- They will not say how many animals they have.
- Little effort is made to adopt out the animals; the main focus is on animal acquisition.
- There is continuing acquisition of the animals in the face of declining health for the existing animals.
- They claim to be able to provide excellent lifetime care for animals with special needs, such as feline leukemia–positive cats or paralyzed animals.
- The number of staff and/or volunteers is inconsistent with the number of animals.
- They only receive animals at a remote location rather than on-site.

Additional warning signs of hoarding among veterinary clients follow:

- There is a constant change in pets, with few, if any, repeat visits (Patronek 2004).
- There are recurrent illnesses that can be related to a stressful or unsanitary environment.
- The veterinarian rarely sees the same animal to old age or for geriatric problems.
- The veterinarian rarely sees the animals for preventative health care; instead, he or she only sees the animals for injury or infectious disease (Patronek, 2004).
- Hoarders tend to use multiple veterinarians, come at odd hours, and travel great distances to the veterinary practice (Patronek 2004).

- Hoarders may seek great heroics in futile cases, especially for a recently acquired animal (Patronek 2004).
- Hoarders are unwilling to say how many animals they have.
- Hoarders refuse home veterinary visits.
- There is a foul odor from the owner, the carrier, or the animal; and the possible use of perfume to mask the odor.
- Hoarders may bring in an animal that is in a severe state of neglect and claim they just rescued the animal (Patronek 2004).
- Hoarders show an interest in acquiring more animals.

Crime Scene Findings

Ideally, the veterinarian should be at the scene of all hoarding cases. General observations of the animals and environmental findings should be documented (Appendix 21). This includes the number of live and deceased animals, obvious signs of disease seen on the animal or in the environment, the conditions of care, any timeline evidence, and the behavior of the animals. The veterinarian should evaluate all medications found, including the indication for their use, if stored correctly, the date of the prescription, the expiration, the name of the veterinarian and hospital, and the amount that has been used.

The environment can directly impact what is found on the physical examination of the animals. The animals are usually suffering from starvation, dehydration, parasites, and infectious diseases. Dead animals often are found lying around, in bags, or buried (Fig. 11.3). Evidence of cannibalism may be present, including the lack of newborn animals. A tremendous amount of insects may be found, both live and deceased. This entomological evidence must be properly identified and collected

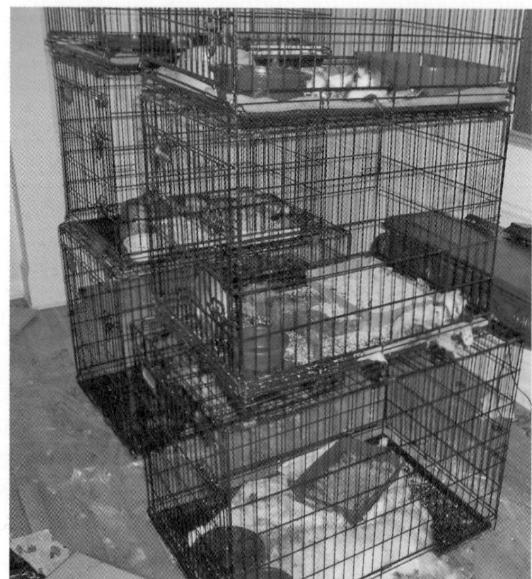

Fig. 11.3 Cat hoarding case with multiple cages containing deceased cats. For color detail, please see color plate section.

for forensic analysis (see Chapter 14). The entomology findings can determine time of death of the animals and give a timeline for the conditions to have been present.

The conditions of the environment usually are extremely unsanitary. Precautions should be taken to wear personal protective gear when investigating the scene. Cockroaches and rodent activity may be present. The availability and conditions of any food and water should be photographed and recorded. There is usually a tremendous amount of feces and urine present on the floors and other surfaces of the home or facility (Fig. 11.4). The presence of feces and rotting food can be a source of infection and spread of disease. This includes intestinal parasites, viruses, Salmonella, and other bacterial infections. The odor and unsanitary conditions are often overwhelming and can cause irritation and injury to animals and humans. This includes injury to the skin, eyes, and respiratory tract. At the scene, a towel or fresh piece of carpet should be laid at the entry to the home for investigators to walk on as they go in and out. When the investigation is complete, this towel or carpet should be bagged in an airtight container to preserve the odor as evidence for court.

The most predominant odor problem is ammonia. Ammonia is considered a toxic gas at certain levels. The pungent odor may be detected by humans at approximately 10 ppm or less. The Occupational Safety and Health Administration standard for ammonia states that anything 50 ppm or higher is considered an extreme irritant. The ammonia gas acts as a chronic stressor to animals at levels less than 100 ppm (Carson 1986). Anything ≥300 ppm is considered a direct threat to health and life. This gas is water soluble and reacts to the moist membranes of the eyes and respiratory tract. Symptoms of toxicosis include epiphora, tachypnea, and clear or purulent nasal discharge. Ammonia causes irritation to the mucosal lining of the entire airway system from the nose to the deep lung tissue. This in turn causes increased secretion of mucus from the respiratory epithelium, tachypnea, bronchiolar constriction, and hyperplasia of the alveolar and bronchiolar epithelium (Carson 1986).

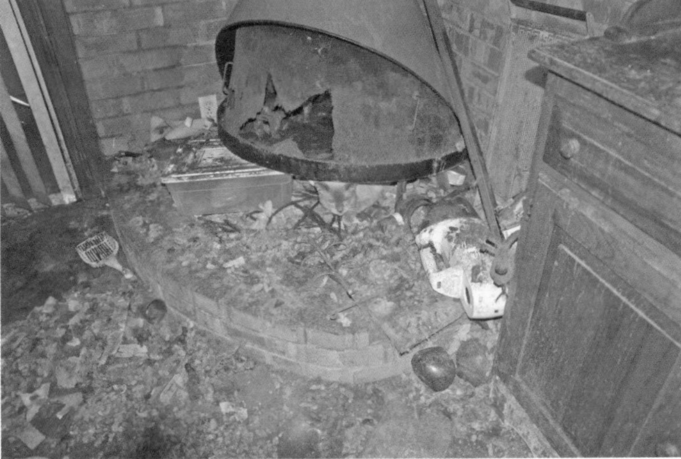

Fig. 11.4 Cat hoarding case with the surfaces covered with urine and feces. For color detail, please see color plate section.

Exam Findings

Animals from hoarding situations are most commonly suffering from neglect. They have been subjected to severe stress from overcrowding, lack of adequate food and water, and unsanitary conditions. This stress compromises their immune system, which makes the animal more susceptible to disease. The presence of a large number of animals also increases the risk of infectious diseases commonly seen in communal situations. The unsanitary environment increases the risk of re-infection among the animals.

When examining the animals, it is important to note what would have been readily apparent to the owner. These animals are usually suffering from prolonged malnutrition, starvation, and dehydration. A body condition score should be recorded. Malnutrition and eating rotting food can cause severe dental disease. The animals are often infested with external and internal parasites, including ear mites. They may have skin conditions secondary to the external parasites. The unsanitary conditions can predispose them to pyoderma. Demodicosis and dermatophyte infections may be seen, especially in severely stressed, immunocompromised animals. The animals may have long, sometimes embedded toenails. The animals may have scars, wounds, or abscesses from fighting among themselves. There may be evidence of alopecia because of stress-induced allogrooming. Their coats may be severely matted with feces and urine around the perineum, causing skin scald. Severe matting can compromise the animal's ability to walk, see, defecate, and urinate. This should be documented, preferable with videography. Any significantly matted fur that is shaved off should be photographed and the fur saved as evidence.

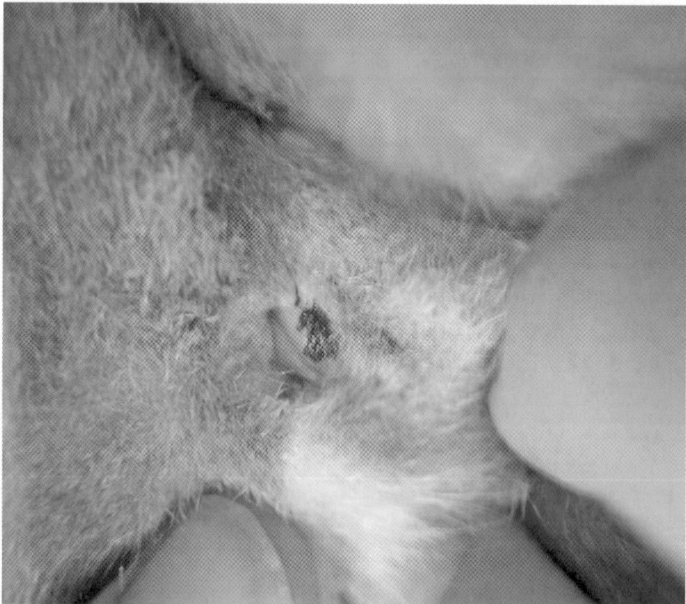

Fig. 11.5 Vulva abrasions found in a cat hoarding case. For color detail, please see color plate section.

The genital area should be examined on every animal. The male animals (cats and dogs) may have infections within the penile sheath and females may have vaginitis or vaginal plugs composed of fur and feces. Hoarding situations involving a large number of intact cats living in a confined area can produce forced mating injuries to the females. Female cats that are in heat may cause arousal of the males to incite them to breed other females. The female cats may be weak and unable to get away from the intact males, regardless of whether or not the female is in heat. Examination may reveal vulva and/or vaginal trauma such as abrasions (Fig. 11.5).

Full blood work and urinalysis should be performed on all animals, including tests for heartworm, parvovirus, feline leukemia, and feline immunodeficiency virus. These animals often have abnormal blood work related to starvation and dehydration (see Starvation). They often have urinary tract infections.

It should be noted that there is a risk of disease outbreak after the animals are removed from the hoarding environment. Initially, the animals may be free of severe infectious disease. The colony of animals has reached a state of stability even though they are carrying disease. Any additional stressor, such as movement from the environment, can cause instability and a disease outbreak. There can be cats that are carriers of calci, and cats that carry Salmonella but do not have any disease. A stressor can cause them to decompensate and break with disease.

The treatment for each condition should be documented in the report. It is important to address all measures the owner could have taken to have prevented the conditions found. Examples include heartworm prevention, flea control, clean environment, ear mite treatment, routine deworming, ivermectin treatment for Demodex, etc. The veterinarian should address the physical and mental stress, and the medical and behavioral effects on the animals living in those conditions.

Heat Stroke

Overview

Heat stroke is a severe pathological state in which the body temperature is extremely elevated. This is considered non-pyrogenic hyperthermia versus pyrogenic hyperthermia, which is caused by a fever (Ruslander 1992). In animal cruelty cases, this may be caused by leaving an animal inside a hot vehicle, a building, or outside without any protection from high environmental temperatures and direct sunlight. The environmental temperature is influenced by relative humidity. As humidity increases, the heat index is actually higher than the recorded temperature.

Heat stroke is commonly seen in animals left in a vehicle. A dog can die in as little as 20 minutes in a car parked in direct sun (Gregory 2004). In 85°F ambient temperature, the temperature inside a car, even with the windows left slightly open, can reach 102° in 10 minutes and 120° in 30 minutes (API 2005). The color of the car does not seem to make a difference to the internal temperature in the passenger compartment, but darker-colored cars have a higher temperature in the trunk. The vehicle being in the shade vs. direct sun does make a difference on the inside temperature. Lowering the windows does not make much of a difference to the inside temperature unless they are fully open (Di Maio and Di Maio 2001).

Heat stroke is not commonly reported in cats. This may be because of lack of detection. When heat stroke is seen, it is usually caused by the cat being subjected to a sudden change in temperature or the cat has been confined in an area in which it cannot escape the extreme temperatures. Cats that are debilitated are more susceptible to heat stroke.

The animal has several ways to dissipate heat from its body. There is radiation of infrared heat waves away from the body. Conduction involves the exchange of heat between two objects that are in direct contact. Convection refers to the removal of heat by air flow over the body. The process of evaporation of water or sweat cools the body. When the body temperature rises above the set point, the body has certain homeostatic mechanisms to bring the body temperature down. These include cutaneous vasodilation, sweating, postural changes, increased respiration, panting, and loss of appetite. Heat stroke occurs then the heat dissipating mechanisms cannot compensate for the heat production such as extreme environmental temperatures.

Dogs with heat stress start to pant. Then they begin to salivate and their tongue hangs out of their mouth. When the rectal temperature reaches 40.5°C, there is loss of equilibrium and uncontrolled hyperpyrexia may occur. The dog becomes excited and starts to bark. At 42.8°C, the dog becomes ataxic with possible abdominal swelling from aerophagia, and collapses (Gregory 2004).

Cats have a limited ability to sweat. They primarily sweat in their pads. The cat will first pant through its nose. When the rectal temperature reaches 39.4°C, the cat starts open-mouthed panting. The cat may groom to spread saliva for evaporation cooling (Gregory 2004).

There are several factors that may predispose an animal to suffer from heat stroke, including high humidity, lack of water, obesity, increase exercise, lack of acclimation to the environment, certain drugs, central nervous disease, brachycephalic breeds, animals with upper airway disease, and previous episodes of heat stroke (Ruslander 1992). Dehydration exacerbates the negative effects of heat stroke. Heat stress in conjunction with dehydration causes conflicting needs. With heat stress, the body needs to vasodilate the peripheral blood vessels for heat dissipation. With dehydration, the body needs to vasoconstrict these vessels to maintain blood volume. These conflicting processes can cause cerebral hyperthermia (Gregory 2004).

Exam Findings

The severe, complex pathological consequences of heat stroke result from direct thermal injury to body tissues. Diagnosis of heat stroke should be considered when the temperature of the dog is 106°F. The critical temperature considered to consistently cause multi-organ deterioration is 109°F (43°C).

The animal may present in a stupor or coma. The central nervous system is affected by the high body temperature. Neuronal injury, neuronal death, cerebral edema, and localized areas of intraparenchymal hemorrhage can lead to seizures, coma, or death (Ruslander 1992). The cerebellum may be permanently affected even in surviving animals. The hypothalamus also may be destroyed or damaged permanently, causing dysfunction of the thermoregulatory center. This dysfunction will subsequently predispose the animal to future heat stroke episodes (Ruslander 1992).

The heart is affected by hyperthermia. The cardiac output is increased. The development of tachyarrhythmias and cardiogenic shock is common, which is likely caused by myocardial ischemia, hemorrhage, and necrosis. There is tissue hypoxia resulting from increased metabolic demand, decreased vascular resistance, and hypovolemia caused by dehydration (Ruslander 1992).

The animal may have acid-base abnormalities such as respiratory alkalosis caused by excessive panting and severe metabolic acidosis caused by excessive muscular activity and shock. The gastrointestinal tract may develop ulceration and present early on with bloody vomiting and diarrhea. This is unrelated to disseminated intravascular coagulation, which may develop later on. Often, the animal subsequently develops endotoxemia.

The liver may have severe and even fatal damage to the parenchyma caused by thermal injury. The kidney may be severely affected from the high temperatures causing acute renal failure, especially in the face of dehydration. Severe thermal injury to the muscle can cause muscle necrosis, resulting in rhabdomyolysis. The urine may be dark brown in color. Rhabdomyolysis may cause further kidney damage resulting from dehydration, hypoperfusion, and pigment deposition (Ruslander 1992).

Hemoconcentration may be seen as a result of dehydration, leukocytosis caused by catecholamine release, anemia from blood loss, and clotting abnormalities. High body temperatures can cause decreased clotting factor synthesis with liver damage and destruction to the clotting factors. Thrombocytopenia is often seen early on caused by increased consumption resulting from gastrointestinal bleeding. The megakaryocytic line is also highly sensitive to thermal damage, causing decreased production, the effects of which may not be seen for a few days. Disseminated intravascular coagulation may be seen early on or within several days of the incident. This may be seen because of the consumption and destruction of clotting factors, lack of platelets, disruption of the vascular endothelium, and sludging of blood secondary to shock (Ruslander 1992).

Gross and Microscopic Findings

The diagnosis of death resulting from heat stroke is often a diagnosis of exclusion and is based on the circumstances surrounding death, including the crime scene findings. As with all necropsy procedures, it is important to consider and rely on the circumstances surrounding death. Every attempt should be made to rule out other causes or contributory factors to death. This should include full-body radiographs, and a full necropsy, as well as collecting tissue and blood samples for testing.

Heat stroke can cause a permanent rigidity of the body, which may be mistaken for rigor mortis. Rigor mortis is a transient condition that occurs postmortem (see Chapter 14). The rigidity caused by heat stroke death is a result of the coagulation of the muscle proteins. This results in the shortening of the muscle, producing rigidity.

With heat stroke death, there may be generalized tissue autolysis, especially in the internal body cavities. This same autolysis can be seen with advanced decomposition

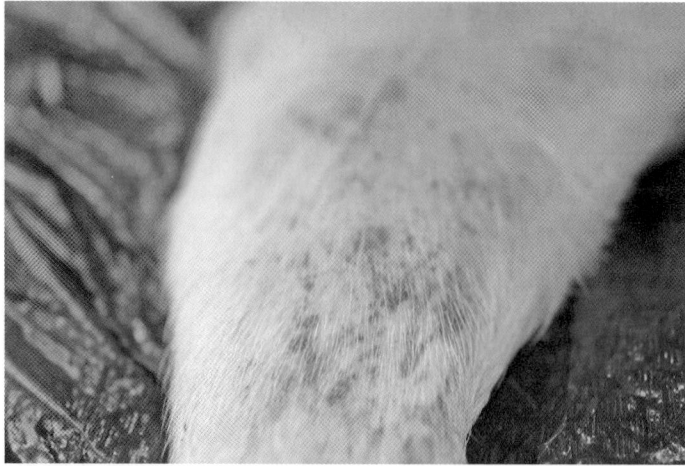

Fig. 11.6 Skin petechiae in a dog that died of heat stroke. For color detail, please see color plate section.

or accelerated decomposition caused by high environmental temperatures. Because of this autolysis it may be difficult to perform additional tests to rule out other causes or contributing factors of death. Tissue autolysis hinders histopathology evaluation. The exceptions are anything that would show up microscopically despite tissue destruction, such as refractile crystals seen in ethylene glycol poisoning. In addition, it is possible to perform viral tests, such as a test for parvovirus, on decomposed tissue from the spleen or small intestines.

Examination may reveal gross evidence of disseminated intravascular coagulopathy (DIC) such as scattered petechiae on the skin, internal body cavities, and on the surface of the internal organs (Fig. 11.6). There may be evidence of cerebral edema and localized areas of intraparenchymal hemorrhage. Stomach ulcerations and bloody intestinal contents may be found. The heart may have evidence of myocardial ischemia, hemorrhage, and necrosis. There may be microscopic evidence of endotoxemia found on multiple tissue samples. Muscle tissue may show evidence of necrosis. The kidney may contain pigment deposition from rhabdomyolysis. Microthrombi of DIC may not be present postmortem because fibrinolysis continues after death. Most microthrombi are lysed within 3 hours of death and thus may not be found if the necropsy is delayed.

Hypothermia

Overview

Hypothermia is usually caused by exposure to low environmental temperatures. It occurs when the body heat loss exceeds heat production. Immersion in cold water can cause more rapid loss of body heat than exposure to cold air temperatures. Animals are more sensitive to the cold if they are not properly acclimated. Cats are much more sensitive to sudden changes in temperatures than dogs. Hypothermia is much less commonly reported in cats most likely caused by lack of detection.

Exam Findings

Animals can have pain from cold stress. There is limb and body stiffness caused by muscle stiffness and increased viscosity of the joint fluid. In severe cases, this muscle rigidity can inhibit breathing. Animals are more sensitive to cold environmental temperatures and have a greater risk of mortality when they are ill. Cold stress can cause weight loss and immune compromise. With starvation and cold stress there are conflicting demands for energy use (Gregory 2004). Animals are more susceptible to hypothermia when they are debilitated or confined to an area from which they cannot escape the extreme temperatures.

The body's initial defense against the cold is vasoconstriction of blood vessels in the skin and muscle to conserve body heat. There is increased heat production through shivering and chemical thermogenesis, which increases the rate of cellular metabolism (Di Maio and Di Maio 2001). As hypothermia progresses, there is a reduction in respiration and heart rate. Eventually, the hypothalamus loses the ability to regulate the body temperature. Cold narcosis develops and there is the abolishment of reflexes (Di Maio and Di Maio 2001). When the core body temperature falls by more than 2°C, the animal's coordination deteriorates. The physical functions are affected and the animal can lose consciousness. If the body temperature drops by more than 5°C it can produce cardiac arrhythmias and death. Death from hypothermia is usually caused by cardiac arrest (Gregory 2004).

In humans, hypothermia can cause hemoconcentration from cold diuresis and leaking of plasma into extracellular spaces (cold edema). Hyperglycemia may be seen in early phases caused by the effects of glucocorticoids and epinephrine on the liver. Eventually, hypoglycemia may develop with possible increased levels of insulin. If a human victim survives for a period of time, he or she may develop hemorrhagic pancreatitis, erosions, and hemorrhage of the gastric mucosa, ileum, and colon. The victim can develop bronchopneumonia, acute renal tubular necrosis, and cardiac muscle degeneration (Di Maio and Di Maio 2001).

In animals, prolonged exposure to cold temperatures or short exposure to severe cold can cause necrosis of the exposed tissue. As in humans, the extremities are the most susceptible to cold damage caused by reduced peripheral circulation and the thin hair coat. The areas most commonly affected in animals include the ears, tail, scrotum, mammary glands, digits, and skin folds in the flank. The affected tissue is pale, hypoesthetic, and cool. Once the tissue is thawed it becomes very painful, hyperemic, and scaly. Cell damage and death occur because of the ice crystals formed in the intracellular and extracellular spaces. If the tissue is non-viable, it undergoes dry gangrene or mummification and subsequently sloughs. The injury is classified as superficial when the skin and subcutaneous tissue are involved. Deep injuries extend beyond the subcutaneous tissues (Hedlund 2002).

Gross and Microscopic Findings

If an animal dies from uncomplicated hypothermia, there may not be any specific lesions found that are associated with hypothermia. It is possible to see petechiae on the surface of the lungs but this is a non-specific finding (Fig. 11.7). In humans, the liver mortis can have a cherry red color caused by increased amounts of oxy-

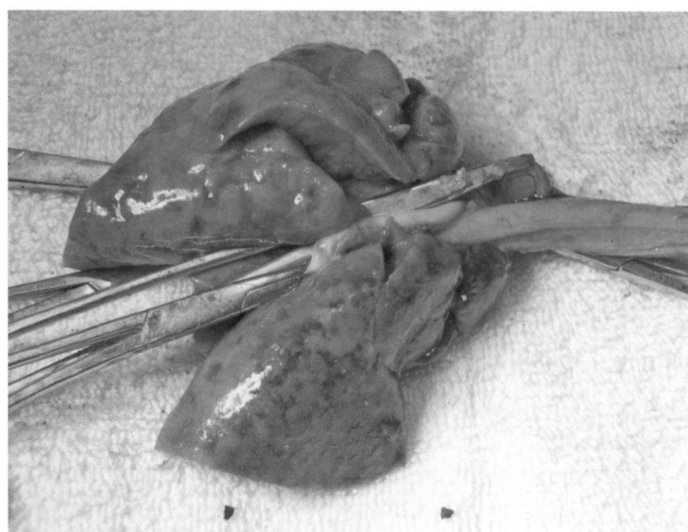

Fig. 11.7 Petechiae on the lung surface in a puppy that died from hypothermia. For color detail, please see color plate section.

hemoglobin. This is caused by the antemortem binding of oxygen to the hemoglobin. In some cases, the liver mortis can appear white (Di Maio and Di Maio 2001).

In lethal hypothermia, Wischnewsky spots may be seen on the gastric mucosa of humans. These are disseminated, blackish-brown spots ranging in diameter from 0.1 to 0.4 cm. Reddish fluid may be found in the stomach, although these spots are not gastric erosions. These spots express immunopositivity with anti-hemoglobin antibody. It is thought that the cool temperatures cause hemorrhage of the gastric glands while the victim is alive or in the agonal period. With subsequent autolysis and erythrocyte destruction, hemoglobin is released and hematinized, causing the typical spots (Tsokos et al. 2006).

Other findings may be related to the complications of hypothermia such as frostbite. Histologically, areas of frostbite have edema and hyperemia of the dermis with occasional foci of inflammatory cell infiltrates.

Embedded Collars

Exam Findings

Depending on the laws and the degree of injury, embedded collar cases may qualify as felony animal cruelty. Because the collar becomes embedded as the animal grows, younger animals are most affected. Embedded collars can cause severe infection and serious disfigurement of the neck. As the collar grows into the neck, there is pressure necrosis of the skin and underlying tissue. Infection develops that can eventually cause sepsis. The constriction of the collar on the vessels causes tissue swelling and edema. This swelling and pressure of the collar can cause pain, difficulty swallowing, and prevent movement of the head and neck. Many animals with embedded collars are also suffering from malnutrition, starvation, and dehydration. It is important to examine the animal for other evidence of abuse. Full-body radiographs should be performed. In addition, a complete blood workup should be done.

When examining the animal it is important to note what must have been obvious to the owner. This includes the odor, purulent discharge, hemorrhage, and physical deformities. Photographs should be taken before and after treatment. The width and depth of the wound should be measured. Cultures of any infection should be taken.

The collar must be collected as evidence. Gloves should be used to remove the collar. The collar should be cut away from the fastened area to remove. It should not be untied or unbuckled to prevent loss of any trace evidence that could be tied to the owner. The circumference of the neck, in an area that is not swollen, should be compared with the circumference of the collar as it was fastened.

Establishing Timelines

It is not uncommon to find maggots infesting the wounds caused by an embedded collar. This is called myiasis. The maggots can be used to give an estimate for the length of time for the embedded collar (see Chapter 14). The maggots are attracted to the smells associated with decay and infection. They lay eggs on live animals with necrotic, bloody, infected wounds. These maggots should be collected, along with appropriate weather data, and submitted to a forensic entomologist.

The wound caused by the embedded collar usually has evidence of attempted healing by the body, i.e. granulation tissue. Bright red, fleshy granulation tissue is formed by new capillaries, fibroblasts, and fibrous tissue. The granulation bed forms 3–5 days after injury. It forms at the edge of the wound at a rate of 0.4–1 mm/day (Hedlund 2002). In general, granulation tissue grows at a rate of 1 mm/day and slows as the lesion ages to 1 cm/month (Reisman 2004). Unhealthy granulation tissue is characterized by a white color and contains an increased fibrous tissue and very few capillaries. Epithelialization commences after a sufficient granulation bed has formed which usually takes 4–5 days (Hedlund 2002).

Demodicosis

Demodicosis deserves special mention because it is often associated with cases of neglect. Demodicosis is usually secondary to a compromised immune system, which occurs in most situations of neglect. When an animal's immune system is suppressed, as seen with starvation, the mites can proliferate and cause skin lesions. These lesions also can become infected over time. It is possible for Demodicosis to spontaneously resolve once the cause of the immunosuppression is corrected. Generalized demodicosis can be fatal if left untreated. It is important to document the relatively simple treatments that were available to the owner such as oral ivermectin.

Untreated Injuries

Some cases of neglect involve untreated injuries. The veterinarian must document the original injury and the results caused by lack of treatment. The degree of pain and the affect on the animal's mobility, appetite, and ability to perform normal functions should be documented. It is important to document the prognosis of regaining full function and the likely outcome of treatment now versus if it had been initiated when the animal was first injured. It may be helpful to give an estimate of the cost of current treatment and follow-up and compare it to what the cost would have been if treatment had been initiated after the injury.

References

Abella, E., E. Feliu, I. Granada, F. Millá, A. Oriol, J.M. Ribera, L. Sánchez-Planell, L. Berga, J.C. Reverter, and C. Rozman. 2002. Bone Marrow Changes in Anorexia Nervosa Are Correlated with the Amount of Weight Loss and Not with Other Clinical Findings. *American Journal of Clinical Pathology* 118(4):582–588.

Allen, T.A., and P.W. Toll. 1995. Medical Implications of Fasting and Starvation. In *Kirk's Current Veterinary Therapy XII Small Animal Practice*, ed. J.D. Bonagura, and R.W. Kirk, pp. 53–59. Philadelphia: W.B. Saunders.

API: Animal Protection Institute. Press release 6/15/05, National Call to Save Dogs from Dying in Cars This Summmer. www.api4animals.org

Burrows, C.F., R.M. Batt, and R.G. Sherding. 1995. Diseases of the Small Intestine. In *Textbook of Veterinary Internal Medicine: Diseases of the Dog and Cat*, vol. 2, 4th ed., ed. S.J. Ettinger, and E.C. Feldman, pp. 1169–1232. Philadelphia: W.B. Saunders.

Carson, T.L. 1986. Toxic Gases. In *Current Veterinary Therapy IX Small Animal Practice*, ed. R.W. Kirk, pp. 203–205. Philadelphia: W.B. Saunders.

Di Maio, V.J., and D. Di Maio. 2001. *Forensic Pathology*, 2nd ed. Boca Raton, FL: CRC Press.

Gregory, N.G. 2004. *Physiology and Behaviour of Animal Suffering*. Oxford, UK: Blackwell Science.

Hargis, A.M., and P.E. Ginn. 2001. Muscle. In *Thomson's Special Veterinary Pathology*, 3rd ed., ed. M.D. McGavin, W.W. Carlton, and J.F. Zachary, pp. 537–599. St. Louis: Mosby.

Hedlund, C.S. 2002. Surgery of the Integumentary System. In *Small Animal Surgery*, 2nd ed., ed. T.W. Fossum, pp. 134–228. St. Louis: Mosby.

HARC: Hoarding of Animals Research Consortium at: www.tufts.edu/vet/cfa/hoarding

Labato, M.A. 1992. Nutritional Management of the Critical Care Patient. In *Kirk's Current Veterinary Therapy XII Small Animal Practice*, ed. J.D. Bonagura, and R.W. Kirk, pp. 117–125. Philadelphia: W.B. Saunders.

Leifer, C.E. 1986. Hypoglycemia. In *Current Veterinary Therapy IX Small Animal Practice*, ed. R.W. Kirk, pp. 982–987. Philadelphia: W.B. Saunders.

Lockwood, R.L. 2006. *Hoarding: Psychology and Punishment.* Presented at Animal Cruelty Cases: Investigations and Prosecutions and Animal Law, Institute of Continuing Legal Education in Georgia, May 19, 2006. Atlanta, Georgia.

Alfonso López. 2001. Respiratory System, Thoracic Cavity, and Pleura. In *Thomson's Special Veterinary Pathology*, 3rd ed., ed. M.D. McGavin, W.W. Carlton, and J.F. Zachary, pp. 125–195. St. Louis: Mosby.

McGavin, M.D., and B.A. Valentine. 2001. Muscle. In *Thomson's Special Veterinary Pathology*, 3rd ed., ed. M.D. McGavin, W.W. Carlton, and J.F. Zachary, pp. 461–498. St. Louis: Mosby.

Miller, C.C., and J.W. Bartges. 2000. Refeeding Syndrome. In *Kirk's Current Veterinary Therapy XII Small Animal Practice*, ed. J.D. Bonagura, and R.W. Kirk, pp. 87–89. Philadelphia: W.B. Saunders.

Patronek, G.J. 2004. Animal Cruelty, Abuse, and Neglect. In *Shelter Medicine for Veterinarians and Staff*, ed. L. Miller, and S. Zawistowski, pp. 427–452. Ames, IA: Blackwell Publishing.

Reisman, R. 2004. Medical Evaluation and Documentation of Abuse in the Live Animal. In *Shelter Medicine for Veterinarians and Staff*, ed. L. Miller, and S. Zawistowski, pp. 453–487. Ames, IA: Blackwell Publishing.

Ruslander, D. 1992. Heat Stroke. In *Kirk's Current Veterinary Therapy XII Small Animal Practice*, ed. J.D. Bonagura, and R.W. Kirk, pp. 143–146. Philadelphia: W.B. Saunders.

Searcy, G.P. 2001. The Hemopoietic System. In *Thomson's Special Veterinary Pathology*, 3rd ed., ed. M.D. McGavin, W.W. Carlton, and J.F. Zachary, pp. 325–379. St. Louis: Mosby.

Sinclair, L., M. Merck, and R. Lockwood. 2006. *Forensic Investigation of Animal Cruelty: A Guide for Veterinary and Law Enforcement Professionals*. Washington, DC: Humane Society Press.

Tsokos, M., M.A. Rothschild, B. Madea, M. Ribe, and J.P. Sperhake. 2006. Histological and Immunohistochemical Study of Wischnewsky Spots in Fatal Hypothermia. *The American Journal of Forensic Medicine and Pathology* 27(1):70–74.

Van Vleet, J.F., and V.J. Ferrans. 2001. Cardiovascular System. In *Thomson's Special Veterinary Pathology*, 3rd ed., ed. M.D. McGavin, W.W. Carlton, and J.F. Zachary, pp. 197–233. St. Louis: Mosby.

Chapter 12
Sexual Assault

Overview

Sexual assault of animals is a sensitive and uncomfortable issue for those involved and is often met with silence and inaction. It is a crime of abuse and cruelty shrouded in sexual violence (Ascione 2005). One cannot ignore the fact that this form of abuse inflicts serious harm and sometimes death on the victim. Sexual abuse of animals encompasses a wide arrange of behaviors, including vaginal or anal penetration; genital fondling; penetration with an object; or the injury or killing of an animal for sexual gratification. It is the eroticization of violence, power, and control (Sinclair, Merck, and Lockwood 2006). A study in the United Kingdom of 448 animal cruelty cases seen by veterinarians found that 6 percent of the cases were sexual abuse. Of the victims 21 were dogs and five were cats. Physical injuries were present in all the animals, with the exception of two cases (Munro and Thrusfield 2001).

To recognize this type of animal abuse it is important to understand the types of sexual abuse the animal may be subjected to and its significance to society. Sexual abuse of animals has also been recognized as one of the early warning signs of psychological dysfunction, including conduct disorder in children and adolescents, and antisocial personality disorder in adults (Beetz 2005a). Sexual abuse of animals has similar characteristics and distinctions as child abuse. A correlation has been found with childhood sexual abuse in some of the cases of animal sexual abuse.

This type of animal abuse also has been linked with violent sex offenders. A connection has been seen between sex with animals and those engaged in sadomasochistic practices (Beetz 2005a). The type of sexual interaction between a human and the animal includes masturbating the animal, receiving oral sex, performing oral sex, performing vaginal intercourse, performing anal intercourse, receiving anal intercourse, sodomy with objects, and the animal as a surrogate for a behavioral fetish such as sadomasochistic practices or sexual murder (Beetz 2005b). Necrophilic tendencies have been seen with the animal first killed during sexual gratification; then the dead body may be used for masturbation, or may be dissected and mutilated (Beetz 2005a). The species of animals that offenders abuse include chickens, dogs, cats, horses, cows, sheep, and goats with either a male or female animal involved.

Invariably, cases of sexual abuse are seen in the practice of veterinary medicine. A study in Germany revealed that 36 percent of surveyed veterinarians had seen animals involved in bestiality (Beetz 2005a). The owner may or may not be aware that the animal has been assaulted; only bringing in the animal if it is injured or has developed an infection. The range of injuries and physical findings of the study by Munro and Thrusfield parallels those found in human sexual assault victims. The findings in dogs and cats from the study include: vaginal trauma, vaginal hemorrhage, recurrent or refractory vaginitis, knife wounds in the vagina, uterine tears near the cervix, cervical scarring, uterine or peritoneal hemorrhage, necrotic anal mucosa, anal dilation, anal tears, ligature around the genitalia (penis or scrotum), necrosis of the scrotum or testicles with a ligature no longer present, castration, and penetrating wounds around the anus, vulva, or perineal area. In addition, intrauterine, intracervical, or vaginal foreign bodies were reported, including a candle, knitting needle, sticks, a broom handle, and a possible tampon (Munro and Thrusfield 2001).

Crime Scene Investigation

As in all cases of suspected abuse, the circumstances surrounding the injury must be considered and it is important to rule out other causes of the injury. Equally important is to show due diligence by performing diagnostics to either support or exclude sexual assault.

At the crime scene, all bedding around the animal and anything he or she could have sat or laid on should be collected for analysis. Semen can leak from an orifice onto other surfaces. If present on the fur, it could have been transferred to the surrounding surface items either by contact or the animal scooting after the event. The scene needs to be examined for evidence the animal may have defecated or urinated after the assault, and the feces or urine must be collected.

General Findings

The injuries from animal sexual abuse parallels that found in child abuse and human forensic pathology. The injuries range from severe and even lethal to the complete lack of any abnormal finding. The injuries may involve the anus, perineal area, rectum, colon, vulva, vagina, uterus, scrotum, or penis. Any abuse that involves injuries to the anorectal region or genitalia by definition qualifies as sexual abuse. The injuries found in sexual assault victims depend on what was used to commit the assault, the type of assault, the size of the object, and the size of the animal. With penetration injuries, the size of the animal may be a factor in the degree of damage sustained.

There may be evidence of acute or chronic abuse. These injuries may be related directly or indirectly to sexual assault or result from a history of repetitive abuse. The animal may have been stunned or physically beaten to gain control over it. There may be evidence of head trauma and other blunt force injuries to the body. It is possible for animal sexual assault victims to have peritonitis from rectal or uterine tears. Examination of the eyes and ears may reveal evidence of trauma, including retinal hemorrhage, retinal detachment, ear canal hemorrhage, ear canal petechiae, or injuries to the pinnae. The ears may show acute or chronic injury if the perpetrator restrained the animal by grabbing the ears. Other injuries may be present on the rest of the body from restraints used on the animal or additional inflicted trauma.

In human cases of sexual assault the most common mechanism of death is asphyxia. This may be the case with animal victims, especially if they were surrogates for sexual murder. With any deceased animal that is thought to be the victim of a sexual assault, the neck should be carefully examined for evidence of strangulation or attempted strangulation (see Chapter 9). The animal's neck may be fractured during the assault or the throat cut (Beetz 2005a).

It is possible to see injuries to the tail, which may or may not produce bruising in the perineal region. The perpetrator may pull the tail and force it up or to the side, causing separation or fractures to the coccygeal vertebrae. This usually occurs in the proximal tail region, close to the pelvis. This is not an area of the tail that lends itself to getting caught in something, which is the most common cause of accidental tail fractures and vertebral separation. This injury causes bleeding in the surrounding tissues, which often dissects ventrally around the anus. This looks like bruising to the perianal region (see Figure 3.1).

Ligatures around the genitalia should not be labeled as just a childish prank. This type of abuse is a common finding in abused male children. In addition to the sadistic injury to the animal, there should be an investigation into why the offender had the idea to inflict the abuse in that manner. This issue should be addressed whenever any sexual assault is perpetrated by a juvenile on an animal.

Examination of the Victim

The initial exam should start with photographic documentation of injuries. In addition, a diagram of all injuries should be made. The external body should be examined carefully with a UV light source to find any trace evidence or bodily fluids, such as semen, saliva, urine, blood, fibers, or pubic hair (see Chapter 2). With deceased victims, the feet should be placed in paper bags and the body wrapped in a clean white sheet or body bag. These items should be examined for obvious evidence after removal from the body and then preserved for further analysis at a laboratory. Fiber and hair found on the body should be collected and swabs taken of any fluids (see Chapter 2). These may be related to the assailant or the victim. In human sexual assault crimes it is common for saliva to be transferred to the victim during the assault. Consider the circumstances surrounding the crime in relation to the injuries to determine where the assailant would have likely deposited saliva on the animal. There may be ejaculate found on or near the animal if the attacker did not wear a condom. To collect samples of dried fluid, first moisten a sterile cotton-tip applicator with sterile water, and then swab the area, which will rehydrate the cells. Next, roll a dry sterile swab on the moistened area. Both swabs should be saved for testing.

After the coat has been inspected with a UV light and evidence collected, the animal should be placed on white roll paper and the fur combed thoroughly to look for embedded trace evidence, such as pubic hair or fibers. During the assault, the animal may have transferred his or her own DNA or fur to the attacker. Samples for DNA (see Chapter 4) and a sample of fur, including one of each color on the coat, should be collected and held for comparison testing.

It is important to consider that the animal may have been drugged by the assailant to facilitate the act. Blood and urine should be collected immediately for toxicology testing. The drugs used on the animal may include illegal substances, human tranquilizers, or similar narcotics. The assailant may have given veterinary tranquilizers such as acepromazine, a commonly prescribed drug for animals that have anxiety related to travel, thunderstorms, or fireworks.

It is possible the victim fought and scratched the attacker during the assault. The feet and legs need to be inspected for evidence of injury, ligature marks, nail injuries, and embedded trace evidence using a magnifying glass and a UV light source. After the collection of evidence, the nails should be scraped and then clipped, saving all scrapings and clippings for analysis. In deceased animals, the nails should be removed using clean instruments to prevent contamination and saved for trace and DNA testing at a crime lab.

Full-body radiographs, including the tail, need to be done on the live and deceased victim, to look for evidence of additional injuries. The external muzzle and oral cavity should be examined for evidence of trauma, foreign material, or trace evidence. It is important to consider what the animal may have done to defend itself during the assault or in response to pain. The mouth of an animal contains certain bacteria that may be linked to any bite wound infection inflicted by the victim to the attacker. The teeth need to be inspected for any tissue or trace evidence caught on the teeth. The oral cavity needs to be swabbed for possible DNA or other potential evidence related to the assailant or the crime. Swabs should be taken from the outside and inside of the lips, under the tongue, inside the buccal mucosa, and along the gums and teeth.

The assailant's DNA may be present in the vagina or anorectal region. A human rape kit may be used to collect samples, which contain sterile swabs, microscope slides, slide holders, labels, gloves, and envelopes for hair evidence. Separate swabs should be taken all around the perineal and genital areas even if there is a lack of visible fluids with the UV light source. Swabs need to be taken of the vagina and rectum. Several rectal swabs should be taken prior to taking the animal's temperature or treatment of a rectal prolapse (see below) to prevent any cross-contamination. Slides should be made and air dried. A wet slide should be made and immediately examined for sperm, making note of any motility. Evaluation of sperm and semen is covered later in this chapter. Separate swabs should be saved for DNA, cultures, trace evidence, and other tests. Swabs should be placed in a cardboard box, allowing the swab to air dry.

The animal's first bowel movement should be collected and preserved for DNA testing (the assailant's DNA). If it is known that the animal had a bowel movement prior to examination, for example, during transport, that fecal sample also should be collected. A urine sample should be obtained in female victims. Because the opening of urethra is inside the vagina in dogs and cats, the assailant's sperm may travel from the vaginal area to the bladder.

When examining the genitalia it is important to know what is normal to be able to recognize what is abnormal. An otoscope may be used for vaginal and anal exams, which are done preferably while the animal is under anesthesia. There is a vaginal speculum that may be used with the Welch-Allyn otoscope base. Colonoscopy may be indicated, especially if blood is found on the fecal swabs or the animal exhibits painful defecation. If there is vaginal or rectal penetration by the perpetrator, there may be severe trauma to these areas, causing deeper lacerations and subsequent peritonitis. If there is evidence of penetration with an object, trace evidence may be present from the object. Evidence from the animal also may be transferred onto the offending object.

In addition to the injuries found in the study by Munro and Thrusfield, findings may include vulva and vaginal edema, abrasions in the perianal or perivulvar region, or along the vaginal mucosa or rectal mucosa. Bruising may be visible in these areas or on the surface of the cervix. Depending on the animal, the vulva folds may be forced inward by the penetrating object, protecting the internal vaginal mucosa. In this case, bruising, abrasion, or laceration injuries may be seen to the outside of the vulva folds and the cervix, if penetration reached that area (Fig. 12.1).

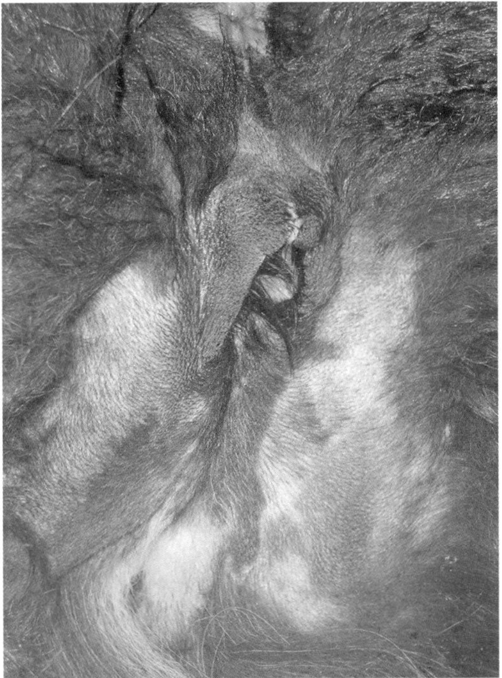

Fig. 12.1 Canine sexual assault victim: perianal subcutaneous hemorrhage resulting from a proximal tail fracture, external vulva abrasions, perivulvar bruising, medial thigh bruising, and cervical bruising (not pictured). For color detail, please see color plate section.

Suspicious Exam Findings

There are certain physical findings that should raise the index of suspicion sexual abuse. These findings may be related to acute or chronic abuse. It is important in every situation to rule out other causes and take appropriate samples for testing. Sexual assault victims often go undetected by the veterinary community.

Vaginal

Penetrating vaginal assault can cause hemorrhage from the vulva caused by vaginal lacerations. Vaginal strictures may be result from previous sexual abuse. Recurrent vaginitis may be indicative of sexual abuse. Vaginitis can occur in sexually intact or neutered bitches, but is rare in queens. It may be caused by bacterial or viral infections, immaturity of the reproductive tract, androgenic stimulation, chemical irritation as with urine, or mechanical irritation. This mechanical irritation may result from neoplasia, anatomical abnormalities of the vagina or vestibule, foreign bodies, or human sexual penetration. The vaginal discharge associated with vaginitis may be mucoid, mucopurulent, or purulent, and rarely contains blood. Cytological findings may be non-septic or septic inflammation without hemorrhage. The vaginitis causes mucosal inflammation, hyperemia, and edema. A concurrent urinary tract infection commonly is found but it is not the cause of the vaginitis. In addition to vaginitis, other causes of vaginal discharge include vulvitis, pyometra, metritis, abortion, uterine stump granuloma or abscess, or retained foreign body. Vaginoscopy is needed to rule out anatomical abnormalities and other mechanical causes (Johnson 2003).

Vaginal prolapse rarely occurs in the bitch or the queen. When seen, it is normally due to tenesmus, dystocia, or forced extraction of the male during the genital tie (Purswell 1995). Vaginal prolapse may be seen in dogs with estrogen stimulation, as seen in proestrus or estrus. It also may recur after parturition or even at the end of diestrus. Vaginal prolapse is primarily seen in young, intact, large breed dogs. The tissue becomes swollen because marked edema. The presence of a vaginal prolapse in a spayed female or without other predisposing causes is highly suspect and the possibility of sexual assault should be thoroughly investigated.

Anus, Rectum, and Colon

There may be injury to the anus, rectum, or colon in sexual assault victims. Anal tears can be caused by anal penetration. Dilation of the anus can be indicative of spinal cord disease, spinal injury, or anal penetration and trauma. However, after death the anus relaxes and can be mistaken as traumatically stretched.

Proctitis is the inflammation of the rectum. This may be seen because of trauma from rectal foreign bodies and sexual assault. It may cause recurrent rectal prolapses. Clinical signs of hematochezia, dyschezia, tenesmus, and pain may be seen with proctitis. Abdominal radiographs, proctoscopy, and colonoscopy should be performed on any animal showing these signs. Rectal foreign bodies can cause rectal fistulas, perirectal abscesses, and peritonitis (Washabau and Brockman 1995). Rectal strictures may be caused by neoplasia or previous sexual assault.

Sexual abuse must be considered as a possible cause for rectal prolapse. Appropriate swabs should be taken prior to treatment until the history is evaluated to determine the cause for the prolapse. Rectal prolapse is usually secondary to straining caused by rectal irritation. This irritation can be secondary to several predisposing factors, including enteritis, diarrhea, colitis, rectal foreign bodies, or sexual assault. Also it may be seen from a blow to the abdomen in which there is a sudden increase in abdominal pressure. Rectal prolapse is generally uncommon in animals with longstanding tenesmus and dyschezia (Washabau and Brockman 1995). Rectal prolapse may be partial, involving the protrusion of the rectal mucosa through the anal orifice, or complete, with the protrusion of all layers of the rectum. It may or may not involve layers of the anal canal. The rectal mucosa exposed increases straining, which aids and promotes further prolapse.

Zoonotic Disease

A consideration for any sexual assault case is the possibility of zoonotic disease transmission during the attack. This pertains to any disease that is unique to the animal that could have been transferred to the perpetrator, such as a bacterial or parasite infection of the genital, intestinal, or urinary tract. Any intestinal parasite that has zoonotic potential, such as roundworms, may be transmitted to the assailant through the fecal–oral route. Because there may be residual fecal material around the genitalia, this transmission may occur through any sexual contact with the animal. To confirm the source of any human infection, perform DNA typing of the parasite found in the human if possible and compare the results with the profile of the parasite carried by the animal.

Several bacteria that the animal may normally carry may cause infection in the assailant. The aerobic bacteria normally found in the vagina have been isolated from 59 healthy, breeding bitches. The bacteria, listed in descending order by percentage of isolates, are as follows: *Pasteurella multocida* (98 percent of dogs), β-hemolytic streptococcus, *E. coli*, unclassified gram-positive rods, unclassified gram-negative rods, *Mycoplasma*, *α-hemolytic* and *non-hemolytic streptococcus*, *Pasteurella*, enterococci, *Proteus mirabilis*, *Staphylococcus intermedius*, corniforms, *coagulase-negative staphylococcus*, and *Pseudomonas st.* (10 percent of dogs) (Nelson and Feldman 1996).

In addition, there are bacteria with zoonotic potential that the animal may carry that can cause infection in the animal, assailant, or both. *Coxiella burnetii* is found in cats. The symptoms of cats may be subclinical, can cause abortions, or stillbirth. Humans can become ill from direct contact through aerosol exposure to birthing fluids passed by parturient or aborting cats. Humans develop symptoms 4 to 30 days post-exposure. These symptoms include fever, malaise, headache, pneumonitis, myalgia, and arthralgia. Approximately 1 percent of infected people later develop hepatic inflammation or valvular endocarditis. *Leptospira* spp. can infect dogs and rarely cats. It can be transmitted to humans via urine from animals, usually by human contact with abraded skin or mucous membranes. The symptoms in dogs can be fever, malaise, inflammatory urinary tract disease, inflammatory hepatic disease, uveitis, and central nervous system disease. Humans have similar symptoms, depending on the serovar of the *Leptospira*. *Brucella canis* is an infection of dogs that causes orchitis, epididymitis, infertility, abortion, stillbirth, vaginal discharge, uveitis, diskospondylitis, fever, and malaise. It is transmitted between dogs primarily by venereal transmission. Humans can be infected by direct contact with vaginal or preputial discharges from the dog. Symptoms in humans are usually fever, depression, and malaise (Lappin 2003).

Evaluation of Assailant's Sperm and Semen

Another special consideration in sexual assault cases is the condition of any recovered sperm. In humans, the motility and condition of the sperm can help establish timelines that enable an estimate of the time of the assault. In human rape cases, the sperm remains motile in live victims up to 6 hours and less often up to 12–24 hours (Di Maio and Di Maio 2001). Sperm can survive longer in the cervical mucus than in the vaginal area. Non-motile sperm with tails can be seen up to 26 hours in living rape victims. Sperm heads without tails from the vaginal area may be seen up to 120 hours later. Sperm has been found 7 days later in a cervical swab (Di Maio and Di Maio 2001). In anal and rectal swabs, sperm with tails are not commonly found, particularly if more than 6 hours have elapsed. Sperm heads were found in anal swabs 45 hours later; in rectal swabs 65 hours later (Di Maio and Di Maio 2001). The sperm survival in deceased victims is shorter because the sperm are destroyed by decomposition. In humans sperm has been found in the vagina up to 2 weeks after death. Any sperm on a piece of material and air dried may be recovered years later (Di Maio and Di Maio 2001).

Sperm may not be present in sexual assault cases. This may be because of the lack of ejaculation, use of a condom, aspermia resulting from a vasectomy or disease, or drainage of the semen out of the vaginal area. Human semen contains high quantities of acid phosphatase for which the swab can be analyzed. The presence of acid phosphatase is usually 8–24 hours after the act, then begins to disappear and is completely gone by 48–72 hours. Because non-motile sperm can be identified 2–3 days later, this test can indicate the act was more recent. P30 is a semen-specific glycoprotein of prostatic origin. It is present in semen only, regardless of the presence of sperm. This P30 can be detected 13–47 hours later. It has been found that there are cases in which the acid phosphatase was negative and the P30 was positive, confirming the sexual act (Di Maio and Di Maio 2001). In cases in which there are no visible sperm it still may be possible to get male DNA from epithelial cells in the ejaculate or premature lysis of sperm. In human cases, the female DNA can overwhelm the quantity of male DNA, causing problems with interpretation of the mixed profile results. In these cases, better results may be obtained by performing DNA tests using Y-chromosome short tandem repeats (Y-STRs). This test may be helpful in compromised sexual evidence of any sexual assault case (Johnson et al. 2005).

References

Ascione, F.R. 2005. Bestiality: Petting, "Humane Rape," Sexual Assault, and the Enigma of Sexual Interactions between Humans and Non-human Animals. In *Bestiality and Zoophilia*, ed. A.M. Beetz, and A.L. Podberscek, pp. 120–129. Ashland, OH: Purdue University Press.

Beetz, A.M. 2005a. Bestiality and Zoophilia: Associations with Violence and Sex Offending. In *Bestiality and Zoophilia*, ed. A.M. Beetz, and A.L. Podberscek, pp. 46–70. Ashland, OH: Purdue University Press.

Beetz, A.M. 2005b. New Insights into Bestiality and Zoophilia. In *Bestiality and Zoophilia*, ed. A.M. Beetz, and A.L. Podberscek, pp. 98–119. Ashland, OH: Purdue University Press.

Di Maio, V.J., and D. Di Maio. 2001. *Forensic Pathology*, 2nd ed. Boca Raton, FL: CRC Press.

Johnson, C.L., R.C. Giles, J.H. Warren, J.I. Floyd, and R.W. Staub. 2005. Analysis of Non-Suspect Samples Lacking Visually Identifiable Sperm Using a Y-STR 10-Plex. *Journal of Forensic Science* 50(5):1116–1118.

Johnson, C.A. 2003. Disorders of the Vagina and Uterus. In *Small Animal Internal Medicine*, ed. R.W. Nelson, and C.G. Couto, pp. 870–881. St. Louis: Mosby.

Lappin, M.R. 2003. Zoonoses. In *Small Animal Internal Medicine*, ed. R.W. Nelson, and C.G. Couto, pp. 1307–1321. St. Louis: Mosby.

Munro, H.M., and M.V. Thrusfield. 2001. 'Battered Pets': Sexual Abuse. *Journal of Small Animal Practice* 42:333–337.

Nelson, R.W., and E.C. Feldman. 1996. *Canine and Feline Endocrinology and Reproduction*, 2nd ed. Philadelphia: W.B. Saunders.

Purswell, B.J. 1995. Vaginal Disorders. In *Textbook of Veterinary Internal Medicine: Diseases of the Dog and Cat*, vol. 2, 4th ed., ed. S.J. Ettinger, and E.C. Feldman, pp. 1642–1648. Philadelphia: W.B. Saunders.

Sinclair, L., M. Merck, and R. Lockwood. 2006. *Forensic Investigation of Animal Cruelty: A Guide for Veterinary and Law Enforcement Professionals*. Washington, DC: Humane Society Press.

Washabau, R.J., and D.J. Brockman. 1995. Recto-Anal Disease. In *Textbook of Veterinary Internal Medicine: Diseases of the Dog and Cat*, vol. 2, 4th ed., ed. S.J. Ettinger, and E.C. Feldman, pp. 1398–1409. Philadelphia: W.B. Saunders.

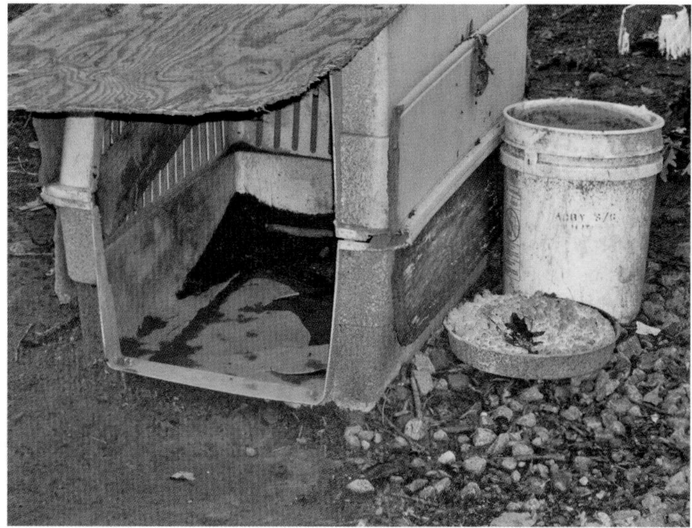

Figure 2.1 Inadequate housing with torn floor, open sides and front; moldy food.

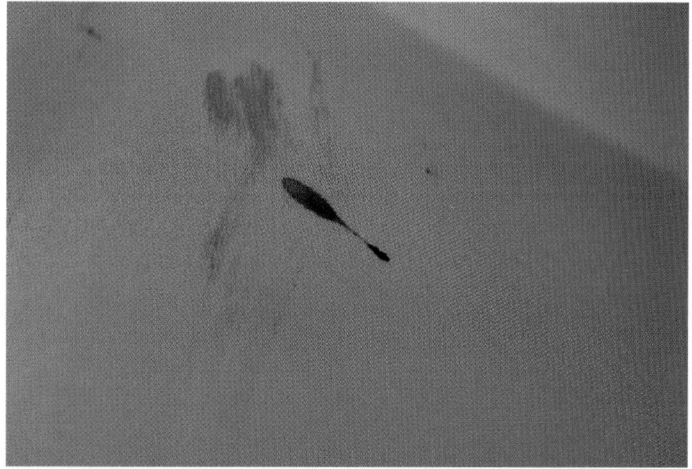

Figure 2.2 Wave cast-off blood spatter.

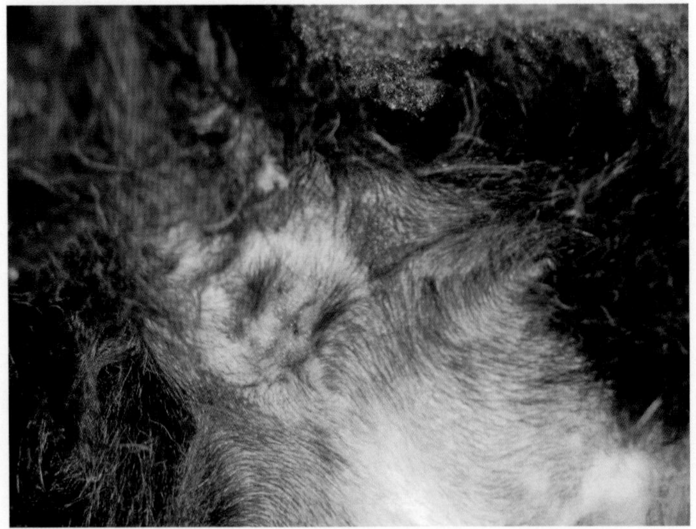

Fig. 3.1 Dissecting subcutaneous hemorrhage around anus resulting from proximal tail fracture and dislocation.

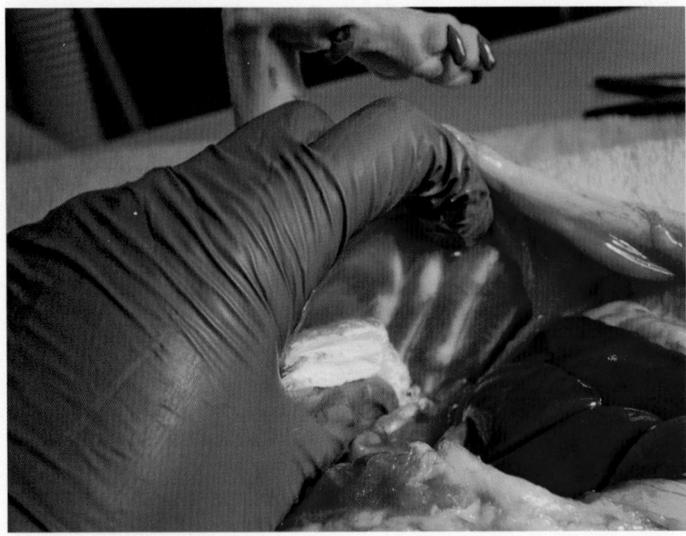

Fig. 3.2 Older, healing rib fracture.

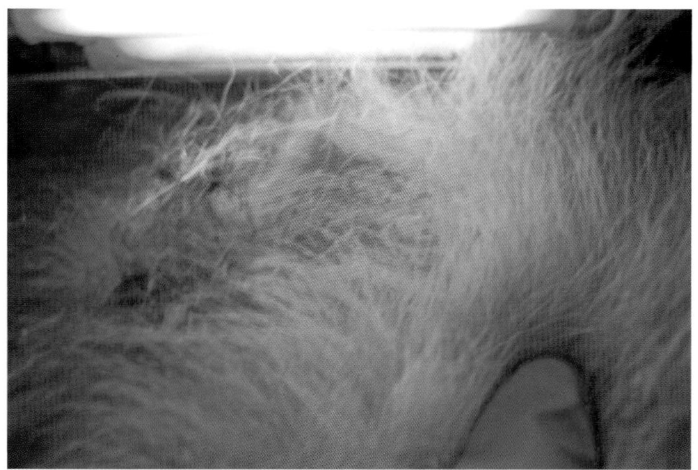

Fig. 4.1 UV light causing saliva on the fur to fluoresce.

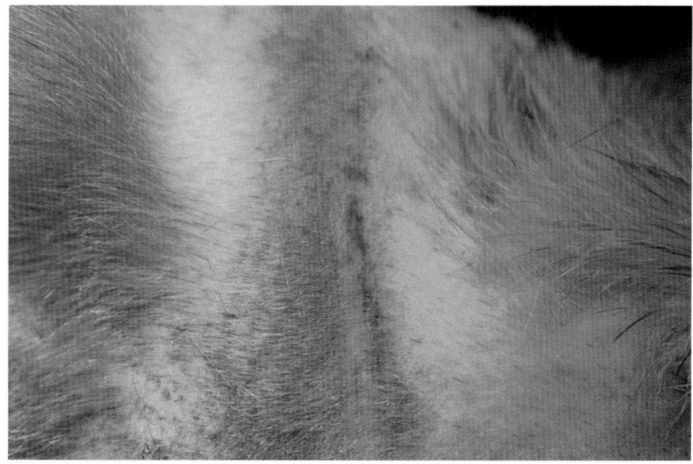

Figure 5.1 Interrupted bruising pattern caused by chain collar *(right)* and bruising from nylon collar below *(left)*.

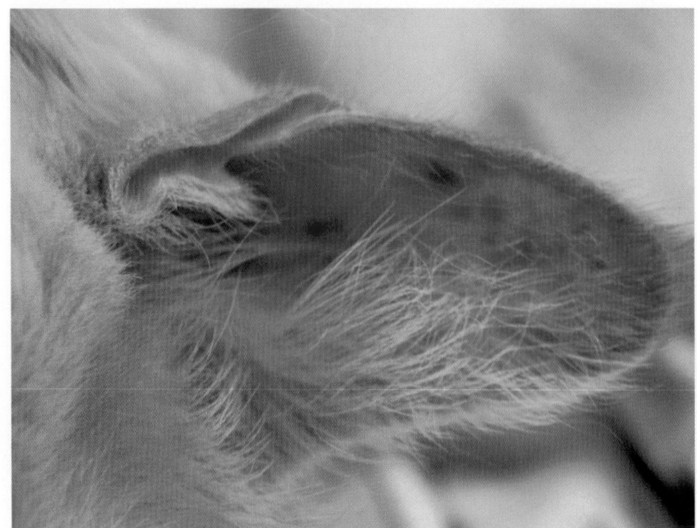

Fig. 5.2 Petechiae on the ear pinna caused by blunt force trauma to the head.

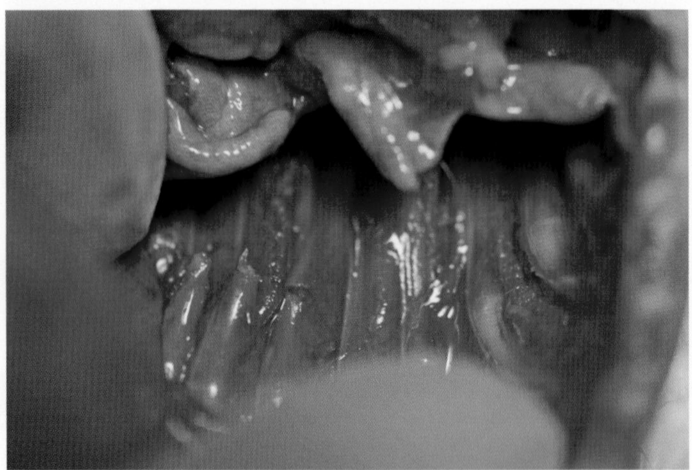

Fig. 5.3 Multiple rib fractures caused by blunt force trauma.

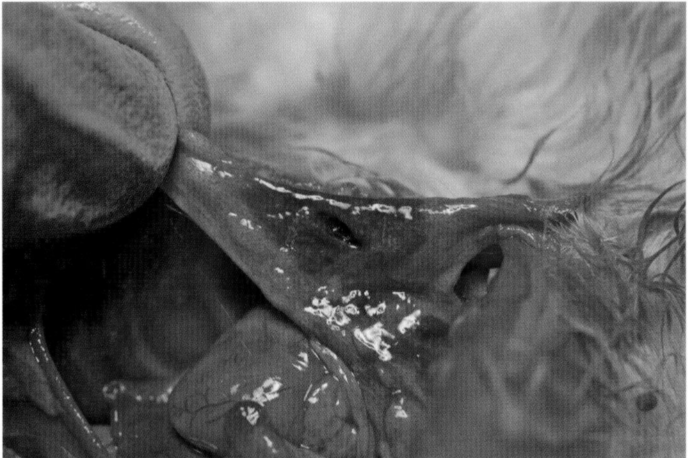

Fig. 5.4 Lung lacerations and contusions secondary to the rib fractures seen in Figure 5.3.

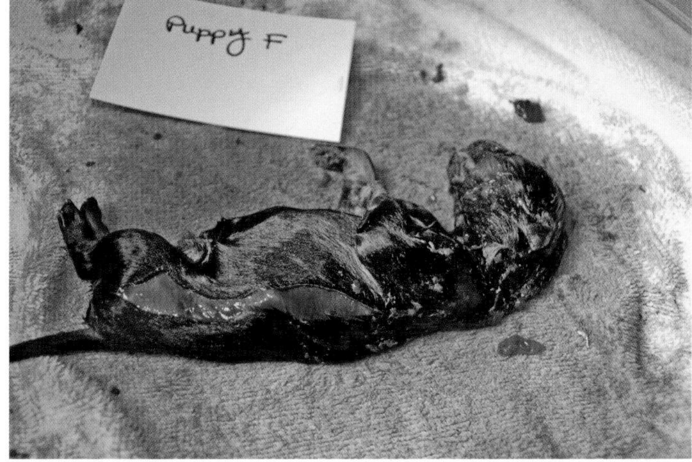

Fig. 6.1 Laceration on puppy caused by blunt force trauma using a barbell weight.

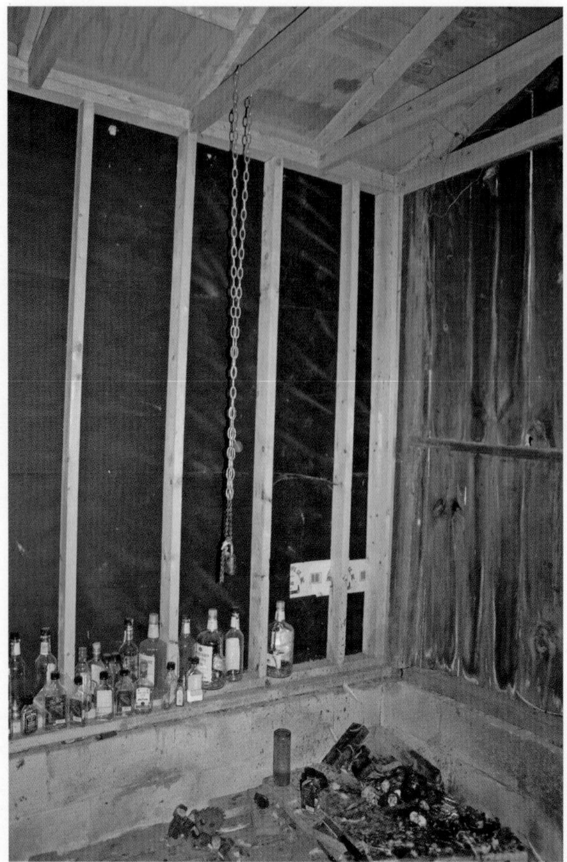

Fig. 6.2 Palo Mayombe ritual site with bottles of alcohol, candles, and a chain to hold the animals while dripping blood on the altar.

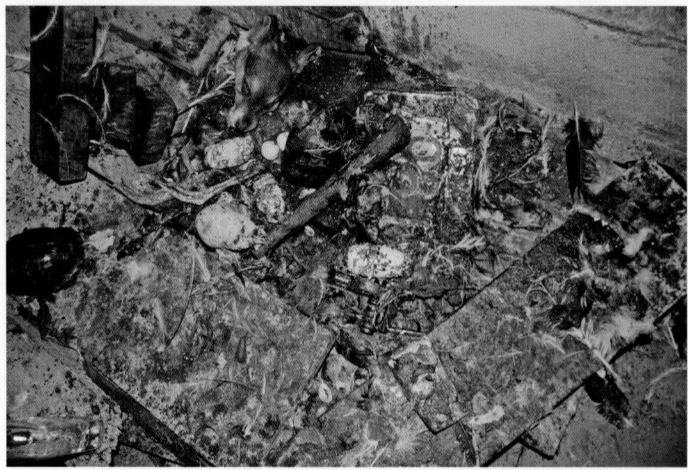

Fig. 6.3 Palo Mayombe inner altar containing bird feet, turtle shells, sea shells, eggs, feathers, animal bones, toy cars, pictures, license plate, and the head of a puppy.

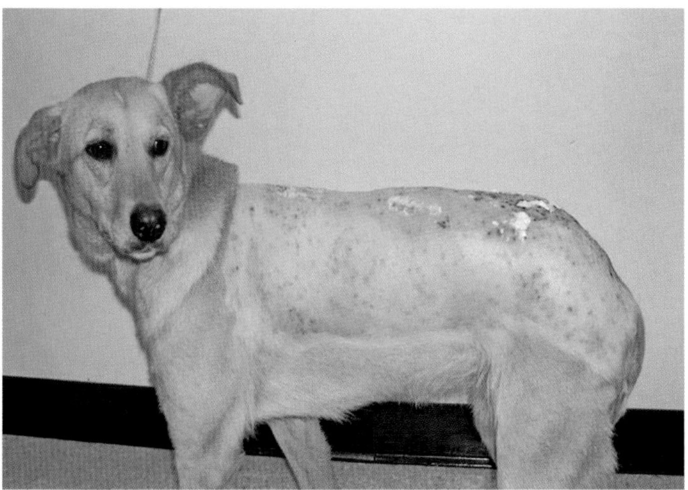

Fig. 7.1 This dog was seen running down the street with her back on fire. The fur was shaved revealing a symmetrical burn pattern on the sides of the torso and caudal pelvis.

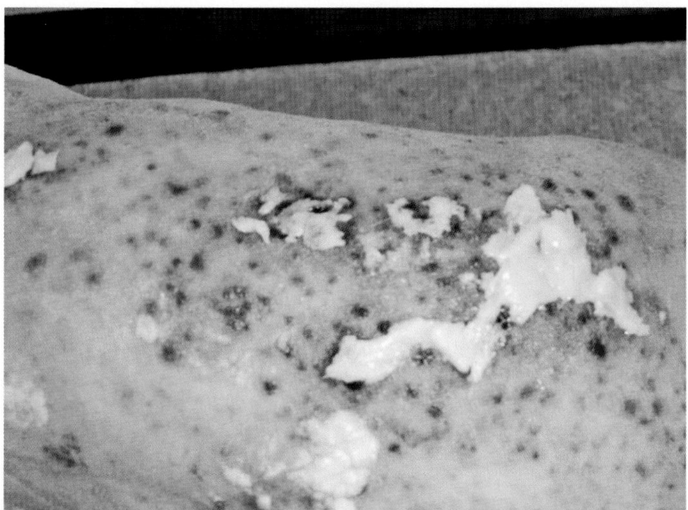

Fig. 7.2 Close-up of dog from Figure 7.1 revealing a few larger and deeper burn areas that have been treated with burn cream. The majority of the body is covered with small, circular burns because the fur acts as a wick for the fire to burn down to the skin.

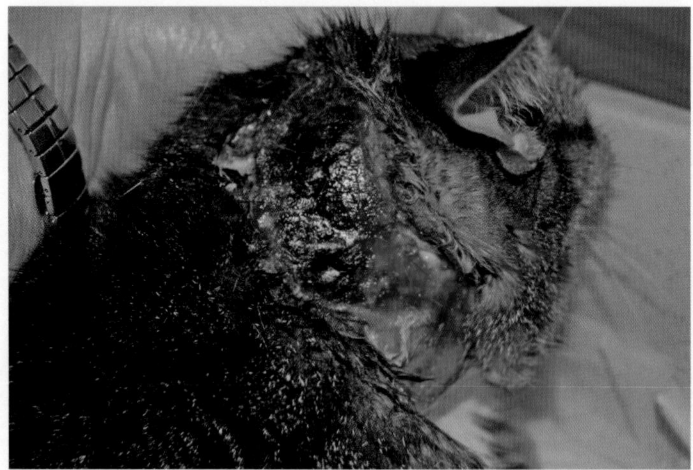

Fig. 7.3 Eschar burn on the neck of a cat caused by a heat lamp.

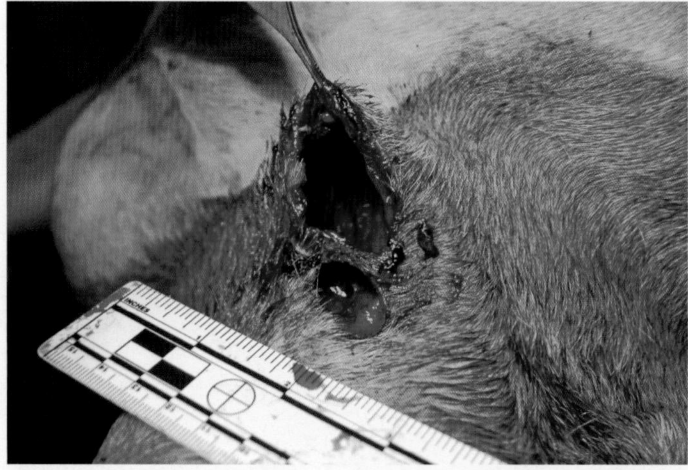

Fig. 8.1 Gunshot entrance wound caused by a slug. The slug entered over a fold of skin, causing the first wound, which is circular; then the slug expanded, causing the larger irregular second wound.

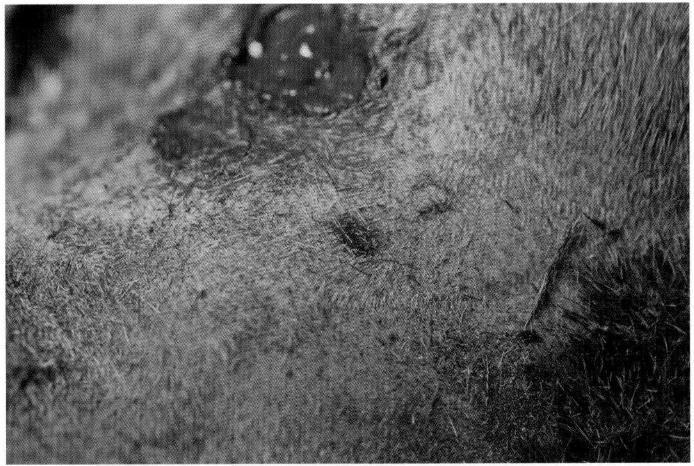

Fig. 8.2 Circular and linear abrasion adjacent to the gunshot wound (see Figure 8.1) from the impact of wadding.

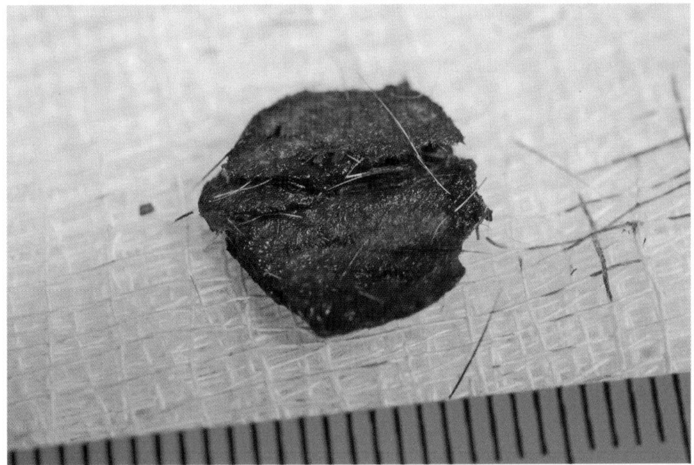

Fig. 8.3 Paper wadding found inside the second entrance wound (see Figure 8.1)

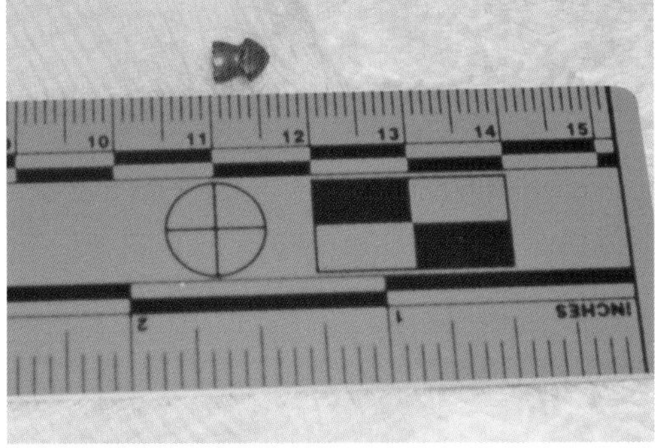

Fig. 8.4 Conical pellet from an air rifle that was fired into the neck of a dog and recovered from the opposite right shoulder (see Figure 8.5).

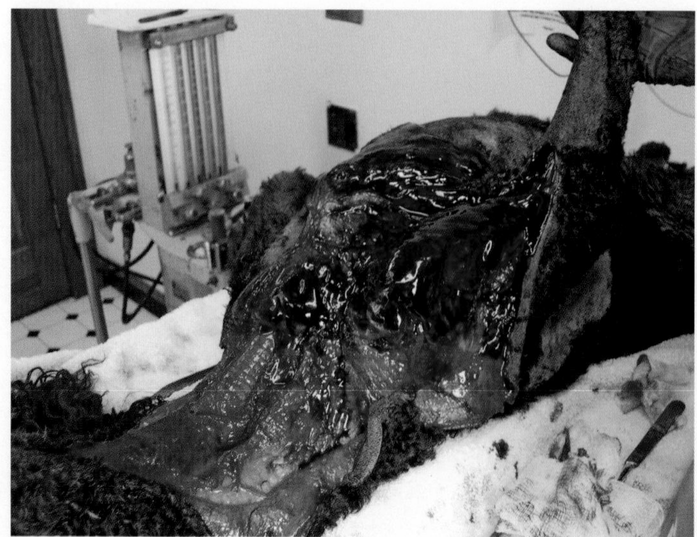

Fig. 8.5 This dog was shot with an air rifle. The pellet entered the left neck, perforated the trachea, punctured the right carotid artery, punctured the right jugular vein, and lodged in the subcutaneous tissue over the right shoulder. The dog died from massive exsanguination into the surrounding tissue and mediastinum.

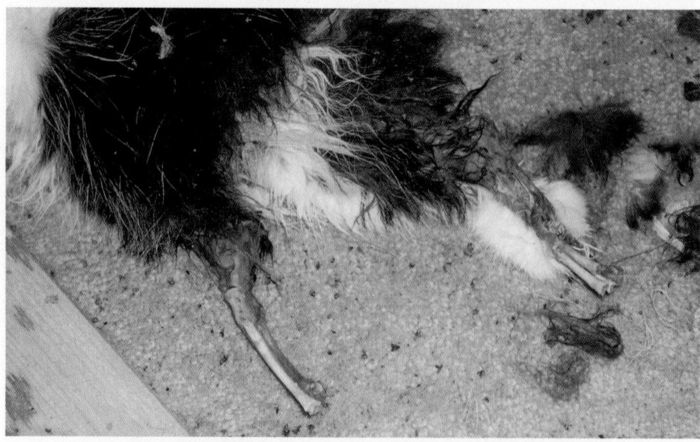

Fig. 11.1 Cat hoarding case with cannibalism of the hind feet of a cat.

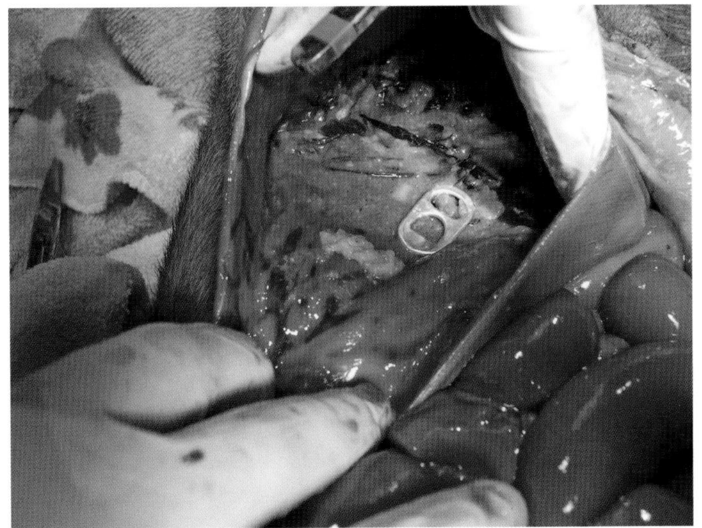

Fig. 11.2 Stomach contents of starving dog with evidence of pica: pieces of plastic, metal tab from soda can, and gastric ulceration.

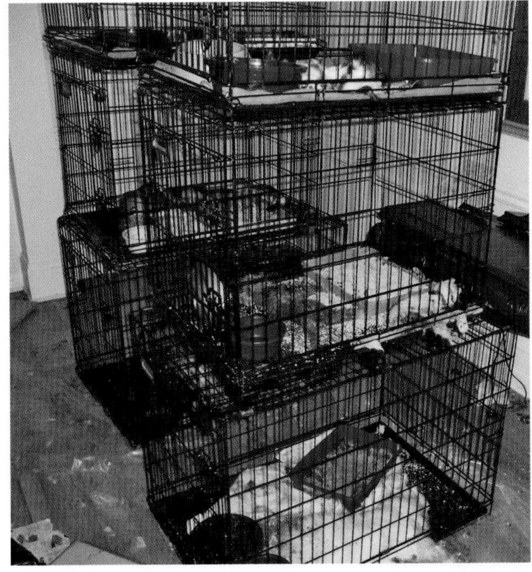

Fig. 11.3 Cat hoarding case with multiple cages containing deceased cats.

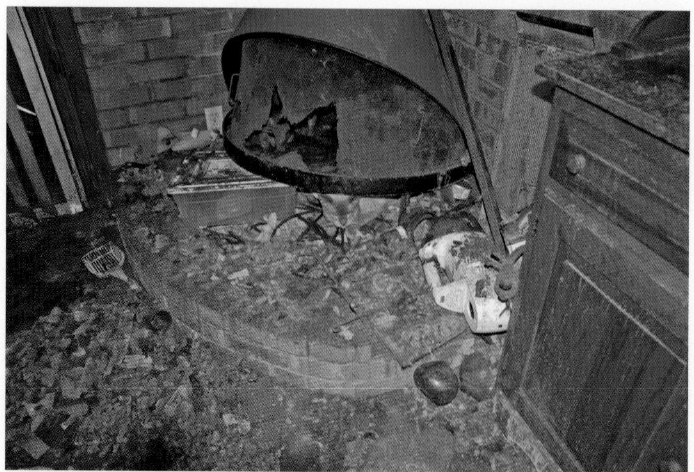

Fig. 11.4 Cat hoarding case with the surfaces covered with urine and feces.

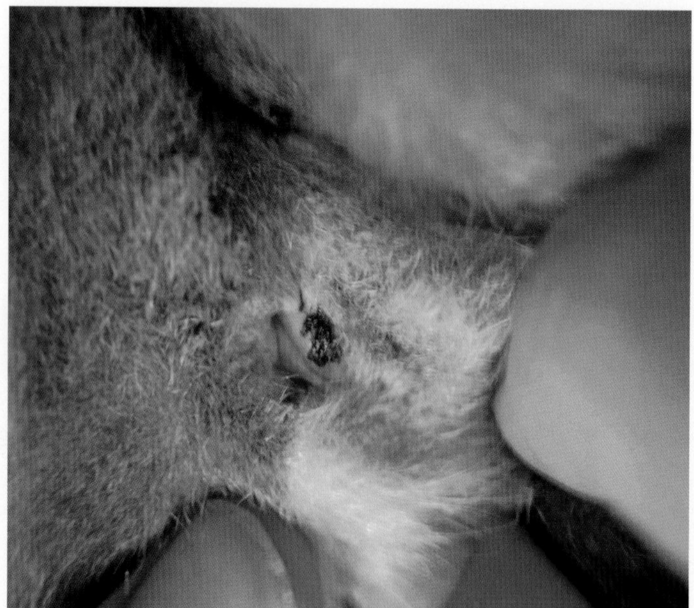

Fig. 11.5 Vulva abrasions found in a cat hoarding case.

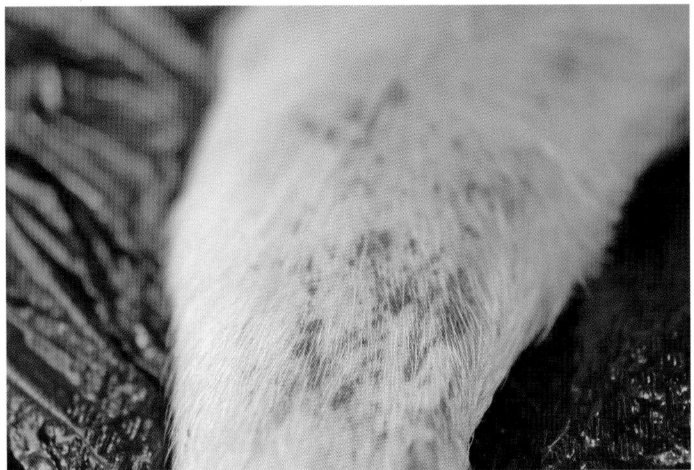

Fig. 11.6 Skin petechiae in a dog that died of heat stroke.

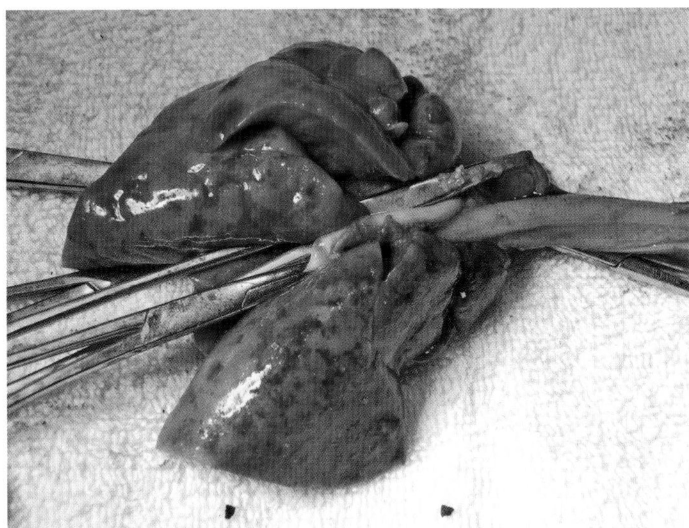

Fig. 11.7 Petechiae on the lung surface in a puppy that died from hypothermia.

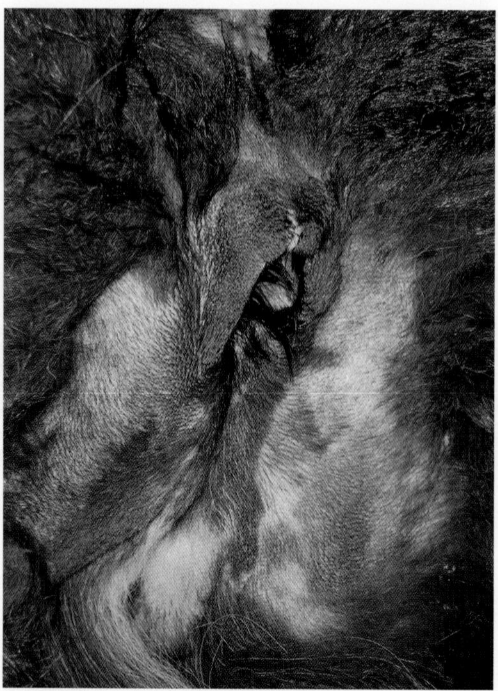

Fig. 12.1 Canine sexual assault victim: perianal subcutaneous hemorrhage resulting from a proximal tail fracture, external vulva abrasions, perivulvar bruising, medial thigh bruising, and cervical bruising (not pictured).

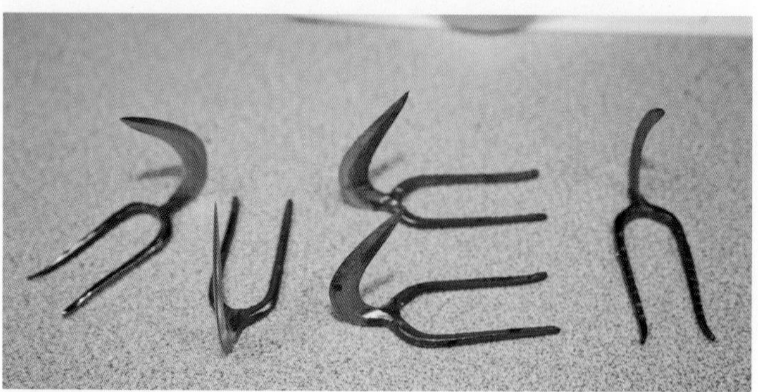

Fig. 13.1 Blades that are tied to the legs of gamecocks for cockfighting.

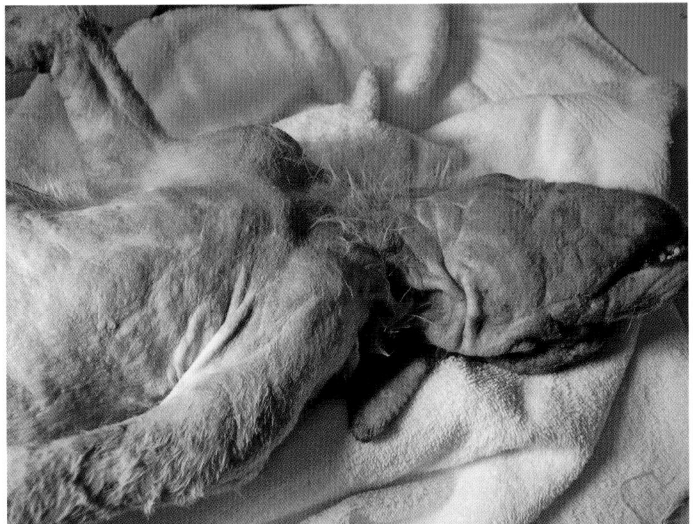

Fig. 14.1 Lividity on the ventral surface of the body.

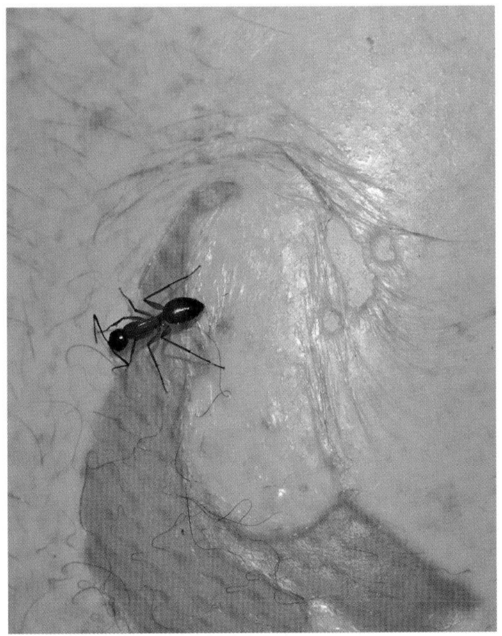

Fig. 14.2 Postmortem ant feeding causing injury artifact on a human body.

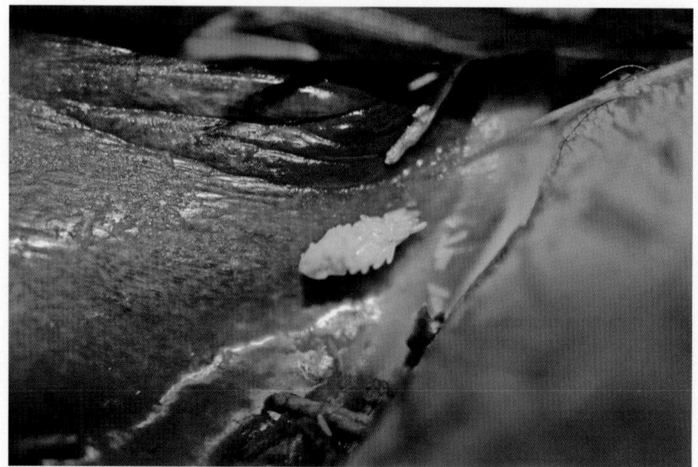

Fig. 14.3 Freshly laid blow fly eggs (maggot eggs).

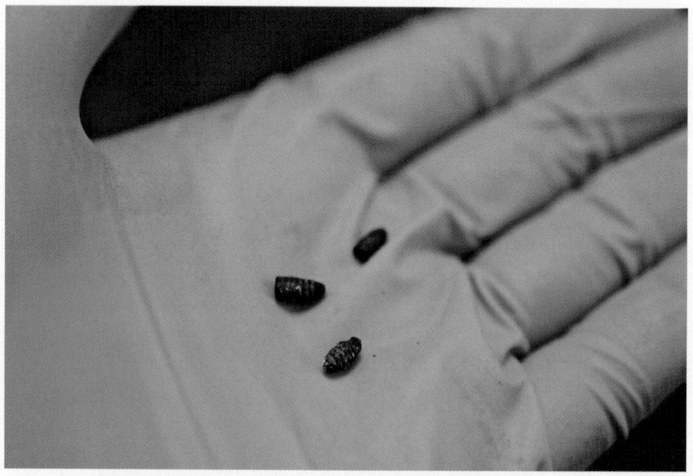

Fig. 14.4 Blow fly puparium and empty pupa case.

Chapter 13
Animal Fighting

Overview of Dog Fighting

Dog fighting is a violent blood sport that is illegal in all 50 of the United States and is a felony in most states. Some states have felony laws for the spectators of dog fighting. In addition to animal cruelty, dog fighting is associated with illegal gambling, drugs, and firearms. Recently, the sport of hog-dog rodeo has become popular. This involves the use of a captured wild hog that one to two pit bulls are released to attack in an enclosed arena. In addition to the same issues associated with traditional dog fighting, there is the issue of the illegal captivity of the wild hog. It is important for the veterinarian to be familiar with all aspects and issues of dog fighting to recognize and interpret evidence found on the animal or at the scene.

The Pit Bull Breed

The pit bull is the most common breed involved in dog fighting. In some areas, other breeds of dogs are being used, such as the Presa Canarios. The original dog used was the bulldog. The breed was ultimately cross-bred with terrier-type dogs selected for characteristics to make them better fighters, producing the Staffordshire bull terrier. The dog needed to have a compact size but maintain its original strength. The bite style of puncture, shake, and tear was desired to inflict the maximum amount of tissue damage. They needed to have excellent agility and athleticism to avoid serious injuries. The dog needed to be highly aggressive toward other animals but not humans. This allowed the handler to safely separate dogs during a fight. These dogs should ignore signs of submission and instead continue to attack. They were selected to not show behavioral cues that an attack was imminent, such as raising hackles or bearing of teeth. Most importantly, these dogs were bred for gameness. Gameness refers to the animal's willingness to continue to fight regardless of the injuries, pain, or suffering the dog is enduring. The term *deep game* or *dead game* refers to a dog's willingness to fight until death (Dinnage, Bollen, and Giacoppo 2004).

Eventually, breeding took place outside of Staffordshire, England, and the breed's name was changed to pit bull terrier because the dog was bred primarily for the pit. Once the dog came to America, there was a breed split by those who liked the breed, but not for fighting. Breeding to select against the aggressive traits was done to produce a family pet (Dinnage, Bollen, and Giacoppo 2004).

Fighting Classifications

There are three categories of fighting dog owners: the professional (serious), the hobbyist, and the street fighter. The professional dog fighter travels all around the county to participate in fights. The owner invests a large amount of money in training, equipment, and purchasing dogs. Their dogs are often given performance-enhancing steroids. They may be on chronic antibiotics for infections resulting from injuries sustained in fighting. The stud fees from these dogs and the stakes for their matches are usually high (Dinnage, Bollen, and Giacoppo 2004).

The hobbyist is someone who enjoys the local fighting circuit. He or she spends the minimal amount of time necessary on training and may not condition the dog. The main focus of the arranged fights is gambling to win back the owner's investment (Dinnage, Bollen, and Giacoppo 2004).

The street fighter uses the dog for more than fighting purposes. The owner is usually involved with gangs and associated with other illegal activity. Drugs may be hidden under the dog's collar, harness, or dog house. The dog is aggressive toward humans and is the most likely fighting dog to cause a fatal dog attack (Dinnage, Bollen, and Giacoppo 2004). Impromptu matches are usually initiated in public areas. Generally, these dogs are kept in neglectful conditions and may have suffered physical abuse. The dogs may have been debarked and declawed to allow them to attack without audible warning.

The Dog Fight Pit

The dimensions and configuration of the pit varies. They are typically 14–16 square feet with walls 2–3 feet high. The floor may be covered with canvas or carpet to improve traction for the dogs. Most pits are portable, with the walls made of wood or chain-link panels, or they may be made from hay bales. The scratch line is a diagonal line in opposite corners for each dog to be held at before they are released to fight. They may be made with duct tape or spray paint. They are usually 12–14 feet apart, depending on the rules. Occasionally, there is a center line on the floor.

Training and Fighting Paraphernalia

Several types of equipment are used to train and condition fighting dogs and also during a fight. The training starts when the dogs are very young. They are exercised daily and conditioned to be aggressive to other animals. They may be given small live animals to use as toys or the animal may be used to entice the puppies to jump up, grab, and hold on. As the puppies age, bait animals may be used, such as cats, rabbits, or weaker dogs. Neighborhood pets may be stolen and used as bait animals.

If the animals survive, they may be found abandoned and injured. In weaker dogs that are used as bait animals, the owner may file or break off the dog's canine teeth to further reduce the animal's ability to fight back and cause injury to the dog in training. These bait dogs have multiple, deep, infected wounds.

For conditioning, the pit bull dog may be forced to run on a treadmill for several hours a day. To entice it, a small bait animal may be suspended at the end of the machine and later given as a reward. A jenny or cat mill may be used for conditioning. This resembles a miniature horse walker in which the dog is harnessed to a projecting spoke and a small bait animal is attached to a leading spoke to entice the dog.

The springpole is used to reinforce the desired bite characteristics for dog fighting. This device consists of a hide, inner tube, tire, or rope suspended from a large spring that has been suspended from a tree limb or rafter. The device also may be found without a large spring attached. The dog is trained to jump up, grab, shake, and hold onto the suspended material. This exercise builds up the leg muscles from jumping and the jaw muscles from gripping the hold.

A breeding stand, also called a rape stand, is used for preventing the male and female dog from fighting. A bite stick is used during the dog fight to separate the dogs. The stick is inserted in the side of the mouth and manipulated to force the dog to release the hold on the other dog.

All training and paraphernalia should be examined for evidence of use. The identity of the dogs that were fought or that used the equipment may be needed for the case. The rape/breeding stand should be checked with UV light for blood, saliva, semen, and swabs should be taken for DNA testing. The bite stick should be swabbed for blood and saliva. The pit should be properly examined for blood evidence (see Chapter 2). Any deceased animals found that were used as bait animals should be checked for microchips and a DNA sample obtained.

It is common to find antibiotics, steroids, and muscle-building supplements at the home. Surgical instruments and suture material may be found that were used to treat wounds or perform ear crop surgery.

Examination of the Animal

General Considerations

Victims of dog fighting may be male or female dogs. These animals should be examined and photographed as soon as possible after they are impounded. For safety, it is imperative that proper restraint be used. The dogs should be examined for injuries and a time estimate given for the injuries. Each wound and scar should be documented and completely described. The ears of these dogs may have been cropped. Often, this surgery was performed by the owner, which can result in additional charges of practicing medicine without a license. All the dogs should have radiographs to detect older or occult injuries. Detection of injuries on exam may be difficult because they have a high threshold of pain. Measurements of the dog should be taken to compare to blood spatter found in the dog pit (see Chapter 3 for specifics). Buccal DNA swabs should be taken of each dog seized for dog fighting.

For common street fighter dogs, exam findings are often related to their substandard care and conditions. These dogs are usually suffering from starvation, dehydration, heartworm disease, intestinal parasites, skin parasites, and infection. Each dog should have a full blood work-up, including heartworm testing and a fecal exam.

The pit bull is predisposed to several health problems that are unrelated to fighting. They are highly susceptible to the parvovirus and have a high rate of being subclinical carriers of *Babesia gibsoni*. They are also prone to demodectic mange, dermatophytosis, flea allergy dermatitis, acral lick granulomas, acute moist dermatitis, pressure calluses, false pregnancy, anterior cruciate ligament rupture, and hip dysplasia (Dinnage, Bollen, and Giacoppo 2004).

A common issue is the disposition of these dogs after the case has been resolved. Because they have been bred to be aggressive toward other animals and humans (street fighters), public safety is a serious issue. It is the general opinion of most authorities that these dogs be humanely euthanized. Currently, there are several studies into the long-term behavior outcome of dogs that were re-homed after initial positive behavioral evaluations.

Types of Injuries

Dogs that were used for animal fighting have characteristic scars and injuries. They are usually located on the face, ears, chest, and legs when associated with fighting. If the dog showed submission, there may be injuries to the groin and abdomen. Scars or punctures that are from bites usually have corresponding marks from the opposing teeth of the attacker. These marks may indicate the upper and lower dental arcade of the attacking dog. Wounds may be in various stages of healing. Another type of injury is a *ring* injury to the leg. This occurs when a dog bites down on the lower leg and pulls, creating a degloving injury partially or fully encircling the leg (Sinclair, Merck, and Lockwood 2006). Depending on the conditions in which the animal was kept, there may be injuries resulting from pens or debris in the area. The ventral neck often lacks hair and is inflamed from the dog pulling against the tie-out.

Special Tests

The dogs used for dog fighting often have been given muscle-building steroids, drugs that have steroid effects, hormones, and diuretics. They may have been given or exposed to illegal drugs, such as methamphetamine. Urine may be tested for the use of anabolic steroids. It is important to get urine samples as soon as possible because of the elimination periods for the steroids. Oral forms may be found in the urine 2–14 days later; injectable anabolic steroids may last up to 30 days; nandrolone may last up to 8–12 months. Clenbuterol is a sympathomimetic that has an anabolic steroid effect. It is a commonly abused drug by humans or it may be used in horses and cattle. Urine is the ideal source to test for anabolic steroids and similar drugs or masking agents used to hide their use. A very large quantity (25 ml) is needed for some laboratories to perform the test. Although not the preferred source, hair may be tested for these drugs. Serum might be used to test for a specific steroid, so samples should be taken and held. The laboratory should be consulted regarding sample handling and submission.

Overview of Cockfighting

Cockfighting is illegal in most of the United States, and is a felony in several of the states. The sport of cockfighting usually involves two or more birds fighting to the death. The cocks are fitted with gaffs, long knives, or short knives on their legs to use during the fight (Fig. 13.1). Heeling is the act of attaching the steel gaffs or knives to the roosters' legs. The stump where the natural spur as been cut off is wrapped in moleskin or tape and the gaff/knife is attached with leather straps and waxed string. The pit usually has a diameter of 15–20 feet with walls 3 feet high. They may be circular or rectangular and made of plywood, cement blocks, bales of hay, canvas, or Plexiglas. There may be smaller pit arenas called drag pits.

The Fighting Gamecock

Gamecocks used in fighting are usually from two main varieties: Spanish gamecocks and Yankee gamecocks (Dinnage, Bollen, and Giacoppo 2004). The birds are often a hybrid of these birds to maximize the aggressive traits. The show standards for exhibition birds are distinct and they are required to be disease tested by the state and wear leg bands at all times (Dinnage, Bollen, and Giacoppo 2004). It is important to note that raising birds for exhibition versus cockfighting are not mutually exclusive.

Often, the wattles, earlobes, and comb have been trimmed (dubbed) to prevent injury during a fight and reduce the bird's overall weight. The natural spur is cut off leaving a 1/2-inch stump to anchor the artificial spurs or gaffs. Some birds have their feathers shaved around the legs and over the dorsal lumbar region. Serious cockfighters put their birds through intensive training and conditioning, called a keep, to improve the birds' strength and endurance prior to a fight.

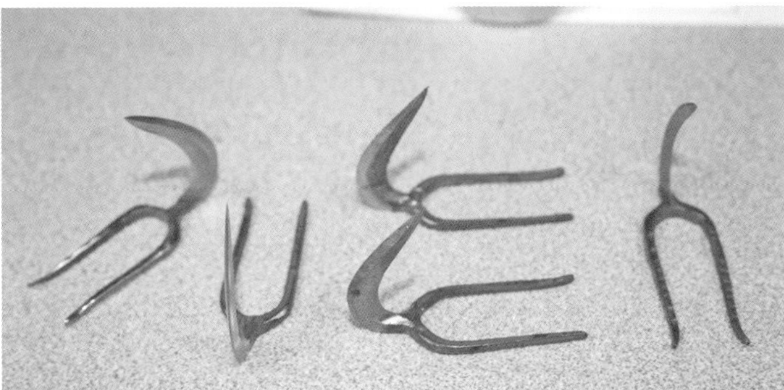

Fig. 13.1 Blades that are tied to the legs of gamecocks for cockfighting. For color detail, please see color plate section.

Examination of the Animal

These birds have wounds that are primarily located on the head. The faces are usually swollen, especially around the eyes. The globe may be pierced but may be difficult to detect because of the swelling. The noses may be covered in blood, causing respiratory difficulty. There may be additional wounds to the body, punctured lungs, and fractures to the legs and wings.

The fighting gamecock often has been given drugs to enhance its performance. These include hormones (testosterone), blood-clotting agents (vitamin K), and stimulants. Strychnine is a stimulant that is often used to increase the rooster's agitation and aggression (Dinnage, Bollen, and Giacoppo 2004). They may also be given digitalis as a heart stimulant. Additional drugs and supplements used in cockfighting include antibiotics, caffeine, methamphetamines, dextrose capsules, vitamin B12, and vitamin B15.

Disease Testing

Each state has specific testing requirements for poultry. This usually includes avian influenza, *Salmonella pullorum*, and exotic Newcastle disease (END). In the past, outbreaks of END in Mexico and the United States have been linked to the illegal smuggling of gamecocks for the purpose of cockfighting.

References

Dinnage, J., K. Bollen, and S. Giacoppo. 2004. Animal Fighting. In *Shelter Medicine for Veterinarians and Staff*, ed. L. Miller, and S. Zawistowski, pp. 511–521. Ames, IA: Blackwell Publishing.

Sinclair, L., M. Merck, and R. Lockwood. 2006. *Forensic Investigation of Animal Cruelty: A Guide for Veterinary and Law Enforcement Professionals*. Washington, DC: Humane Society Press.

Chapter 14
Time of Death

Overview

Determining the time of death is very important in animal cruelty cases. The time of death is determined by the postmortem interval. The time of death may be used to determine the charges in the case. For example, some state felony statutes require that the defendant "knowingly and maliciously" committed animal cruelty. In a hoarding case, time of death was used to meet the felony statute. Using forensic entomology the time of death was determined on the numerous dead animals in the home. In addition, it was discovered that the defendant then obtained more animals *after* the death of the others. It was viewed as a "knowledgeable and malicious" act to bring more animals in to a home in which dozens were already dead, qualifying as a felony animal cruelty charge.

Determining the postmortem interval may be used to support or refute the defendants or witness statements. It also may be used to invalidate a suspect's alibi. The author had one case in which a dog was shot and killed. The main suspect was arrested and put in jail the same day that gunshots were heard. The time of death was determined by the use of forensic entomology and it was proved that the dog died *prior* to the suspect's arrest.

Another consideration is the possible time lapse from the fatal injury to the time of death. In these cases, time of death does not equal the time of the fatal injury. This time lapse may be a short period of time or an extended period if death was slow to come, and is called the survival period. An animal may have suffered injuries and subsequent maggot infestation of the wounds. By using forensic entomology, the time of injury may be determined.

The environmental observations must be recorded to estimate the postmortem interval. When at the scene it is important to know if the air conditioning or furnace is on and at what setting. Confirmation must be made that the power is on and that the heating and air conditioning are working. Often the windows or doors have been opened at the scene to allow dissipation of the foul odor, thereby changing the temperature inside. These windows and doors must be closed, the temperature allowed to stabilize, and then a temperature reading recorded. If heating or air conditioning unit has been turned off or the power has been disconnected, the inside temperature must be taken in addition to the outside temperatures. The times of any temperature readings must be noted.

Determining the Postmortem Interval

The time of death is made by determining the postmortem interval (PMI). Unless the death was witnessed, determining the time of death is an estimate at best. One must take into account all examination, crime scene, forensic tests, and investigative findings to arrive at the estimate. It is critical that investigators interview witnesses and determine when the animal was last seen alive. As a general rule, the longer the PMI, the less precise will be the time of death estimate. No single observation or exam finding is a reliable or accurate indicator of the PMI. Forensic entomology has the greatest ability to give an accurate time of death. By using a variety of methods in conjunction with examination findings, the window of time for the PMI may be narrowed.

Examination of the Body

After an animal dies, the body undergoes a variety of changes. These postmortem changes include livor mortis, rigor mortis, algor mortis, and decomposition. Certain things that do not change may assist with time of death determination, such as gastric emptying time.

Livor Mortis

Livor mortis, also referred to as hypostasis or lividity, is the pooling of blood because of gravity in dependent body sites after the heart stops beating. Lividity is most useful in determining the body position at time of death and whether the body was moved. It is usually visible in light-colored skin, the buccal mucosa, and the sclera (Fig. 14.1). It is also found on the internal body surfaces and internal organs, where it is most noticeable on the surface of the lungs. Lividity on internal organs can be mistaken for congestion. The color of lividity is usually reddish purple to violet, but may vary because of blood oxygen content or certain poisonings. The color is more cherry red, with any condition causing increased oxygenated hemoglobin: carbon monoxide poisoning resulting carboxyhemoglobin, cyanide, hypothermia, or cold environmental temperatures at time of death (Di Maio and Di Maio 2001). In humans, brown lividity has been seen in deaths caused by potassium chlorate or nitrobenzene poisoning (Dix and Graham 2000). The presence and interpretation of lividity may be obscured by the color changes caused by decomposition.

In humans, lividity may be visible from 30 minutes to 2 hours after death, becoming fixed in 8–12 hours. If the body is moved prior to the fixation, livor will shift, responding to gravity (Di Maio and Di Maio 2001). There will be slight discoloration from lividity in the new dependent areas. Livor mortis can speed up with accelerated decomposition or slow down with cool ambient temperatures, becoming fixed 24–36 hours in humans (Di Maio and Di Maio 2001). Lividity is considered fixed when blood shifting and drainage no longer occur because the blood had leaked out of the blood vessels resulting from hemolysis and breakdown of the blood vessel walls from decomposition. To determine if

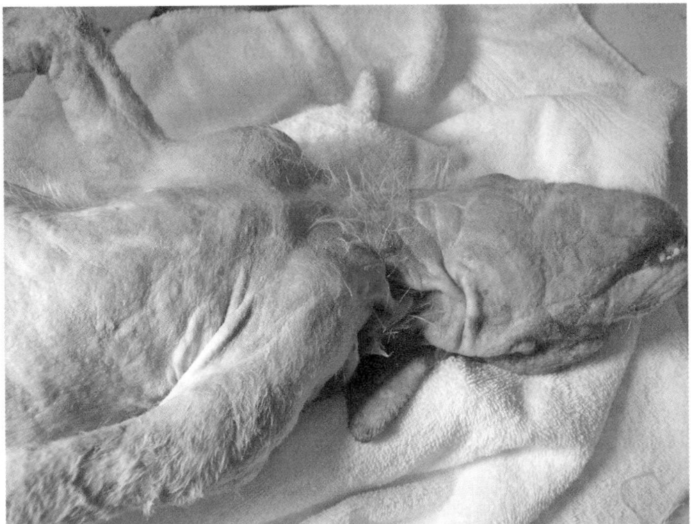

Fig. 14.1 Lividity on the ventral surface of the body. For color detail, please see color plate section.

hypostasis has become fixed, apply pressure to the area; it will not blanch if fixation has occurred. The presence of fixed lividity in non-dependent areas indicates the body was moved after death. Areas that are pressed against a firm surface do not have lividity because the compression of blood vessels does not permit the blood to pool in that area. This allows the veterinarian to determine if the body was moved and reconstruct the body's position after death. The same applies for any constricting material or device on the body. These constricted areas may reveal a pattern related to the item that was used on the body. Lividity may be mistaken for bruising. When pressure is applied to the area there is not any blanching. To differentiate between bruising and lividity, incise the area in question. A bruised area has diffuse hemorrhage into the soft tissues, whereas lividity is characterized by blood confined within the blood vessels (Di Maio and Di Maio 2001).

The pooling of blood can overwhelm the blood vessels and leak out, causing postmortem petechiae, called *Tardieu* spots, or larger purpura. In humans, this can take 18–24 hours and indicates rapidly approaching decomposition. It may occur in as little as 2–4 hours in cases in which the limbs are hanging over something or the body is suspended (Di Maio and Di Maio 2001). As decomposition progresses, the blood vessels can break down and the blood hemolyzes, leaking into the surrounding tissue. The only indicator of antemortem versus postmortem hemorrhage is their location. The petechiae and purpura are located in the dependent areas if they occurred postmortem. Lividity in the region of the head can make evaluation of injuries difficult. As decomposition progresses, hemolyzed blood can leak from the blood vessels into the soft tissues of the scalp, which may be confused as the bruising from head trauma that can occur without abrasions or lacerations. This leakage of blood below the scalp can be difficult to distinguish from antemortem bruising

(Di Maio and Di Maio 2001). Leakage can occur inside the brain into subarachnoid or subdural spaces also, creating a very thin, localized blood film coating the surface. The brain needs to be examined closely for other signs of hemorrhage to rule out postmortem changes. Human drowning victims can show confusing postmortem "hemorrhage" on the scalp where the head was floating down. In addition, a small amount of blood seepage may be seen in the anterior soft tissues and muscles of the neck (Di Maio and Di Maio 2001).

Rigor Mortis

Rigor mortis is postmortem muscle contraction, which immobilizes the joints of the body. Rigor mortis occurs because of the depletion of adenosine triphosphate (ATP), which causes the muscle proteins actin and myosin to stay locked together until decomposition breaks them down. ATP is a source of energy for muscle contractions and needs to be replenished. ATP is used up faster with exercise or exertion, and the consumption of ATP continues after death. Three metabolic systems supply ATP: the phosphagen system, glycogen–lactic acid system, and aerobic system (Di Maio and Di Maio 2001). Rigor sets in faster, sometimes in minutes, if prior to death there was exercise, violent struggle, convulsions, or high body temperature (as seen with sepsis). Rigor occurs in all muscles at the same time, but is noticeable in the smaller muscle groups first, primarily the jaw. It may be forcibly broken by stretching the limbs and will not reform if rigor was fully developed. Rigor recurs if this happens prior to full development, although it is less than the expected stiffness. It is important to know how the body was handled and transported prior to examination. Once rigor has occurred, it then dissipates in the same apparent order of formation. In rare cases rigor is instantaneous at the time of death; this is called cadaveric spasm. This can be seen also with cases of electrocution (Dix and Graham 2000). The body's position frozen in rigidity can help determine if the body was moved as well.

Rigor mortis disappears with decomposition, although it is possible for both decomposition and rigor to still be present in cold drowning cases (Di Maio and Di Maio 2001). Cold body or ambient temperatures slows down and may stop the formation and disappearance of rigor, whereas high temperatures speed it up. If a body is placed in refrigeration prior to the development of rigor, it may slow down or stop. Rigor may be difficult to evaluate in cases in which the body was frozen in cold weather. In humans, rigor may appear 2–4 hours after death and reach full formation in 6–12 hours, depending on perimortem factors, cause of death, and temperature conditions. It may disappear in 36 hours in temperate conditions, but may last up to 6 days. In hotter conditions, rigor may come and go in 24 hours or less (Di Maio and Di Maio 2001). Poisons that cause convulsions or any antemortem condition that causes increased body temperature will speed up rigor. It is important to consider if there was a violent struggle prior to death, as one would expect in drowning victims, which would speed up formation of rigor mortis. Rigor may be delayed or be very mild in emaciated bodies (Di Maio and Di Maio 2001). The onset of rigor is faster and of shorter duration in animals that have decreased glycogen levels, as seen with starvation and exhaustion.

Algor Mortis

Algor mortis refers to the cooling of the body after death. It cools from the normal internal temperature to the surrounding environmental temperature. It also may increase if the environment is hotter than the internal temperature at death or if the body is exposed to direct sunlight. Algor mortis is much more accurate in the first 24 hours after death but is affected by numerous variables. The animal's temperature may be taken rectally or in the liver. A special thermometer is needed to register extremely high and low temperatures. To take the liver temperature, a small incision is made in the skin and the thermometer is inserted into the liver or under a lobe to avoid iatrogenic damage. The place from which the temperature reading is taken can affect the numbers, i.e. rectum or liver. One study in humans found that rectal temperature actually can elevate in the early postmortem period and return to normal in 4 hours, possibly because of continued metabolic activity of bowel bacteria and the body (Di Maio and Di Maio 2001).

To approximate time of death, the temperature at the time of death and rate of cooling must be estimated. It is important to keep in mind that "normal" body temperature is an average of that species. One must also consider that death does not always occur immediately following the precipitating injury or event, and the effects of this on body temperature prior to death. It is important to consider things that would affect body temperature at time of death, such as brain dysfunction from either trauma or disease, which can either raise or lower the body temperature if the thermoregulatory center is affected.

The process of heat loss is affected by: conduction, which is the loss of heat through transfer to objects in contact with the body; convection, which is the movement of air over the body causing cooling; and radiation, which is the loss of heat from the body through infrared heat rays. In addition to ambient temperature, the rate of cooling is affected by the body condition score because fat acts as an insulator and slows down heat loss. The position of the body can affect the rate of heat loss (e.g. a curled body position slows down heat loss). It is also affected by the type and temperature of the surface on which the body is laying, the presence of any covering, whether the body becomes wet, and the weather conditions (e.g. dry, humid, and windy). Smaller animals cool faster because they have a larger surface area compared with mass. The density of the hair coat as an insulator must be considered as well. To complicate matters further, the conditions found at the scene are most likely variable since the time of death, such as ambient temperatures, which rise and fall in a 24-hour period. In addition, weather conditions may change, and the cover over the animal may change with the movement of the sun.

The animal's temperature should be taken at the scene. If sexual assault is suspected, take rectal swabs prior to taking rectal temperature. This should be done multiple times over a 3- to 6-hour period to establish the rate of cooling. The body temperature will keep cooling until it reaches ambient temperature or, if on a cooler surface, until it reaches the temperature of the surface on which it is laying. In humans, the average rate of heat loss is 1.5°F loss per hour with 70–75°F environmental temperatures.

$$\text{Time since death (hr)} = [\text{Normal body temp (°F)} - \text{rectal temp (°F)}] \div 1.5$$

There is the possibility of an initial temperature plateau during the early postmortem period that does not take into account changing environmental conditions. This is possibly a result of the time it takes to establish a temperature gradient. Therefore, a plateau is more likely to occur if the environmental temperature is relatively high, there is body and/or surface insulation (which slows down conduction and convection heat loss), and/or the body is large with a greater amount of external body fat (Henssge et al. 1995). It is recommended to add 1–2 hours to the postmortem interval estimate in cases in which the plateau was likely to have occurred (Henssge et al. 1995). It makes sense to apply this rule to animal cases as well.

Decomposition

Overview

Decomposition involves the two processes of putrefaction and autolysis. Autolysis is a chemical process by the intracellular enzymes that causes the breakdown of tissue and organs. Heat accelerates autolysis, whereas cold slows it down. Freezing can stop the process and in some cases significant heat can inactivate the intracellular enzymes. Organs that have higher enzymes undergo autolysis faster, such as the liver and pancreas. Decomposition usually occurs in 6–36 hours, depending on the condition of the animal and the environmental conditions of the exposed body. Microscopic exam may reveal autolysis of the tissues with no immune or inflammatory reaction. However, the presence or absence of an inflammatory reaction to an area of injury can help determine a time interval between injury and death. Depending on the cause of death or type of injury hemorrhage, neutrophils, and/or edema fluid may be present within hours of the injury. The inflammatory responses may be affected by the age of the animal, tissues affected, medications, and health of the animal. An injury without an inflammatory response is indicative that it occurred in close proximity to death. The nature of any inflammatory response may also determine a time interval, such as in the case of peritonitis resulting from intestinal rupture caused by blunt force trauma. The microscopic examination may have evidence of chronic inflammation, including fibroblasts and hemosiderin (Dix and Graham 2000).

Putrefaction involves bacteria and fermentation and is often used interchangeably with the term decomposition. After death, bacteria from the gastrointestinal tract spread throughout the body. Putrefaction is accelerated in animals that are septic prior to death, and this process may continue even with refrigeration of the body. In addition to the body, the development of putrefaction is dependent on the environment. In high temperatures the rate of decomposition is accelerated and the body can reach an advanced state of putrefaction within 24 hours (Di Maio and Di Maio 2001). The rate slows down in cold temperatures, and may even stop in extreme cold. Even under refrigeration, a non-septic body may still continue to decompose. If the body is constricted in any way decomposition may be delayed. If the animal is overweight, has a heavy fur coat, or is wrapped in something to retain heat, putrefaction may be accelerated. Decomposition may be asymmetrical, occurring more rapidly in areas of injury. Decomposition may progress to skeletonization in only one part of the body because of insect feeding in areas of injury (Dix and Calaluce 1999).

Sequence of Decomposition Changes

The sequence of decomposition in humans begins with a greenish discoloration of the abdomen usually in the first 24–36 hours. This discoloration then develops on the head, neck, and shoulders along with bacterial gas formation, causing bloating of the face. Marbling occurs in these areas because of hemolysis of the blood within the vessels and the hemoglobin reacting to hydrogen sulfide, developing a greenish-black discoloration along the blood vessels at the surface of the skin. In 60–72 hours, the body develops generalized bloating in which the eyes may bulge and the tongue protrude from the mouth. This is followed by development of vesicles on the skin, skin and hair slippage, and the color of the body becoming pale green to green-black. The weight of the internal organs actually decreases with decomposition. A red-colored decomposition fluid, known as purge fluid, drains from the mouth and nose and may be found in the body cavities. This may be mistaken as being secondary to an injury, but the amount of fluid is usually small in the body cavities. Decomposition also causes hemolyzed blood to leak out of the broken down blood vessels into the surrounding tissue (imbibition) usually within 12–24 hours after death. This can be mistaken for antemortem bruising, so careful examination of lividity and concurrent injuries must be done to differentiate the two (Di Maio and Di Maio 2001). Microscopically this is represented by hemolysis of erythrocytes in the blood vessels, whereas the hemorrhage from antemortem bruising is represented by erythrocytes outside the vessels in the surrounding tissues.

Changes in the eyes are difficult to interpret and depend on whether the eyes are open or closed. In humans with closed eyes, a white scummy deposit develops on the cornea, making it cloudy by 24 hours postmortem. If the eye is open and exposed to the air, occasionally a brown to black band may form on the sclera because of drying called *tache noire* (Di Maio and Di Maio 2001).

Following the wet decomposition, the surface tissues begin to dry, collapse, and darken developing a leathery texture. The organs and tissues become desiccated and shrink. Then the body may become mummified or skeletonized. The time frame for skeletonization of the body depends on environmental conditions, insect activity, and scavengers. In humans, if the body is exposed to the elements and available to insects and scavengers, skeletonization can occur within 9–10 days. The last two organs to decompose are the uterus and prostate in humans (Di Maio and Di Maio 2001).

Mummification can occur in hot, dry conditions when the body rapidly dehydrates. The skin appears brown or black and leathery. Decomposition continues with the internal organs turning blackish brown with a putty-like consistency (Di Maio and Di Maio 2001).

Adipocere is a grayish-white to brown, firm, wax-like material made up of the fatty acids oleic, palmitic, and stearic acids. It is found primarily in the subcutaneous tissue and other fatty deposit areas. When a body is found immersed in water or in a damp, warm environment, adipocere formation may occur. It may be seen also in bodies that have been placed in bags. In these warm moist environments, fat undergoes hydrolysis by endogenous lipases and bacterial enzymes to free fatty acids. These are then converted to hydroxyl fatty acids by bacterial enzymes, primarily *Clostridium perfringens*. Adipocere formation can take weeks to several months to develop and is resistant to chemical bacterial destruction.

Flow Cytometry

Flow cytometry has been investigated as a possible instrument to determine time of death in the early postmortem period in humans. The test involves looking at the degradation of nuclear DNA using flow cytometry and comparing it to the degradation in known controls. The percentage of degradation is then correlated to the postmortem interval in hours. The spleen, peripheral blood, and liver have been looked at as possible sources for testing. Research has shown that hepatocyte degradation has a linear correlation with the time elapsed since death. The presence of hepatic neoplasia does not alter the findings. In addition, hepatic tissue is ideal because of the ease of obtaining samples through a biopsy needle (Di Nunno et al. 2002).

Vitreous Humor

Overview

The potassium concentration in the vitreous humor has been used in human forensics to aide in the determination of the postmortem interval. After death, autolysis starts when cell metabolism stops and subsequently the integrity of all tissues throughout the body are lost. Selective cell membrane permeability and the active cell membrane transport ceases. In turn, this causes ions to diffuse across the membranes, depending on the gradients. The vitreous humor is more isolated than other structures in the body and more resistant to bacterial degradation resulting from decomposition. It is relatively more stable postmortem compared with blood or cerebrospinal fluid. The potassium gradient reverses postmortem and diffuses from the lens and retinal blood vessels into the vitreous humor. There may be different levels in the anterior, central, and posterior layers of the vitreous until equilibrium has been reached. As much vitreous as possible should be removed to eliminate the problem of concentration variation in the layers (Henssge et al. 1995). In large animals, the aqueous is sampled for electrolyte testing. The laboratory should be contacted regarding sample collection and submission.

Sampling and Testing

Sampling technique of the vitreous is important. The sample should be aspirated carefully with a syringe and small needle, applying gentle pressure to minimize contamination. Only a clear, colorless sample should be used. The sample is centrifuged and then the supernatant is tested. The sample may be frozen and held prior to testing. A sample from each eye should be taken. It is normal to have up to a 10 percent difference between the right and left eye in humans. Although there are differences between the individual eye measurements, the mean value does not change and the regression lines used for analysis are the same (Henssge et al. 1995).

The relationship of potassium concentration and postmortem interval is linear up to 120 hours. The equation used by Henssge is:

$$PMI = 5.26 \times K^{+} \text{ Concentration} - 30.9$$

The 95 percent confidence level of the formula is 20–100 hours postmortem. The estimate for PMI may be undervalued by 0.3 hour, with a standard deviation of 19 hours (Henssge et al. 1995). A study by James et al. on postmortem vitreous potassium levels was conducted on 100 human bodies that came to the forensic center in which the PMI was known. The study showed similar results to the formula from Henssge (Ross, Hoadley, and Sampson 1997).

The vitreous potassium is of more value after the first 24 hours after death because other measurements are accurate in that postmortem interval (Henssge et al. 1995). The vitreous potassium increases as postmortem time increases, but there is great variability, which increases the longer the postmortem interval. Potassium levels are controlled by the rate of decomposition, so anything that affects this rate also affects the rise in potassium levels (Di Maio and Di Maio 2001).

Gastric Emptying Time

Gastric emptying time and the gastric contents are helpful in human cases to help narrow down the postmortem interval. In an animal, when it is known what and when it last ate, it may be possible to use that information. Gastric emptying time is affected by many factors, including solid or liquid food, the fat and caloric content of the food, water intake, volume of food ingested, and whether the animal was fed meals or free-choice. It can be affected by the age and size of the animal, although in cats increasing age does not slow down the gastric emptying time as it does in humans. Table 14.1 is a compilation of maximum and minimum reported times in dogs and cats. For any determination of the postmortem interval, gastric emptying time must be placed in context with all the other postmortem findings.

Determining the PMI: Forensic Entomology

Overview

Forensic entomology involves the analysis of insects for legal cases, primarily to help determine the postmortem interval. With appropriate collection and documentation, forensic entomology can provide the most accurate time of death. The foundation for the use of forensic entomology is that the time of colonization, rate of growth, and stages of insect succession can be determined by analyzing climate data. Because maggots, with rare exception, only colonize a body after death, this time determination represents the time of death, or the minimum postmortem interval.

Table 14.1. Gastric emptying times.

Dogs	Solids 4.7–15 h	Liquid 0.5–3.5 h
Cats	Solids 4.7–12.5 h	Liquid 1 h

Average Normal for dogs and cats: <14 h.

The veterinarian, as part of the death investigation team, must become knowledgeable in forensic entomology to properly recognize evidence, and collect, preserve and ship the entomological samples. The deceased body of an animal serves as a food source for insects. The decomposition of an animal attracts insects of certain species at different times, depending on season and weather conditions. The changing composition of the body biologically, physically, and chemically alters which insects are attracted over time; this continues until no more food source remains or the environment conditions change to prevent further feeding.

Insects have additional forensic value because they may be analyzed for drugs that were present in the body at the time of death. Certain drugs can affect the rate of larval development, so the presence of any known drugs should be documented for the entomologist's consideration. It is possible to assay the gut contents of maggots for DNA from the body on which they were feeding. This has been used in cases in which a body was moved and maggots that were not even observed on the body were linked by DNA testing. Maggots can help determine the presence of wounds and whether or not the body has been moved or disturbed postmortem. The analysis of insects should be conducted by a forensic entomologist. All samples collected should be shipped immediately to the entomologist. It is recommended to always contact the entomologist prior to shipment to discuss the case and verify that someone will receive the samples and handle them accordingly.

Myiasis refers to the colonization by maggots of a live body. This is usually found on injured or debilitated animals in which blood or excrement is present, which attracts flies. Forensic analysis of the maggots can help determine the time of injury. Myiasis may create confusion forensically on a deceased body when determining the postmortem interval. It always should be noted when examining the body if there are conditions that may have caused myiasis prior to death, such as injuries that may not have resulted in immediate death; then the time frame must be taken into consideration. In severe neglect cases in which the animal may have had excrement on the body for a period of time prior to death, it is possible for myiasis to have been present. Because blow flies are attracted to decomposition, the wounds of an animal may not be colonized until infection and dead organic matter are present.

Numerous insects are of forensic importance, including blow flies, flesh flies, muscoid flies, skipper flies, dung flies, black scavenger flies, small dung flies, minute scavenger flies, soldier flies, humpbacked flies (scuttle flies), month flies, sand flies, owl midges, carrion beetles, skin beetles, leather beetles, hid beetles, carpet beetles, larder beetles, rove beetles, clown beetles, checkered beetles, hide beetles (family Trogidae), scarab beetles, and sap beetles. In addition, venomous arthropods are forensically important in that they can be the underlying cause of death. Scavenging insects are important in that they can feed off the animal and cause postmortem damage to the tissue, which may be misinterpreted as other types of injury (Fig. 14.2). These insects include paper wasps, yellowjacket wasps, ants, cockroaches, pillbugs, and sowbugs. Pillbugs and sowbugs are usually found in the protected area underneath the remains next to the soil. Fire ants can cause tissue damage that resembles burns antemortem. Acrobat ants feed on fly eggs and maggots affecting the initial colonization, sometimes causing a time delay for 2–3 days (Byrd and Castner 2001).

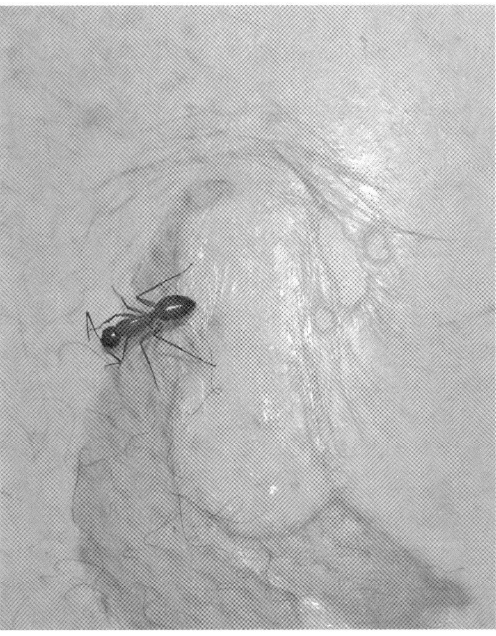

Fig. 14.2 Postmortem ant feeding causing injury artifact on a human body. For color detail, please see color plate section.

Blow Fly Life Cycle Stages

The blow fly is the first insect to colonize on the body after death. It is important for the veterinarian to understand the life cycle of the blow fly to recognize various life cycle stages and collect appropriate samples. The developmental rate of the blow fly species present on the body is used to determine time of death in a fresh body or the first few weeks after death, because it is usually the first insect to colonize on the remains. Additional insect species continue to colonize in a sequential pattern, and these insects help determine time of death when the victim has been dead for weeks, months, or even years. The blow fly first deposits eggs on the body, which hatch and develop to first-, second-, and third-instar larvae (maggots), commonly referred to as instars. They then pupate into adult flies through a process called metamorphosis. This developmental sequence is influenced by species, temperature, weather conditions, and season. It may be affected also by how fresh or decomposed the body and the covering of the animal are, as well as how easily the flies may reach the animal to lay their eggs.

The blow fly eggs hatch into first-stage larvae that are small, vulnerable, and require a liquid protein meal. Because they are unable to penetrate skin, the eggs are usually deposited around a wound or orifice that will provide the liquid meal or allow them to feed on the softer mucosal layers. The larvae may drown in wet areas, so the eggs are usually deposited around the edges of the openings. These eggs are laid in large numbers as an egg mass, which in turn attracts other flies to lay eggs (Fig. 14.3). These eggs hatch after a predictable amount of time, which is valuable in the early postmortem interval when there is little to no maggot activity. Blow flies may continue to lay eggs even after maggots are present. It should be noted that the eggs are usually laid on the body in a preferential order, starting with the facial orifices first. The dating of colonization from the head region and comparing with the posterior region may narrow down time of injury and time of death. If maggots or eggs are found on the extremities of the body it may be indicative of injury. As a rule, blow flies are not active at night and no oviposition occurs.

The blow fly eggs hatch into larvae (maggots) that go through three stages: first-, second-, and third-instar development. The first instars are 1–2 mm in length. They leave behind the egg shells or cast chorions, which can be seen on or around the body. The larvae feed for a period of time, and then molt into their subsequent instar stages, continuing to second and then third instar. They shed the outer layer, the lining of the tracheal system, and the internal cephalopharyngeal skeleton or mouth parts. Each stage has a new set of spiracular slits and mouth parts that are the most diagnostic feature for identification (Anderson and Cervenka 2002). As the number of maggots increases, they form a large mass, which raises the temperature of the body, and within the mass itself. The temperature reading inside the maggot mass is important to obtain for the entomologist. The maggot mass temperatures fluctuate diurnally, so a daytime temperature is representative of the maximum temperature (Anderson and Cervenka 2002).

After a period of time, the maggots enter a pre-pupal stage, a wandering stage, and they are commonly referred to as post-feeding maggots. They leave the area, usually completely leaving the body (although there are some species exceptions), looking for a protected area to pupate, such as soil, clothing, hair, or carpet, and sometimes traveling a significant distance, especially on a hard, exposed surface. In wet environments, they may climb up on higher surfaces, including tree trunks. Some species may pupate on or near the body.

In the next stage of maggot development, the pre-pupal maggot pupates. It hardens the outer cuticle, which darkens in color to form the puparium, also called the

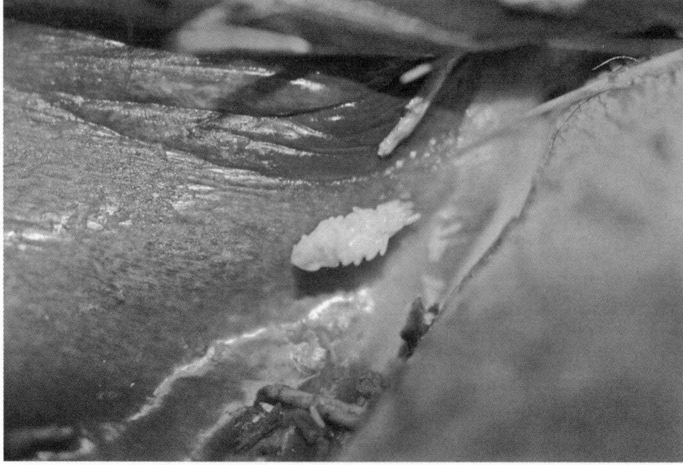

Fig. 14.3 Freshly laid blow fly eggs (maggot eggs). For color detail, please see color plate section.

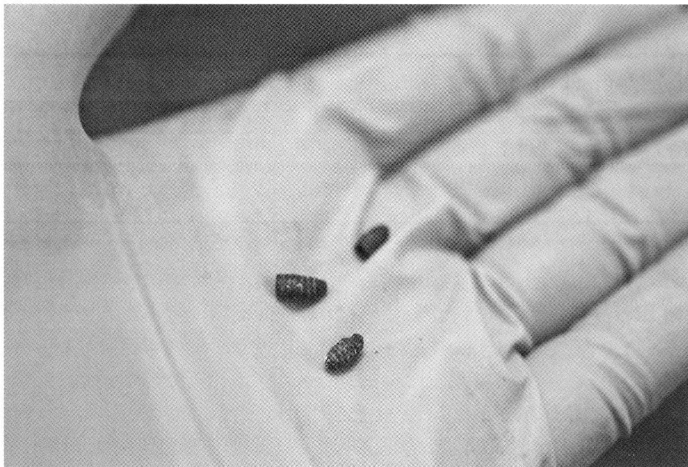

Fig. 14.4 Blow fly puparium and empty pupa case. For color detail, please see color plate section.

pupa case, which now contains the live pupa. Together they are referred to as the *pupa* and the later discarded puparium as the *pupa case* (Fig. 14.4). These puparia are often mistaken for rat droppings, although they have segmental lines that are not found on rat droppings. Initially, the pupa is pale in color and darkens to a red, brown, or black color. The age can be precisely determined at this stage, so photographs should be taken. The subsequent color changes should be noted prior to shipping. If pupa are found at the scene, then a search for pupa cases should be made to determine if the pupa stage represents the oldest stage present, or others have fully developed and hatched into adults.

Once the pupa has completed its metamorphosis to an adult fly, it breaks out of the puparium by forcing the operculum off, splitting the ecdysial cap in half. One-half contains discarded respiratory horns, and the other half contains the third instar mouth parts, which can be used to identify the species of fly. The newly emerged adult fly is spindly, dark, and dull in color, with crumpled wings. It cannot immediately fly. It is fragile, vulnerable, and tends to run and hide very fast. It is often mistaken for a spider. The fly can take up to 24 hours to become fully pigmented and expanded and appear like any other fly, whereas the newly emerged adult blow fly is clearly associated with the maggot activity on the body.

Documentation and Collection of Entomological Evidence

Initial Documentation at the Crime Scene

A trained forensic entomologist will most likely never be at the scene at which the crucial initial assessment, data collection, and sample collection should be done. For this reason, veterinarians should be ready to perform these duties at the crime scene. Entomology logs and data forms are helpful to use (see Appendices 22–24). The very process of collecting insect samples often turns up additional small forensic evidence. If for any reason insect samples cannot be collected, then a written and photographic record of the insects should be taken with a size reference scale in the photo.

The entomological investigation at the scene begins with assessment of the general scene. The physical surroundings and location and placement of the remains should be documented with written notes, photographs, and diagrams or sketches. Special attention should be paid to the position of the body (e.g. curled, prostrate) and the exposure of the head because this is the first area of colonization. A photo log should be kept for all pictures, noting the time they were taken. A route of ingress and egress to the body should be established. The remains should not be disturbed to minimize the impact on both crawling and flying insect activity, and any approach to the body should be careful and slow. Initial observations should start several feet from the body to determine the type of insects present, major areas of insect infestation, and location of insect activity near the body or on the ground. The stages of insects (eggs, larvae, puparium, or adult) and any insect predators should be noted, such as carrion and rove beetles, ants, or wasps (Haskell et al. 2001). Note and measure any insect activity away from the body within 10–20 feet. Note any alterations on the body that could be naturally occurring, from scavengers, or man-made, including trauma, covering, burial, or dismemberment. The exact position of the body should be noted, including position of the extremities and head. What parts are in sunlight and shade should be noted, and what area is in contact with the substrate (Haskell et al. 2001).

Climate and Weather Documentation

After the initial observations, climatological data should be recorded. While these data are being collected, insect sampling and collection can begin. Climatological data are critical to estimate the postmortem interval using forensic entomology and for analysis of other postmortem findings. The time of colonization and life cycle development are largely dependent on temperatures and may be influenced by other factors such as rainfall, sun exposure, and snow. All temperature readings should be done with shading the sensing element of the thermometer to protect it from the influence of direct sun rays.

Ideally, several temperature readings should be taken at the scene in close proximity to the body: ambient air temperature at 1- and 4-foot heights; ground surface temperature on top of surface ground cover; body surface temperature on the upper surface of the body; under-body interface temperature, sliding the thermometer between the ground surface and the body; maggot mass temperatures at the center of the mass; soil temperatures beneath the body immediately after the body is removed; and additional soil temperatures 3–6 feet from the body starting at the ground cover, 4 inches deep, and 8 inches deep. If the body was buried, soil temperatures should be recorded at the depth of burial.

An estimate of the body's exposure to direct sunlight, broken sunlight, or shade during the daylight hours should be made by looking at the surrounding vegetation and structures (Haskell et al. 2001). Blowflies do not like to lay their eggs in direct sunlight.

In addition to data collected at the scene, data must be obtained from the nearest weather station to the scene and for the previous 1–2 weeks or longer in severely decomposed remains. This information is used to evaluate temperatures prior to the discovery of the body. This information is usually available from nearest the National Weather Service station, through a local university, or from a qualified climatologist or meteorologist. In some cases, only the highs and lows and any precipitation accumulation for the time period are available. In some cases hourly readings are needed. Often, this information is only available through a climatologist or meteorologist. The forensic entomologist compares this information to readings taken at the scene.

All effort should be made to collect entomological evidence at the scene. If this cannot happen, then temperature data must be documented every time the animal's body changes environment and/or location. The time and temperatures at the scene are still taken as described. The temperature of the transport vehicle's holding area for the body must be taken and the time recorded for transport in that environment. If the body is placed in a cooler, the time and temperature readings must be documented. This documentation protocol is repeated until the entomology samples are collected. Failure to keep this documentation can cause problems with the subsequent forensic analysis.

Collection of Entomological Evidence at the Scene

All preparation for entomological collection should be done distant from the remains. When collecting insect samples there should be minimal disturbance to the body and any unavoidable disturbance should be documented and photographed. Every effort should be made to get a sample of live flies at the scene where maggots or maggot eggs are present for species identification. Collection of any flying or fast-crawling adult insects is best done with an aerial insect net. One technique is to perform several sweeps over the body, reversing the opening 180 degrees after each pass, ending with a reversal to seal the flies inside the net. This should be repeated three to four times to ensure that a representative sample of flies has been collected. The surrounding vegetation should be swept because the flies may be resting in plants or grasses 10 to 20 feet away. Another technique is to hold the bottom of the net vertically with the mouth of the net over the body using a downward swatting motion. The flies will naturally fly up and into the net.

After the capture of the flies, the end of the net with the insects may be placed in a kill jar for 2 to 5 minutes. Kill jars, made of ethyl acetate and gypsum cement, are commercially available and inexpensive. After the insects are immobilized, they can be transferred to vials of 75 percent ethyl alcohol using a small funnel. An alternative is carefully transferring the netted insects into 75 percent ethyl alcohol by holding the end of the net upward and reaching in and up with the jar of alcohol toward the flies, which have a natural tendency to walk upward, tapping them from the net into the vial. Any ground-crawling adult insects may be collected with forceps or fingers. They should be preserved in the same way as flying insects (Haskell et al. 2001).

Blow fly egg masses should first be photographed and their location documented. Using forceps, break a small piece of egg mass off approximately the size of a dime, taking care to collect from the center as the eggs at the edge may be desiccated and no longer viable. Each egg mass collected from each location on the body should be kept separate. The mass collected should be broken in half and one-half placed in 75 percent ethyl alcohol. The other half should be placed in a larval-rearing pouch. These pouches are made taking a piece of aluminum foil and folding it to create a three-dimensional rectangular pouch, crimping the corners together. A small piece of beef or pork liver should be placed inside as a feeding substrate should the larvae hatch. The top should be crimped together sealing the sample. This pouch then should be placed inside a plastic container for shipment with approximately 1 inch of soil or vermiculite in the bottom and small air holes punched into the plastic top. This substrate absorbs any fluids that leak from the pouch and, for late-stage larval samples, provides a burrowing substrate.

Two labels should be created for the larval feeding pouch with the date and time, case number, location of the sample collected, and sample number. These should be filled out in pencil to avoid any destruction of the writing. There should always be a double labeling system used in which one label is placed inside the plastic container and the other affixed to the outside of the container. For all samples, note the time they were placed in the container and when they were shipped.

When collecting maggots for analysis, it is important to look for the oldest (largest) larvae because they are the ones that first hatched and in turn were the first eggs laid. At first, the body and surrounding area should be examined for pre-pupal maggots (post-feeding). These will be found most likely off the body but may be found in the fur, carpet, the first 3–5 cm of soil, or up to 50 meters from the body. If none are found, then samples of the largest instar larvae should be collected, noting their location on the body. Temperature recordings and time of collection should be documented as described.

A sample of the collected maggots should be preserved at the scene. Place a sample of the largest maggots and some of the next size down into hot or boiling water for 5 minutes to kill and blanch them, documenting the time of blanching. They should then be transferred to a vial of 70–85 percent isopropyl alcohol. They may be placed in 70–85 percent isopropyl alcohol at the scene if hot water is not available for blanching. The vial should be double-labeled as described with egg masses, with one label in the liquid and another affixed to the outside. Another live sample of the maggots should be preserved for examination using the larval-rearing pouches. Do not put too many maggots in the pouch because they need air and too many could cause the majority or all of them to die. Fold over the foil, leaving air above and seal the edges well.

The migratory larvae and puparia may be found usually within 20–30 feet of the body, depending on the species. They may be found under surface debris, in the top few inches of soft soil, vegetation, under rocks, or on tree trunks. The soil and surface debris should be sifted to find migratory larvae or puparia. These samples are post-feeding and do not require a food substrate. They should be placed in the plastic container with vermiculite or sand on the bottom and a damp paper towel to prevent desiccation.

The presence of the empty pupa cases indicates that a complete blow fly life cycle has taken place on the body and indicates a minimum elapsed time since death. These casings are often mistaken for rat droppings. They may be found in the same areas as the pre-pupal maggots and pupae. It is important to look for the ecdysial caps to assist with species identification. These caps are tiny, delicate, and easily missed. They may be found separate from the pupa cases or still attached. The pupa cases and caps should be placed in a dry vial with tissue paper for cushion.

A soil sample from underneath the body, adjacent, and up to 3 feet away, should be collected and placed in a separate container with a solid lid, filling it half full to allow for air if any insects hatch from the soil. Litter samples (leaves, bark, and grass) and any other debris on the ground surface close to the remains should be collected and placed in plastic containers for later examination for insect evidence.

Newly emerged adult flies should be collected in dry vials and a description of their appearance noted, as it will change by the time it reaches the forensic entomologist.

As time goes on, there is sequential colonization of the remains by other insects. The succession of arthropods can be used to determine the minimum and maximum postmortem interval (Wells and Lamotte 2001). Analyses of these later-appearing insects can help with the estimate of the postmortem interval. The successive colonization is dependent on season, weather, and other environmental conditions. The presence of any insect evidence may be forensically important because some insects parasitize others. These insects may be on, below, or flying above the body. All insect evidence should be collected and preserved separate from the maggot samples. Live adult insects should be placed in 70–85 percent isopropyl alcohol and larvae treated the same as blow fly larvae. A soil sample should be collected as with blow fly collection.

Collection from the Body

Collection of entomological samples from the body during examination follows the same basic rules of collection. The time, temperature, and location should be documented for each sample, keeping each location separate. The hand bags, body bags, or any cloth wrapping should be inspected for insect evidence, noting the adjacent body location. If the body was in a cooler and any maggot mass is present, the temperature of the center mass should be taken to see if there was any temperature decrease and if so, by how much. Any botanical evidence may contain hidden insect evidence and should be carefully inspected (Haskell et al. 2001). The areas of insect activity on the body start preferentially around the head, followed by wounds and the urogenital-anal area. The presence of any unhatched eggs may be significant and should be documented. In dried or mummified remains, there may be the accumulation of insect feces (frass). This mass of material can appear like sawdust or pencil shavings (Haskell et al. 2001).

With submerged bodies, there is the possibility of aquatic insects colonizing the remains. This may occur in conjunction with terrestrial insects if part of the body was floating for a sufficient period of time. These aquatic insects can help determine the postmortem submersion interval. Usually only the immature stages of the aquatic insect are found. Care should be taken when removing the body from the water to use a sheet or fine-weave mesh under and around the body to prevent the loss of these insects. They can be very small and fragile, with some having been mistaken for fiber trace evidence (Haskell et al. 2001). The collected specimens should be preserved in 70–80 percent ethyl alcohol for examination. For live rearing, a forensic entomologist should be contacted for current recommendations.

Entomological Evidence in Enclosed Structures

Enclosed structures present several problems. The flies may have limited access into the structure and may be found outside the structure or very few inside. The internal temperature may be very different than the outside temperature. An adjustment can be made if temperature readings are taken from inside the structure over 3–5 days during the peak times and compared with data from the National Weather Service. Often, the first responder opens the windows or doors because of the odor, changing the original inside temperature. First, it must be determined if the air conditioning or heat was on; that temperature setting may be used by the entomologist. To verify this, the windows and doors should be closed and the inside temperature allowed to stabilize. If it is a programmable thermostat, the previous week's program may be retrieved for temperature readings.

The migratory larvae and puparia may be found under carpeting, rugs, or other covering. Dark fly specks, which are fecal spots, may be found on the floors, walls, or ceilings from the flies. Food regurgitation spots that are lighter in color may be found in these same areas. The density of this spotting can indicate the relative size of the fly population attracted to the remains (Haskell et al. 2001).

Determining the PMI: Examination of the Crime Scene

Several types of evidence can be found at the crime scene or on the animal's body that can help determine the time of death. All findings, including examination findings, must be analyzed together to reach the most accurate time of death.

Blood Stains

It is possible to evaluate blood stain findings at the scene to assist in the estimation of time of death. The blood may be fresh or clotted, and the serum separated or dried. It may be in a large pool, or there may be blood spatter. The amount of blood loss should be calculated to help determine if death was caused by exsanguination. Blood can continue to seep from the body after death because of gravity. By recording the blood loss, condition of the blood stains, and environmental factors, scientists can help determine the postmortem interval. Using these findings, they can perform experiments to determine the length of time for that quantity of blood to clot, the serum to separate, or the blood to dry on similar surfaces under similar environmental conditions.

Scene Markers

Other findings at the scene may assist in estimating the time of death. Investigators need to question neighbors to find out when the last person saw the animal alive and the condition of the animal. If the animal was abandoned in a home, the investigator needs to look for signs of when the owner was last there, such as newspapers and mail. The animal's environment and housing should be inspected for clues as to time. It is important to look for what is present as well as what is not present that one would normally expect to find. These may include cobwebs on the body or shelter, fresh urine or feces, lack of fresh urine or feces, botanical evidence, debris build-up around the entrance to a run or crate if the animal was confined, and the presence of mold on the body, feces, or food.

Forensic Botany

Forensic botanists can analyze plant evidence found at the scene and on the body to help determine the postmortem interval, whether the body was moved, and the original location of the body (see Chapter 4). The time frames for the postmortem interval are often months, years, or seasons. The plant specimens may include leaves, twigs, roots, pollen, fungi, and algae that can be analyzed. These plant specimens may be found on the body or in the gastric contents.

Final Analysis: The Report of Exam Findings

The reports generated for an animal cruelty case are very important. These reports are legal documents and are examined throughout the legal process of the case. They are submitted to the investigating and prosecuting agency. As the case progresses, the report is examined by the defense counsel, the defendant, their expert witness, and the judge. It is from these reports that decisions are made by both sides, including whether or not to prosecute and how to charge the defendant. The report may be used to determine plea bargains or sentencing. It is used to map out defense and prosecution strategies.

The contents of the report should be laid out in a logical, factual manner. Often, a report is needed prior to the receipt of all test results and final determination of conclusions. In these cases, a verbal report may be given to the investigating officer or a preliminary report issued. Any preliminary reports should be written with great caution and should not contain anything other than known facts, confirmed findings, and pending tests. If any changes are made in the final report, a valid explanation must be given in the final report. Both the preliminary and final reports should be kept for comparison later. They are both considered evidence and part of discovery to be turned over to the defense attorney. In addition, all notes taken at the scene or during the examination, laboratory results, photographs, radiographs, and any treatment or medical records must be preserved as evidence for the case.

The reports for animal cruelty should be titled "Examination Report" or "Necropsy Report" for a live or deceased victim, respectively. There are report forms from the ASPCA that may be filled out (see Appendices 4–19) or the report may be created as a Word document (see Appendices 20). The following format has been developed by the author in conjunction with medical examiners. It has some variation from the human autopsy report because of the nature of animal forensics. This report format has been well liked by investigators and prosecutors because of its completeness and ease of reading. Those who receive the report tend to read the top, skim the middle, and then read the bottom, so it is important to place all pertinent information in these areas.

Report Format

Heading

The top of the report needs to have information about the investigating agency, lead investigating officer, case number, and animal identification number. This should be followed by information about the examining veterinarian, including the name, address, phone number, fax number, and date of the exam.

Subject of Exam

This section should contain a full description of the animal, including the breed, sex, whether spayed or neutered, estimated age, all coat coloring, and any distinguishing marks.

Reason for Exam

This section should contain a sentence describing the reason for the examination. It may be that the animal was a known victim of cruelty, suspected victim, or deceased animal in which the cause of death or circumstances surrounding the death is unknown.

Crime Scene/Forensic Findings

This section should contain any crime scene or forensic findings. These may be from personal observations during on-scene investigation work or information provided by the investigator. If the information is provided by the investigator, it should be noted, such as "According to Officer (name) . . ." and list the findings that were reported verbally or in the officer's report. All environmental temperatures should be documented here, including the time of the readings. Forensic findings discovered at the scene or conducted by investigators separate and prior to the examination of the animal should be documented. The crime scene and forensic findings are taken into account during the exam and when interpreting all findings and results.

Medical History

There may be cases in which the animal was treated at another hospital for injuries of suspected abuse prior to the official forensic examination. It may be that the victim was initially treated at the examining veterinarian's hospital, and then died later, requiring a necropsy. All medical history related to the victim's injuries should be described in this section, including initial examination findings, response or lack of response to treatment, all medications given, radiographic findings, and whether the animal died or was euthanized.

Examination Findings

This section may have several subsections depending on the nature of the injuries, type of exam, and whether radiographs were taken.

External Exam

This section should begin with a description of the physical status of the animal, including coat condition, body weight, and body condition score. All findings related to decomposition, including rectal temperature, state of rigor, bloating, discoloration of lividity, and distribution of lividity should be listed. In addition, the following should be described: the appearance of the eyes (dried corneas, evidence of trauma); any unusual appearance to the face, ears, nose, legs, or feet; condition of the teeth, presence of tartar, or evidence of oral trauma; presence of vomitus in the nostrils, mouth, or on the fur; evidence of old injuries; evidence of disease; any ectoparasites; presence of urine or feces on the perineum or elsewhere on the body; and any identifying marks, such as tattoos.

Evidence of Medical and/or Surgical Intervention

This section should contain any external findings of medical and/or surgical intervention, including intravenous catheters or chest tubes.

Radiographic Interpretation

If radiographs were taken, the views should be listed and the findings described.

Internal Exam

All necropsy findings are described in this section. Subdivisions of this section are by major organ systems and body cavities. The subdivisions are: head, thoracic cavity, abdominal cavity, neck, respiratory tract, cardiovascular system, gastrointestinal tract, biliary tract, pancreas, spleen, adrenals, urinary tract, reproductive tract, and musculoskeletal system.

Evidence of Injury

In this section, all injuries found, whether major or minor, should be described. If possible, the age of the lesions should be estimated. It is not necessary to repeat the descriptions in the external or internal exam sections. The injuries may be broken down into external and internal evidence of injury. Gunshot and stab wounds should be described in this section, but separate from external and internal evidence subheadings. Gunshot injuries should include a description of the wounds, whether they were exit or entrance wounds, their dimensions, their location related to a landmark, a determination of the gunshot range, the organs penetrated and injured, a description of the missile path such as "front to back and sharply downward," and a description of the bullet, including the approximate caliber if known. Stab wounds should be treated similarly. The description of the wounds should include which edge of the wound was created by the cutting edge of the knife, their dimensions, the wound depth, and the type of weapon used is possible. If there are a large number of wounds, it may be necessary to handle them in groups rather than separately.

Procedures and Results

All evidence collected and tests conducted should be listed in this section. Evidence includes all blood, fluids, tissue samples, swabs, and trace evidence collected from the animal. Any tests that were run on the samples should be listed, including histopathology, toxicology, and DNA testing. Any treatment initiated for a live animal should be documented as well.

Entomology Findings

All entomological evidence collected should be described in this section. The location on the body from which the evidence was retrieved should be noted. The weather data submitted with the samples, if submitted by the veterinarian, should be kept as evidence in the case file. The results reported by the forensic entomologist should be listed in this section.

Summary of Findings

All the pertinent findings should be listed in this section. This should include exam findings, test results, and a summary of the injuries. This section should be written in lay terms as much as possible.

Survival Period

If any findings indicate that the animal survived for a period of time prior to death, then the estimated time should be noted in this section.

Time of Death

The known or estimated time of death should be noted in this section. There should be a description of the indicators that made this determination possible, including the forensic entomology findings.

The next section is known as the "Death/Injury Statement." The final determinations regarding the death or injury are made in this section. For each category, the word *death* may be replaced with *injury* for the live examination report.

Mechanism of Death

This refers to the biochemical or physiological abnormality that resulted in death; for example, shock, septicemia, cerebral edema, ventricular fibrillation, and cardiorespiratory arrest.

Cause of Death

This refers to the injury or disease that began a sequence of events that ultimately led to the death of the animal; for example, gunshot wounds, stab wounds, and blunt force trauma. The cause of death may be proximate or immediate.

Contributory Cause

This refers to any condition the animal had that could have contributed to death; for example, a contributory cause of death in penetrating wounds, in which the mechanism of death was exsanguination and hypovolemic shock, might be a clotting disorder that contributed to the hemorrhage.

Manner of Death

This refers to the circumstances surrounding the death. Traditionally, the classifications in humans are homicide, suicide, accident, natural, or undetermined. In animals, the classifications are non-accidental, accidental, natural, or undetermined.

Conclusions

This section should contain the veterinarian's opinion of all the evidence. It is important to use lay terms to make it easier for all to understand.

References

Anderson, G.S., and V.J. Cervenka. 2002. Insects Associated with the Body: Their Use and Analyses. In *Advances in Forensic Taphonomy*, ed. W.D. Haglund, and M.H. Sorg, pp. 173–200. Boca Raton, FL: CRC Press.

Byrd, J.H., and J.L. Castner. 2001. Insects of Forensic Importance. In *Forensic Entomology: The Utility of Arthropods in Legal Investigations*, ed. J.H. Byrd, and J.L. Castner, pp. 43–79. Boca Raton, FL: CRC Press.

Di Maio, V.J., and D. Di Maio. 2001. *Forensic Pathology,* 2nd ed. Boca Raton, FL: CRC Press.

Di Nunno, N., F. Costantinides, S.J. Cina, C. Rizzardi, C. Di Nunno, and M. Melato. 2002. What Is the Best Sample for Determining the Early Postmortem Period by On-the-Spot Flow Cytometry Analysis? *The American Journal of Forensic Medicine and Pathology* 23(2):173–180.

Dix, J., and R. Calaluce. 1999. *Guide to Forensic Pathology*. Boca Raton, FL: CRC Press.

Dix, J., and M. Graham. 2000. *Time of Death, Decomposition and Identification: An Atlas*. Boca Raton, FL: CRC Press.

Haskell, N.H., W.D. Lord, and J.H. Byrd. 2001. Collection of Entomological Evidence during Death Investigations. In *Forensic Entomology: The Utility of Arthropods in Legal Investigations*, ed. J.H. Byrd, and J.L. Castner, pp. 81–120. Boca Raton, FL: CRC Press.

Henssge, C., B. Knight, T. Krompecher, B. Madea, and L. Nokes. 1995. *The Estimation of the Time Since Death in the Early Postmortem Period*, ed. B. Knight. New York: Oxford University Press.

Ross, J.A., P.A. Hoadley, and B.G. Sampson. 1997. Determination of Postmortem Interval by Sampling Vitreous Humour. *The American Journal of Forensic Medicine and Pathology* 18(2):158–162.

Wells, J.D., and L.R. Lamotte. 2001. Estimating the Postmortem Interval. In *Forensic Entomology, The Utility of Arthropods in Legal Investigations*, ed. J.H. Byrd, and J.L. Castner, pp. 263–285. Boca Raton, FL: CRC Press.

Appendices

Appendix 1	Evidence Log	267
Appendix 2	Cruelty Case Samples Packaging Record	268
Appendix 3	Cruelty Case Samples Receipt Record	269
Appendix 4	Live SOAP Form	270
Appendix 5	Weight Change	272
Appendix 6	Body Condition Assessment	273
Appendix 7	Skin Condition: Cat	274
Appendix 8	Skin Condition: Dog	275
Appendix 9	Condition of Haircoat and Nails: Cat	276
Appendix 10	Condition of Haircoat and Nails: Dog	277
Appendix 11	Physical Care Scale: Haircoat and Nails	278
Appendix 12	Necropsy History	279
Appendix 13	Necropsy Worksheet	280
Appendix 14	External Wounds: Cat	283
Appendix 15	External Wounds: Dog	284
Appendix 16	Fixed Tissue Histology Checklist	285
Appendix 17	Preliminary Veterinarian Statement	286
Appendix 18	Final Veterinarian Statement	287
Appendix 19	Medical Record Certification	288
Appendix 20	Exam/Necropsy Report	289
Appendix 21	Tufts Animal Care and Condition Scale	291
Appendix 22	Forensic Entomology Data Form	293
Appendix 23	Entomology Specimen Disposition/ID Log	294
Appendix 24	Entomological Sample Log Sheet	295
Appendix 25	Forensic Specialists and Laboratories	296
Appendix 26	Animal Cruelty Forensic Kits	308
Appendix 27	Webliography	310

Appendix 1
Evidence Log

Agency: ______________________________

Case Number: __________ **Animal Description:** ________

Notes: ______________________________

____

Items Of Evidence	Collector's Name	Date collected	Disposition

Item: ____________________ Transferred to: ____________________
Received from: ____________ By: ____________________
Date: ____________________ Time: ____________________

Item: ____________________ Transferred to: ____________________
Received from: ____________ By: ____________________
Date: ____________________ Time: ____________________

Item: ____________________ Transferred to: ____________________
Received from: ____________ By: ____________________
Date: ____________________ Time: ____________________

Item: ____________________ Transferred to: ____________________
Received from: ____________ By: ____________________
Date: ____________________ Time: ____________________

Item: ____________________ Transferred to: ____________________
Received from: ____________ By: ____________________
Date: ____________________ Time: ____________________

Appendix 2

Cruelty Case Samples Packaging Record

These samples are part of an animal cruelty investigation.

Agency: ____

Case number: ____

Animal ID number: _____________________________________

Date packaged: ____________________ Time: ______________

By whom (print & sign)

____

____

Carrier: _________________________ Date sent: ____________

Tracking number: _______________________________________

Shipment destination: ____________________________________

Samples included in this shipment: _________________________

____

____

____

____

How samples are packaged (Be as detailed as possible including size and color of any sample containers, ice pack(s) included, in baggies, what type of box used, quantity of each item placed in package, how box was sealed, signature across seal, etc.): ____________________

____

____

____

____

____

Appendix 3

Cruelty Case Samples Receipt Record

To whomever receives and opens this package: Chain of custody is a priority with these samples. To ensure samples have not been tampered with, please fill out this form and fax it back to: ___________ immediately upon receipt of the samples. Please keep the original on file.

Case Agency: ___________________________

Case number: ___________________________

Animal ID number: ___________________________

Carrier: ___________________________

Receiving Agency: ___________________________

Date: _______________ Time: _______________

Person receiving package (print & sign)

____

____

Samples included in this shipment: ___________________________

____

____

____

Package description: (Be as detailed as possible including size and color of any sample containers, ice pack(s) included, in baggies, what type of box used, quantity of each item placed in package, was the box open or sealed, if samples were cool, warm or hot, etc.) ___________________________

____

____

____

____

____

Appendix 4

Live SOAP Form

Medical Evaluation of Neglect/Abuse case

Medical History

Exam	**T**	**P**	**R**	**Weight #**

Behavior - Assess strength, activity and interaction with people and animals

Sensorium N Abn	**Integ.** N Abn	**Ears** N Abn	**Heart** N Abn	**MuscSkel** N Abn
Pain Yes No	**L. nodes** N Abn	**Nose** N Abn	**Lungs** N Abn	**Neurol.** N Abn
Hydration N Abn	**Eyes** N Abn	**Mouth** N Abn NE	**Abdomen** N Abn	**Urogen.** N Abn

Body Condition: Ideal **(1)** Underweight/Lean **(2)** Thin **(3)** Very Underweight **(4)** Emaciated **(5)**

Record abnormal findings below

Attach skin/haircoat forms if appropriate ☐ *Physical Findings continued on second page* ☐

Assessment

Plan

CBC/Chem ☐ **UA** ☐ **Fecal** ☐ **Dog - DAG** ☐ **Cat - FeLV/FIV** ☐ **Microchip** ☐

Rabies / / **DHPP** / / **B. bronchisep.** / / **FVRCP** / /

ASPCA

Medical Evaluation of Neglect/Abuse case

Continuation of physical findings

Assessment and Plan - see first page

ASPCA

Appendix 5
Weight Change

Weight Change

Weight (#)

Date / / ______________

Date / / ______________

Date / / ______________

Date / / ______________

Date / / ______________

Date / / ______________

Date / / ______________

Date / / ______________

Date / / ______________

Appendix 6
Body Condition Assessment

Body Condition Assessment

After Dr. G. Patronek, Tufts Care and Condition Scoring Scales, American Humane Association, 1998.

Body condition is determined by both looking at the animal and feeling the animal

☐ 5	Emaciated	No palpable fat Obvious loss of muscle mass All bony prominences evident from a distance Severe abdominal tuck and extreme hourglass shape
☐ 4	Very Underweight	No palpable fat Some loss of muscle mass Ribs, lumbar vertebrae and pelvic bones easily visible Prominent abdominal tuck. Hourglass shape to torso
☐ 3	Thin	No palpable fat Minimal loss of muscle mass Ribs easily palpated (may be visible) Tops of lumbar vertebrae visible Pelvic bones becoming prominent Obvious waist and abdominal tuck
☐ 2	Underweight/Lean	Waist visible from above. Abdominal tuck evident Ribs easily palpable with minimal subcutaneous fat No muscle loss May be normal for lean breeds such as sighthounds
☐ 1	Ideal	Abdomen tucked slightly when viewed from the side Waist visible from above, just behind the ribs Ribs palpable without excess subcutaneous fat

ASPCA

Appendix 7
Skin Condition: Cat

Condition of Skin: Cat

1) Show location, size, and distribution of skin wounds or lesions (Describe on diagram or in Comments section)

2) External parasites Yes No (Describe in comments section or next to diagram. Include estimate of numbers)

COMMENTS **separate page for description of hair and nails**

ASPCA

Appendix 8
Skin Condition: Dog

Condition of Skin: Dog

1) Show location, size, and distribution of skin wounds or lesions (Describe on diagram or in Comments section)

2) External parasites Yes No (Describe in comments section or next to diagram. Include estimate of numbers)

COMMENTS **separate page for description of hair and nails**

ASPCA

Appendix 9
Condition of Haircoat and Nails: Cat

Condition of Haircoat and Nails: Cat

Physical care scale (see definitions next page)

1) Adequate **2) Lapsed** **3) Borderline** **4) Poor** **5) Terrible**

After Dr. G. Patronek, Tufts Care and Condition Scoring Scales, American Humane Association, 1998.

COMMENTS

ASPCA

Appendix 10
Condition of Haircoat and Nails: Dog

Condition of Haircoat and Nails: Dog

Physical care scale (see definitions next page)

1) Adequate **2) Lapsed** **3) Borderline** **4) Poor** **5) Terrible**

After Dr. G. Patronek, Tufts Care and Condition Scoring Scales, American Humane Association, 1998.

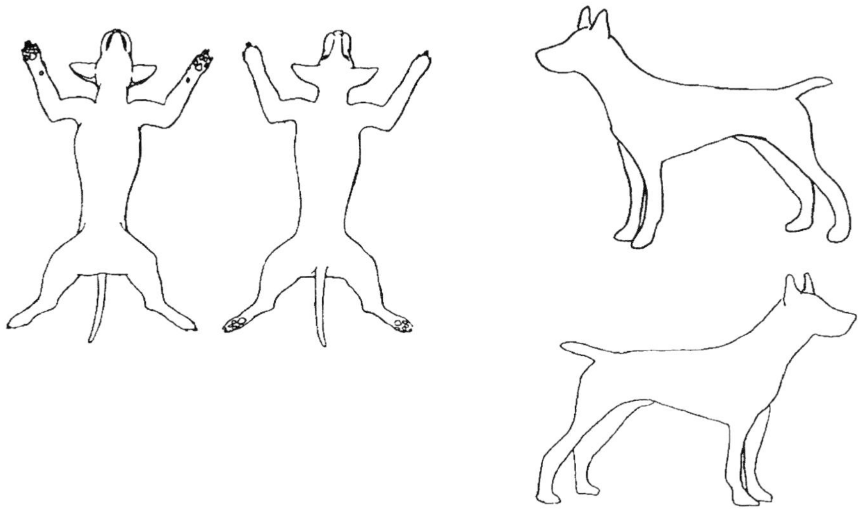

COMMENTS

ASPCA

Appendix 11

Physical Care Scale: Haircoat and Nails

Physical Care Scale: Haircoat and Nails

After Dr. G. Patronek, Tufts Care and Condition Scoring Scales, American Humane Association, 1998.

☐ 5 Terrible	Haircoat a single mat that prevents normal movement and interferes with vision. Soiling of hind end and legs with trapped urine and feces. A complete clipdown required. Nails extremely overgrown into circles and may be penetrating pads causing pain and infection. Nails interfering with normal gait.
☐ 4 Poor	Substantial matting of haircoat. Large sections of hair matted together. Occasional foreign material embedded in mats. Much of the hair will need to be clipped. Fecal and urine soiling of hind end and legs. Long nails that interfere with normal gait.
☐ 3 Borderline	Numerous mats, but animal can still be groomed without a total clip down. No significant fecal or urine soiling. Nails are overgrown which may alter gait.
☐ 2 Lapsed	Haircoat may be somewhat dirty or have a few mats present that are easily removed. Remainder of coat can be easily brushed or combed. Nails need a trim.
☐ 1 Adequate	Dog clean. Hair can be easily brushed or combed. Nails okay.

ASPCA

Appendix 12
Necropsy History

Necropsy of Neglect/Abuse Case

History

Time of necropsy	:	AM PM	/ /
Time dog last seen alive	:	AM PM	/ /
Time animal found dead	:	AM PM	/ /

Describe circumstances of death below

Preliminary conclusion ***Physical Findings on following pages***

Histopathology pending? **Y N**

Toxicology pending? **Y N**

ASPCA

9/24/2003

Appendix 13
Necropsy Worksheet

Gross Examination Worksheet - Necropsy

PROSECTOR: Date: Time: _____ a.m. p.m.

GENERAL CONDITION: (Nutritional condition, physical condition)

Neonates: examine for malformations (cleft palate, deformed limbs etc)

Weight: ___________ #

Body condition
Ideal **(1)** Underweight/Lean **(2)** Thin **(3)** Underweight **(4)** Emaciated **(5)**

SKIN: (haircoat, skin, pinna, feet, subcutaneous fat and subcutaneous bruising)

Attach separate sheet for wound/injury and distribution Yes No

MUSCULOSKELETAL SYSTEM: (Bones, joints, and muscles)
Radiographs: Yes (see separate form) No

BODY CAVITIES: (Fat stores, abnormal fluids)
Neonates: assess hydration (tissue moistness)

After Munson - http://www.vetmed.ucdavis.edu/whc/Necropsy/AppIIe.html 1

Necropsy Worksheet (*continued*)

HEMOLYMPHATIC: (Spleen, lymph nodes, thymus)

RESPIRATORY SYSTEM: (Nasal cavity, larynx, trachea, lungs, and regional lymph nodes)
Neonates: Did breathing occur (i.e., do the lungs float in formalin)? Yes No

CARDIOVASCULAR SYSTEM: (Heart, pericardium, and great vessels)

DIGESTIVE SYSTEM: (Mouth, teeth, esophagus, stomach, intestines, liver, pancreas, mesenteric lymph nodes).
Diarrhea ________________________________
Intestinal parasites ________________________________
Feces submitted for ova and parasites? Yes
Neonates: is milk present in stomach? Yes No

URINARY SYSTEM: (Kidneys, ureters, urinary bladder, and urethra)

After Munson - http://www.vetmed.ucdavis.edu/whc/Necropsy/AppIIe.html 2

(continued)

Necropsy Worksheet *(continued)*

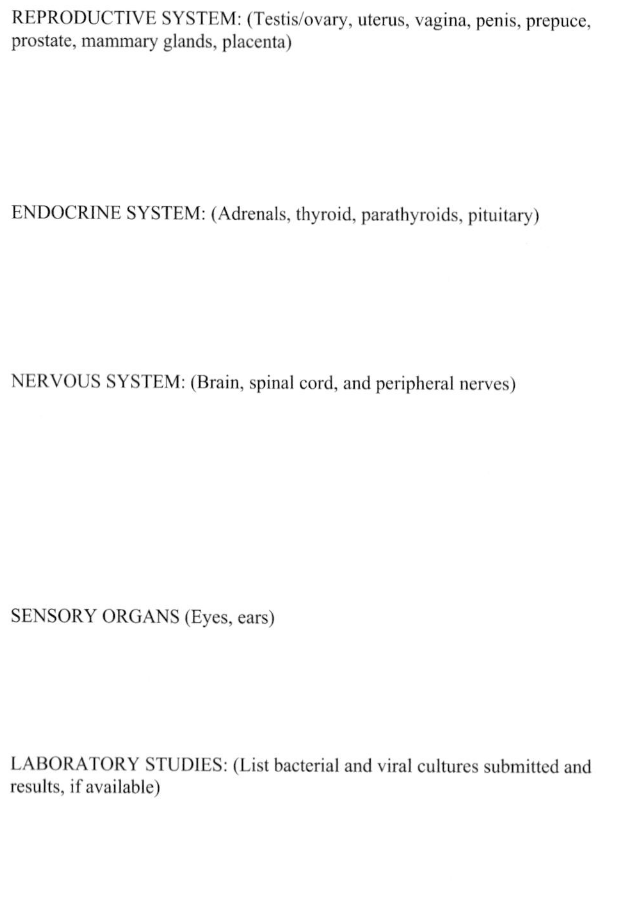

REPRODUCTIVE SYSTEM: (Testis/ovary, uterus, vagina, penis, prepuce, prostate, mammary glands, placenta)

ENDOCRINE SYSTEM: (Adrenals, thyroid, parathyroids, pituitary)

NERVOUS SYSTEM: (Brain, spinal cord, and peripheral nerves)

SENSORY ORGANS (Eyes, ears)

LABORATORY STUDIES: (List bacterial and viral cultures submitted and results, if available)

Attach sample submission checklist

After Munson - http://www.vetmed.ucdavis.edu/whc/Necropsy/AppIIe.html 3

Appendix 14

External Wounds: Cat

Necropsy: External Wounds/Lesions: Cat

1) Show location, size, and distribution of skin wounds or lesions (Describe on diagram or in Comments section)

2) External parasites Yes No (Describe in comments section or next to diagram. Include estimate of numbers)

COMMENTS

Appendix 15

External Wounds: Dog

Necropsy: External Wounds/Lesions: Dog

1) Show location, size, and distribution of skin wounds or lesions (Describe on diagram or in Comments section)

2) External parasites Yes No (Describe in comments section or next to diagram. Include estimate of numbers)

COMMENTS **separate page for description of hair and nails**

Appendix 16

Fixed Tissue Histology Checklist

Preserve the following tissues in 10% buffered formalin at a ratio of 1 part tissue to 10 parts formalin. Tissues should be no thicker than 1 cm.
INCLUDE SECTIONS OF ALL LESIONS AND SAMPLES OF ALL TISSUES ON THE TISSUE LIST.

____ **Salivary gland**
____ **Oral/pharyngeal mucosa and tonsil:** plus any areas with erosions, ulcerations, or other lesions
____ **Tongue:** cross section near tip, including both mucosal surfaces
____ **Lung:** sections from several lobes, including a major bronchus
____ **Trachea**
____ **Thyroid/parathyroids**
____ **Lymph nodes:** cervical, mediastinal, bronchial, mesenteric, and lumbar. Cut transversely.
____ **Thymus**
____ **Heart:** sections from both sides, including valves
____ **Liver:** sections from three different areas, including gall bladder
____ **Spleen:** cross sections, including capsule
____ **Gastrointestinal tract:** 3-cm-long sections of:
  Esophagus
  Stomach: multiple sections from all regions of the lining
  Intestines: multiple sections from different areas
____ **Omentum:** ~3-cm square
____ **Pancreas:** sections from two areas
____ **Adrenal:** entire gland with transverse incision
____ **Kidney:** cortex and medulla from each kidney
____ **Urinary bladder, ureters, urethra:** cross section of bladder and 2-cm sections of ureter and urethra
____ **Reproductive tract:** entire uterus and ovaries with longitudinal cuts into lumens of uterine horns. Both testes (transversely cut) with epididymis. Entire prostate, transversely cut.
____ **Eye**
____ **Brain:** cut longitudinally along midline
____ **Spinal cord:** (if neurological disease) sections from cervical, thoracic, and lumbar cord
____ **Diaphragm and skeletal muscle:** cross section of thigh muscles
____ **Opened rib or longitudinally sectioned femur:** marrow must be exposed for proper fixation
____ **Skin:** full thickness of abdominal skin, lip, and ear pinna
____ **Neonates:** umbilical stump, including surrounding tissues

After Dr. L. Munson - http://www.vetmed.ucdavis.edu/whc/Necropsy/AppIIb.html

Appendix 17
Preliminary Veterinarian Statement

Preliminary Veterinarian Statement - NECROPSY

On / / I evaluated a ______________________________ (*age, breed, species*)

I found the ______________ (*species*) to be (*general appearance, temperament etc.*), ____________

List specific findings below

Attach external wound form ***Y NA*** Radiology ***Y NA*** Histopathology ***Y NA***

Body condition at presentation: Ideal **(1)** Underweight/Lean **(2)** Thin **(3)** Very Underweight **(4)** Emaciated **(5)**

Description of body condition on next page

Pending Histopathology ***Y N*** Radiographs ***Y N*** Toxicology ***Y N***

Preliminary Conclusion

The above statement is an accurate summary of my findings

Stamp of veterinarian Signature of veterinarian / / Date

ASPCA

Appendix 18

Final Veterinarian Statement

Final Veterinarian Statement - NECROPSY

On / / I performed a post-mortem evaluation on a ______________________ (*age, breed, species*)

I found the ______________ (*species*) to be (*general appearance*), ______________________________

List specific findings below

Attach External wound form ***Y NA*** *Internal wound form* ***Y NA*** *Histopathology results* ***Y NA***

Attach Radiology interpretation ***Y NA*** *Radiology consult* ***Y NA*** *Toxicology results* ***Y NA***

Body condition at presentation: Ideal (1) Underweight/Lean (2) Thin (3) Very Underweight (4) Emaciated (5)

Description of body condition on next page **Weight at Presentation ___________ #**

Conclusion

The above statement is an accurate summary of my findings

Stamp of veterinarian Signature of veterinarian / / Date

ASPCA

Appendix 19
Medical Record Certification

Certification of Medical Record

I, *Dr. Robert Reisman*, the Medical Coordinator of Abuse Cases at, the Henry Bergh Memorial Hospital of The American Society for the Prevention of Cruelty to Animals, 424 East 92nd Street, New York, New York, 10128, certify that the attached document is a true and accurate copy of the medical record of;

ANIMAL IDENTIFICATION

Humane Law Enforcement **AO200**________________________________

Bergh Memorial Animal Hospital ________________________________

Animal Placement **A01**________________________________

I also certify that this record was made in the regular course of business of this Hospital. That, it is the regular business of this Hospital to make and keep such a record, and that the record was made upon the dates set forth or within a reasonable time of the condition, act, transaction, occurrence, or event.

Signature: ______________________

Date: ______________________

Appendix 20

Exam/Necropsy Report

Agency:
Officer:
Case:

Examining Veterinarian:

Date of Exam:

EXAM/NECROPSY REPORT

SUBJECT OF EXAM:

REASON FOR EXAM:

CRIME SCENE/FORENSIC FINDINGS:

MEDICAL HISTORY:

EXAMINATION FINDINGS:
External Exam:
Weight:
Coat Condition:
Body Condition Score:
Decomposition:
Ectoparasites:
Head:
Chest:
Abdomen:
Legs:
Feet:

Evidence of Medical/Surgical Intervention:

(continued)

Exam/Necropsy Report *(continued)*

Radiographic Interpretation:

Internal Exam:

- Head:
- Thoracic Cavity:
- Abdominal Cavity:
- Neck:
- Respiratory Tract:
- Cardiovascular System:
- Gastrointestinal Tract:
- Biliary Tract:
- Pancreas:
- Spleen:
- Adrenals:
- Urinary Tract:
- Reproductive Tract:
- Musculoskeletal System:

Evidence of Injury:

PROCEDURES AND RESULTS:

ENTOMOLOGY FINDINGS:

SUMMARY OF FINDINGS:

SURVIVAL PERIOD:

TIME OF DEATH:

MECHANISM OF DEATH:

CAUSE OF DEATH:

CONTRIBUTORY CAUSE:

MANNER OF DEATH:

CONCLUSIONS:

Appendix 21

Tufts Animal Care and Condition Scale

Tufts Animal Care and Condition* (TACC) scales for assessing body condition, weather and environmental safety, and physical care in dogs

*A tool developed for veterinarians, animal control officers, police, and cruelty investigators by Tufts Center for Animals and Public Policy. Published in: Patronek, GJ. Recognizing and reporting animal abuse ~ a veterinarian's guide. Denver, CO:American Humane Association, 1997.

I. Body condition scale (Palpation essential for long-haired dogs; each dog's condition should be interpreted in light of the typical appearance of the breed)

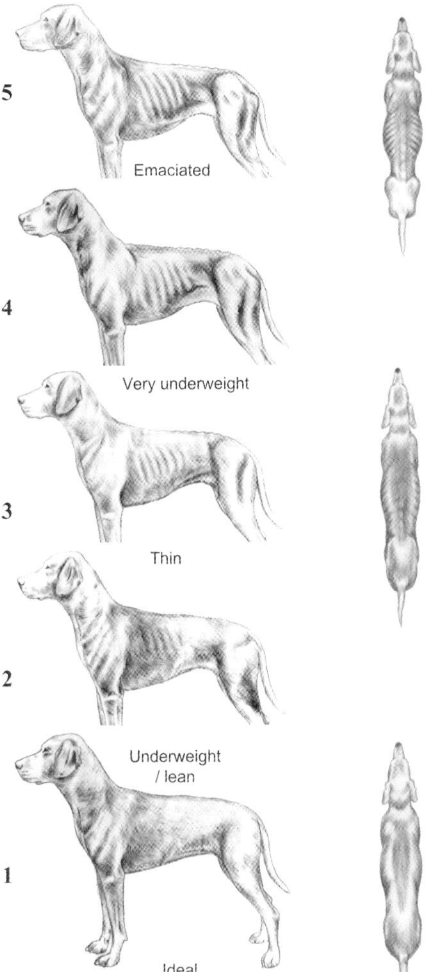

- All bony prominences evident from a distance
- No discernible body fat
- Obvious loss of muscle mass
- Severe abdominal tuck and extreme hourglass shape

- Ribs, lumbar vertebrae, and pelvic bones easily visible
- No palpable body fat
- Some loss of muscle mass
- Prominent abdominal tuck and hourglass shape to torso

- Tops of lumbar vertebrae visible, pelvic bones becoming prominent.
- Ribs easily palpated and may be visible with no palpable fat
- Obvious waist and abdominal tuck
- Minimal loss of muscle mass

- Ribs easily palpable with minimal SQ fat
- Abdominal tuck evident
- Waist clearly visible from above
- No muscle loss
- May be normal for lean breeds such as sighthounds

- Ribs palpable without excess SQ fat
- Abdomen tucked slightly when viewed from the side
- Waist visible from above, just behind ribs

Body condition scale adapted from Laflamme, DP. Proc. N.A. Vet Conf 1993, 290-91; and Armstrong, PJ., Lund, EM. Vet Clin Nutr 3:83-87; 1996. Artwork by Erik Petersen.

(continued)

Tufts Animal Care and Condition Scale *(continued)*

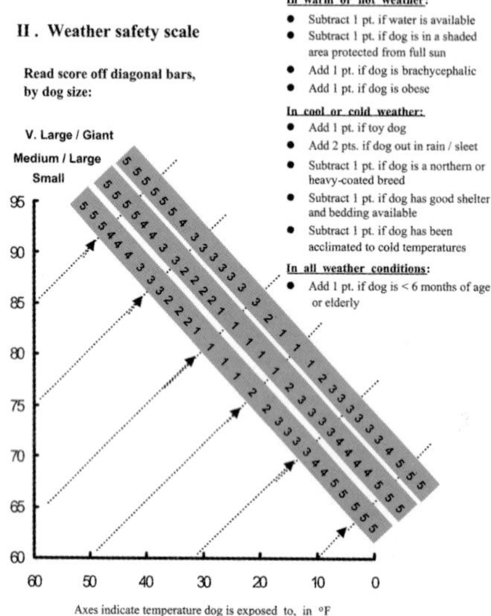

To determine score, draw a line up from the current temperature and parallel to the dotted lines, and read score on bars. Common sense must be used to take into account the duration of exposure to any given temperature when assessing risk; even brief periods of high heat can be very dangerous, whereas a similar duration of exposure to cold temperatures would not be life-threatening.

III. Environmental health scale

5 **Filthy** - many days to weeks of accumulation of feces and / or urine. Overwhelming odor, air may be difficult to breathe. Large amount of trash, garbage, or debris present; inhibits comfortable rest, normal postures, or movement and / or poses a danger to the animal. Very difficult or impossible for animal to escape contact with feces, urine, mud, or standing water. Food and / or drinking water contaminated.

4 **Very unsanitary** - many days of accumulation of feces and / or urine. Difficult for animal to avoid contact with waste matter. Moderate amount of trash, garbage, or clutter present that may inhibit comfortable rest and / or movement of the animal. Potential injury from sharp edges or glass. Significant odor makes breathing unpleasant. Standing water or mud difficult to avoid.

3 **Unsanitary** - several days accumulation of feces and urine in animal's environment. Animal is able to avoid contact with waste matter. Moderate odor present. Trash, garbage, and other debris cluttering animal's environment but does not prohibit comfortable rest or normal posture. Clutter may interfere with normal movement or allow dog to become entangled, but no sharp edges or broken glass that could injure dog. Dog able to avoid mud or water if present.

2 **Marginal** - As in #1, except may be somewhat less sanitary. No more than 1-2 day's accumulation of feces and urine in animal's environment. Slight clutter may be present.

1 **Acceptable** - Environment is dry and free of accumulated feces. No contamination of food or water. No debris or garbage present to clutter environment and inhibit comfortable rest, normal posture and range of movement or pose a danger to or entangle the animal.

"Environment" refers to the kennel, pen, yard, cage, barn, room, tie-out or other enclosure or area where the animal is confined or spends the majority of its time. All of the listed conditions do not need to be present in order to include a dog in a specific category. The user should determine which category best describes a particular dog's condition.

Interpretation of the TACC score from scales I - IV:

The Tufts Animal Condition and Care (TACC) score is assessed from the number of points read off either the **Body Condition, Weather Safety, Environmental Health**, or **Physical Care** Scale. When multiple scales are evaluated, the highest score on any scale should be used to determine the risk of neglect. Multiple high scores are indicative of greater neglect, risk, or inhumane treatment than a single high score.

Score	Body condition, physical care, environ. health scales	Weather safety scale
≥5	Severe neglect and inhumane treatment. An urgent situation that justifies an assertive response to protect the animal.	Potentially life-threatening risk present. Immediate intervention to decrease threat to the animal required (provide water, shelter).
4	Clear evidence of serious neglect and / or inhumane treatment (unless there is a medical explanation for the animal's condition). Prompt improvement required.	Dangerous situation developing. Prompt intervention required to decrease risk (e.g. provide water, shade, shelter, or bring indoors). Warn owner of risk and shelter requirements.
3	Indicators of neglect present. Timely assessment; correction of problems and/or monitoring of situation may be required.	Indicators of a potentially unsafe situation, depending on breed, time outdoors. Inform owner of risk and proper shelter requirements.
2	A lapse in care or discomfort may be present. Evaluate, and discuss concerns with owner. Recommend changes in animal husbandry practices, if needed.	Risk unlikely, but evaluate the situation, and if warranted, discuss your concerns and requirements for proper shelter with the owner.
≤1	No evidence of neglect based on scale (s) used	No evidence of risk

Disclaimer: The TACC score is intended to be a simple screening device for determining when neglect may be present, for prioritizing the investigation of reported animal cruelty cases, and as a system for investigative agencies to use to summarize their case experience. The TACC score is not intended to replace definitive assessment of any animal by a veterinarian or law enforcement agent. A low TACC score does not preclude a diagnosis of abuse, neglect, or a dog requiring veterinary care upon more careful examination of an animal and its living situation.

IV. Physical care scale

5 **Terrible** - extremely matted haircoat, prevents normal motion, interferes with vision, perineal areas irritated from soiling with trapped urine and feces. Hair coat essentially a single mat. Dog cannot be groomed without complete clipdown. Foreign material trapped in matted hair. Nails extremely overgrown into circles, may be penetrating pads, causing abnormal position of feet and make normal walking very difficult or uncomfortable. Collar or chain, if present, may be imbedded in dog's neck.

4 **Poor** - substantial matting in haircoat, large chunks of hair matted together that cannot be separated with a comb or brush. Occasional foreign material embedded in mats. Much of the hair will need to be clipped to remove mats. Long nails force feet into abnormal position and interfere with normal gait. Perineal soiling or irritation likely. Collar or chain, if present, may be extremely tight, abrading skin.

3 **Borderline** - numerous mats present in hair, but dog can still be groomed without a total clip down. No significant perineal soiling or irritation from waste caught in matted hair. Nails are overdue for a trim and long enough to cause dog to alter gait when it walks. Collar or chain, if present, may be snug and rubbing off neck hair.

2 **Lapsed** - haircoat may be somewhat dirty or have a few mats present that are easily removed. Remainder of coat can easily be brushed or combed. Nails in need of a trim. Collar or chain, if present, fits comfortably.

1 **Adequate** - dog clean, hair of normal length for the breed, and hair can easily be brushed or combed. Nails do not touch the floor, or barely contact the floor. Collar or chain, if present, fits comfortably.

All of the listed conditions do not need to be present in order to include a dog in a specific category. The user should determine which category best describes a particular dog's condition. This scale is not meant for assessment of medical conditions, e.g., a broken limb, that clearly indicate a need for veterinary attention.

Appendix 22

Forensic Entomology Data Form

FORENSIC ENTOMOLOGY DATA FORM

DATE: ______________ **CASE NUMBER:** ________________________

COUNTY/STATE: ______________________ **AGENCY:** ______________________

DECEDENT: ________________________________ **AGE:**_______ **SEX:** _____

Last Seen Alive: ______________________ **Date and Time Found:** ___________________
Date Reported Missing: ________________ **Time Removed from Scene:** ___________________

Site Description:
____
____
____

Death Scene Area:

Rural: forest_______ field_______ pasture_______ brush_______ roadside_____
barren area_______ closed building_______ open building_______
other____

Urban/suburban: closed building_______ open building_______
vacant lot_______ pavement_______ trash container_______
other____

Aquatic habitat: pond_______ lake_______ creek_______ small river_______
large river_______ irrigation canal_______ ditch_______ gulf_______
swampy area_______ drainage ditch _______ salt water_______
fresh water_______ brackish water_______
other____

Exposure: Open air_______ burial/depth _______________________________
clothing entire_______ partial_______ nude_______
portion of body clothed_______________________________________
description of clothing ______________________________________
type of debris on body_______________________________________

Stage of decomposition: fresh_______ bloat_______ active decay_______
advanced decay_______ skeletonization _______ saponification_________
mummification_______ dismemberment_____________________________
other: ____

Evidence of scavengers:
____

Possible traumatic injury sites: (Comment or draw below)
____

Scene temperatures: ambient:_______ ambient (1ft) _______ body surface_______
ground surface_______ under-body interface_______ maggot mass________
water temp, if aquatic_______ enclosed structure_______ AC/Heat- on/off_______
ceiling fan- on/off_______ soil temperature- 1in_______ 2in_______

Number of preserved samples ________________ **Number of live samples** ________________

NOTE: Record all temperatures periodically each day at the site for 3-5 days after body recovery.

Appendix 23

Entomology Specimen Disposition/ ID Log

Case # :	Date:
Agency:	

Date Obtained	Sample Number	Location on Body	Specimen Lengths (Range)	Number of Specimens	Stage/ Instar	Family/ Species

IDENTIFIER: ______________________________

Appendix 24

Entomological Sample Log Sheet

Case Number:	Agency:	Date:

NUMBER OF SAMPLES

Preserved:	Live:

WEATHER DATA

SUN	□ Full		□ Partly		□ None
CLOUDS	□ Completely	□ Mostly	□ Partly	□ Scattered	□ None
RAIN	Current Rainfall: □ Heavy □ Light		□ None	Approx. 24 hr total:	
WIND	Direction:		Approx. speed:	Gusts:	
SNOW	Current Snowfall: □ Heavy □ Light		□ None	Approx. 24 hr total:	

SAMPLE INFORMATION

SAMPLE 1:	Date:	Time:	METHOD: □ Aerial □ Hand
Location on Body:		Type: □ Maggots; □ Adult Flies; □ Puparia; □ Beetles.	
		□ Preserved	□ Live for rearing
SAMPLE 2:	Date:	Time:	METHOD: □ Aerial □ Hand
Location on Body:		Type: □ Maggots; □ Adult Flies; □ Puparia; □ Beetles.	
		□ Preserved	□ Live for rearing
SAMPLE 3:	Date:	Time:	METHOD: □ Aerial □ Hand
Location on Body:		Type: □ Maggots; □ Adult Flies; □ Puparia; □ Beetles.	
		□ Preserved	□ Live for rearing
SAMPLE 4:	Date:	Time:	METHOD: □ Aerial □ Hand
Location on Body:		Type: □ Maggots; □ Adult Flies; □ Puparia; □ Beetles.	
		□ Preserved	□ Live for rearing
SAMPLE 5:	Date:	Time:	METHOD: □ Aerial □ Hand
Location on Body:		Type: □ Maggots; □ Adult Flies; □ Puparia; □ Beetles.	
		□ Preserved	□ Live for rearing
SAMPLE 6:	Date:	Time:	METHOD: □ Aerial □ Hand
Location on Body:		Type: □ Maggots; □ Adult Flies; □ Puparia; □ Beetles.	
		□ Preserved	□ Live for rearing
SAMPLE 7:	Date:	Time:	METHOD: □ Aerial □ Hand
Location on Body:		Type: □ Maggots; □ Adult Flies; □ Puparia; □ Beetles.	
		□ Preserved	□ Live for rearing
SAMPLE 8:	Date:	Time:	METHOD: □ Aerial □ Hand
Location on Body:		Type: □ Maggots; □ Adult Flies; □ Puparia; □ Beetles.	
		□ Preserved	□ Live for rearing

Appendix 25
Forensic Specialists and Laboratories

American Academy of Forensic Sciences
Contact Lists of Forensic Specialists
PO Box 669
410 North 21st Street
Suite 203
Colorado Springs, Colorado 80901
www.aafs.org

Entomology Analysis:

American Board of Forensic Entomologists

Gail Anderson, Ph.D., Diplomate
School of Criminology
Simon Fraser University
Burnaby, British Columbia V5A 1S6 Canada
Phone (604) 291-3589
Fax (604) 291-4140
Pager (604) 252-5785
ganderso@sfu.ca

Mel Bishop
Member of Entomological Society of America and The North American Forensic Entomology Association
(434) 531-7780
(352) 843-4127
maggotmel@yahoo.com
maggot1@bigred.unl.edu

Jason H. Byrd, Ph.D., Diplomate
Department of Criminology, Law and Society
College of Liberal Arts and Sciences
University of Florida
201 Walker Hall
PO Box 115950
Gainesville, Florida 32611-5950
jhbyrd@forensic-entomology.com

Val Cervenka, M.S., Diplomate
Invasive Species Unit
Minnesota Department of Agriculture

90 West Plato Boulevard
St. Paul, Minnesota 55107
Phone (651) 296-0591
Fax (651) 296-7386
valerie.cervenka@state.mn.us

M. Lee Goff, Ph.D., Diplomate
Chair, Forensic Sciences Program
Chaminade University of Honolulu
3140 Waialae Avenue
Honolulu, Hawaii 96833
(808) 948-6741
lgoff@chaminade.edu

Robert D. Hall, Ph.D., J.D., Diplomate
Associate Vice Provost for Research
205 Jesse Hall
University of Missouri
Columbia, Missouri 65211
Phone (573) 882-9500
Fax (573) 884-8371
HallR@missouri.edu

Neal H. Haskell, Ph.D., Diplomate
425 Kannal Avenue
Rensselaer, Indiana 47978
Phone (219) 866-7824
Fax (219) 866-7628
blowfly@technologist.com

K.C. Kim, Ph.D., Diplomate
Department of Entomology
501 ASI Building
Pennsylvania State University
University Park, Pennsylvania 16802
kck@psu.edu

Ryan K. Kimbirauskas, Member
Department of Entomology
Michigan State University
East Lansing, Michigan 48824
(517) 355-4665
(517) 353-4354 facsimile
kimbira1@msu.edu

Wayne D. Lord, Ph.D., Diplomate
Forensic Science Unit
Laboratory Division
FBI Academy
Quantico, Virginia 22135
(703) 640-6131
duckislandair@earthlink.net

Richard W. Merritt, Ph.D., Diplomate
Department of Entomology
Michigan State University
East Lansing, Michigan 48824
(517) 355-8309
(517) 353-4354 facsimile
merrittr@msu.edu

Jeffery K. Tomberlin, Ph.D., Diplomate
Texas Cooperative Extension
Texas A&M University
1229 North U.S. Highway 281
Stephenville, Texas 76401
JKTomberlin@ag.tamu.edu

Animal DNA Testing

DNA Diagnostic Center
Veterinary Diagnostic Center
One DDC Way
Fairfield, Ohio 45014
Fax (513) 881-4069

DNA Diagnostics
PO Box 455
626 Bear Drive
Timpson, Texas 75975
(936) 254-2228
info@dnadiagnostics.com

QuestGen
29280 Mace Boulevard
Davis, California 95616
(530) 758-4254
questgen@zoogen.biz

Therion International, LLC
35 Phila Street
Saratoga Springs, New York 12866
(518) 584-4300
therion@theriondna.com

Veterinary Genetics Laboratory
Forensic DNA Testing
Old Davis Road
Davis, California 95616
(530) 752-2211
forensics@vgl.ucdavis.edu

Bone Marrow Fat Analysis

Diagnostic Center for Population and Animal Health
Michigan State University, PO Box 30076
Lansing, Michigan 48909-7576
Director: Reed, Willie M.
Phone (517) 353-0635
Fax (517) 353-5096

Diatom Identification

California Academy of Sciences
Department of Invertebrate Zoology & Geology
875 Howard Street
San Francisco, California 94103-3009
Phone (415)321-8300
Fax (415)321-8615
www.calacademy.org

Animal Forensic Laboratories

US Fish and Wildlife Service
National Fish and Wildlife Forensics laboratory;
1490 E. Main
Ashland, Oregon 97520
Dr. Richard K. Stroud DVM MS
Senior Veterinary Medical Examiner
(541) 482-4191.
Dick_Stroud@fws.gov

General Forensic Laboratories

Aegis Sciences Corporation
345 Hill Avenue
Nashville, Tennessee 37210
Phone (800) 533-7052
Fax (615) 255-3030
www.aegislabs.com

Veterinary Diagnostic Laboratories

Several diagnostic laboratories offer toxicology testing on-site. Check with your local laboratory for more information

Arkansas Livestock and Poultry Diag. Lab
PO Box 8505
Little Rock, Arkansas 72215
Director: Norris, Paul E.
Phone (501) 907-2430
Fax (501) 907-2410

Arizona Veterinary Diagnostic Lab
2831 North Freeway
Tucson, Arizona 85705
Director: Glock, Robert D.
Phone (520) 621-2356
Fax (520) 626-8696

Animal Health Branch
1767 Angus Campbell Rd.
Abbotsford, British Columbia V3G 2M3
Canada
Director: Lewis, Ronald J.
Phone (604) 556-3003
Fax (604) 556-3010

California Animal Health & Food Safety Lab System
PO Box 1770, University of California, Davis
Davis, California 95617
Director: Ardans, Alex
Phone (530) 752-8700
Fax (530) 752-5680

Colorado State University
Veterinary Diagnostic Lab
Fort Collins, Colorado 80523
Director: Powers, Barbara E.

Phone (970) 297-1281
Fax (970) 491-0320

Department of Pathobiology & Veterinary Science
University of Connecticut, Unit 3089
61 North Eagleville Road
Storrs, Connecticut 06269-3089
Director: Van, Herbert
Phone (860) 486-3736
Fax (860) 486-2794

Animal Disease Laboratory
Florida Department of Agriculture
PO Box 458006
Kissimmee, Florida 34745
Director: Miguel, Betty
Phone (321) 697-1400
Fax (321) 697-1467

Athens Diagnostic Laboratory
College of Vet Med, University of GA
Athens, Georgia 30602
Director: Miller, Doris
Phone (706) 542-5568
Fax (706) 542-5977

University of Georgia Veterinary Diagnostic and Investigational Laboratory
43 Brighton Road
Tifton, Georgia 31793-3000
Director: Baldwin, Charles A.
Phone (229) 386-3340
Fax (229) 386-3399

Analytical Sciences Laboratory
University of Idaho
2222 W. Sixth Street
Moscow, Idaho 83844-2203
Phone (208) 885-7900
Fax (208) 885-8937
asl@uidaho.edu

College of Veterinary Medicine
Veterinary Diagnostic Laboratory, 2001 S. Lincoln
Urbana, Illinois 61802-6199
Director: Andrews, John J.
Phone (217) 333-1620
Fax (217) 244-2439

Illinois Department of Agriculture
Centralia Animal Disease Laboratory
9762 Shattuc Road
Centralia, Illinois 62801
Director: Niles, Gene
Phone (618) 532-6701
Fax (618) 532-1195
gniles@agr.state.il.us

Illinois Department of Agriculture
Galesburg Animal Disease Laboratory
2100 South Lake Storey Road
PO Box 2100X
Galesburg, Illinois 61402
Director: Webb, Dale M.
Phone (309) 344-2451
Fax (309) 344-7358
dwebb@agr.state.il.us

Purdue Animal Disease Diagnostic Lab
Purdue University, School of Vet Med
406 South University Street
West Lafayette, Indiana 47907
Director: Hendrickson, Linda
Phone (765) 494-7448
Fax (765) 494-9181

Veterinary Diagnostic & Production Animal Medicine
Iowa State University
1600 South 16th Street
Ames, Iowa 50011
Director: Hoffman, Lorraine
Phone (515) 294-1950
Fax (515) 294-3564

Kansas Veterinary Diagnostic Laboratory
Kansas State University
1800 Denison Avenue, Moiser Hall
Manhattan, Kansas 66506
Director: Anderson, Gary A.
Phone (785) 532-5650
Fax (785) 532-4039

Livestock Disease Diagnostic Center
1429 Newtown Pike
Lexington, Kentucky 40512
Director: Harrison, Lenn
Phone (859) 253-0571
Fax (859) 255-1624

Vet Diagnostic and Research Center
Murray State University
PO Box 2000 North Drive
Hopkinsville, Kentucky 42240
Director: Cox, M. Douglas
Phone (270) 886-3959
Fax (270) 886-4295

LA Veterinary Medical Diagnostic Lab
PO Box 25070
Baton Rouge, Louisiana 70894
Director: Taylor, H.W.
Phone (225) 578-9777
Fax (225) 578-9784

Diagnostic Center for Population and Animal Health
Michigan State University
(toxicology testing available)
PO Box 30076
Lansing, Michigan 48909-7576
Director: Reed, Willie M.
Phone (517) 353-0635
Fax (517) 353-5096

Veterinary Diagnostic Laboratory
1333 Gortner Avenue
St. Paul, Minnesota 55108
Director: Collins, James E.
Phone (612) 625-8707
Fax (612) 624-8707
mvdl@umn.edu

Mississippi Vet Diagnostic Lab
PO Box 4389
Jackson, Mississippi 39296
Director: Pace, Lanny W.
Phone (601) 354-6089
Fax (601) 354-6097

Veterinary Medical Diagnostic Lab
University of Missouri
PO Box 6023
Columbia, Missouri 65205
Director: Bermudez, Alex
Phone (573) 882-6811
Fax (573) 882-1411

State of Montana Diagnostic Laboratory Division
Box 997
Bozeman, Montana 59771
Director: Layton, Arthur W.
Phone (406) 994-4885
Fax (406) 994-6344

Veterinary Diagnostic Center
Fair Street
E. Campus Loop
University of Nebraska
Lincoln, Nebraska 68583-0907
Director: Steffen, David
Phone (402) 472-1434
Fax (402) 472-3094

New Mexico Department of Agriculture
PO Box 4700
Albuquerque, New Mexico 87106
Director: Taylor, R. F.
Phone (505) 841-2580
Fax (505) 841-2518

New York State College of Veterinary Medicine
Vet Diagnostic Lab
Cornell University
Ithaca, New York 14853
Director: Torres, Alfonso
Phone (607) 253-3900
Fax (607) 253-3943

North Carolina Department of Agriculture
Rollins Animal Disease Diagnostic Lab
2101 Blue Ridge Road
Raleigh, North Carolina 27607
Phone (919) 733-3986
Fax (919) 733-0454

Vet Diagnostic Lab
North Dakota State University
Van Es Hall
Fargo, North Dakota 58105
Director: Dyer, Neil
Phone (701) 231-8307
Fax (701) 231-7514

Animal Disease Diagnostic Lab
8995 E. Main Street
Building 6
Reynoldsburg, Ohio 43068
Director: Byrum, Beverly
Phone (614) 728-6220
Fax (614) 728-6310

Oklahoma Animal Disease Diagnostic Lab
Oklahoma State University
College of Veterinary Medicine
PO Box 7001
Stillwater, Oklahoma 74074-7001
Director: Edwards, William C.
Phone (405) 744-6623
Fax (405) 744-8612

University Of Guelph, Animal Health Laboratory
PO Box 3612
Guelph, Ontario N1H 6R8 Canada
Director: Maxie, Grant
Phone (519) 824-4120
Fax (519) 821-8072

Oregon State Veterinary Diagnostic Lab
Oregon State University
PO Box 429
Corvallis, Oregon 9733-0429
Director: Heidel, Jerry R.

Pennsylvania Animal Diagnostic Laboratory System
Department of Agriculture
Pennsylvania Veterinary Laboratory
2305 N. Cameron Street
Harrisburg, Pennsylvania 17110-9408
Director: Acland, Helen M.
Phone (717) 787-8808
Fax (717) 772-3895

Clemson Veterinary Diagnostic Center
PO Box 102406
Columbia, South Carolina 29224-2406
Director: Parnell, Pamela G.
Phone (803) 788-2260
Fax (803) 788-8058

Animal Disease Research and Diagnostic Laboratory
South Dakota State University
PO Box 2175
North Campus Drive
Brookings, South Dakota 57007
Director: Zeman, David Henry
Phone (605) 688-5171
Fax (605) 688-6003

CE Kord Animal Disease Diagnostic Lab
PO Box 40627
Nashville, Tennessee 37204
Director: Wilson, Ronald B.
Phone (615) 837-5125
Fax (615) 837-5250

Texas Veterinary Medical Diagnostic Laboratory
PO Box 3200
Amarillo, Texas 79116-3200
Director: Sprowls, Robert W.
Phone (806) 353-7478
Fax (806) 359-0636

Texas Veterinary Medical Diagnostic Laboratory
PO Drawer 3040
College Station, Texas 77841-3040
Director: Gayle, Lelve
Phone (979) 845-9000
Fax (979) 845-1794

Washington State University
Animal Disease Diagnostic Lab
PO Box 2037
Pullman, Washington 99165-2037
Director: McElwain, Terry
(509) 335-9696
waddle@vetmed.wsu.edu

Wisconsin Veterinary Diagnostic Laboratory
University of Wisconsin
6101 Mineral Point Road
Madison, Wisconsin 53705
Director: Shull, Robert
Phone (608) 262-5432
Fax (608) 262-5005

Wyoming State Veterinary Lab
1174 Snowy Range Road
Laramie, Wyoming 82070
Director: O'Toole, Donal
(307) 721-2051

Appendix 26
Animal Cruelty Forensic Kits

Animal Cruelty Forensic Kits:
for on-scene work for law enforcement and veterinarians

(Kits may be ordered from ASPCA catalogue or Tri-Tech, Inc.)
Evidence tags
Nylon cable ties for body bags
Evidence marking flags
Evidence stickers/labels
Evidence roll tape
Evidence bags, plastic and paper
Smaller paper envelopes for evidence
Plastic evidence jars
Metal evidence collection containers
Swab boxes
Swab protectors
Sterile swabs
Swab evidence labels
Presumptive blood tests
Vinyl photo scales
ABFO L-shaped scale
Measuring tape, metal and soft vinyl
Evidence markers
Plastic disposable tweezers
UV light, long wave, max wattage
UV spectacles
Tyvek suit and boots
Tongue depressors to scoop up samples
Entomology collection tools/jars
Chain of custody/evidence log
Digital thermometers that can register extreme temps
White sheets to wrap bodies
Bagging kit for hands

Animal Cruelty Forensic Kits: for animal examination by veterinarians

Same as above plus . . .
Solid sample metal evidence for collecting accelerants
Trace evidence lifters
White folded paper for trace evidence collection
Magnifying glass
Mikrosil casting putty kit, brown
Trajectory rods
Rape kit

Additional Items Needed: (to which officers/veterinarians usually have access)

Exam gloves
Caps, masks, shoe covers
Digital camera
Large plastic bags
Flashlight

Appendix 27
Webliography

www.aafs.org
American Association of Forensic Science. Source of the Journal of Forensic Science.

www.aavld.org
American Association of Veterinary Laboratory Diagnosticians. From this site you can access the full list of accredited laboratories in the United States.

www.abarbour.net
Website about forensic toxicology.

www.acfei.com
American College of Forensic Examiners. Source for the Forensic Examiner journal.

www.aldf.org
Animal Legal Defense Fund

www.animalforensics.com
The site of Joy Halverson, DVM, MPVM offers forensic animal DNA testing

www.animallaw.info
Michigan State University-Detroit College of Law. This site has case law regarding animals in the United States and the world.

www.animallegalreports.com
Site for the latest legal rulings in cases regarding animals.

www.animalnews.com
Latest news reports on issues regarding animals.

www.api4animals.org
Animal Protection Institute.

www.aspca.org
American Society for the Prevention of Cruelty to Animals.

www.barnsteadthermolyne.com

From this site you can order the ERT 600 thermometer for approximately $16. It has a digital display, is waterproof, can switch from degrees Centigrade to degrees Fahrenheit, and has a 5-inch probe. This thermometer can measure from −58°F to approximately 302°F. You can also reach the company via telephone: (800) 446-6060 or by mail: PO Box 797, 2555 Kerper Boulevard, Dubuque, Iowa 52004

www.bloodspatter.com
You can take a bloodstain tutorial at this site.

www.bvda.com
BVDA forensic supply company.

www.calacademy.org
California Academy of Sciences. Perform diatom identification and testing.

http://canadianveterinarians.net/animal-abuse.aspx
Canadian website with section on animal abuse.

www.crime-scene.com
Arrowhead Forensics. Forensic supply company.

www.crime-scene-investigator.net
This site has links to articles and information.

www.dnacenter.com/forensic/animal.html
DNA Diagnostic Center for animal DNA testing.

www.dnadiagnostics.com
DNA Diagnostics dba Shelterwood Laboratories. This company specializes in animal DNA forensic testing.

www.evidentcrimescene.com
Site to order crime scene and evidence collection products.

www.fbi.gov/hq/lab/fsc/current/index.htm
FBI Forensic Science Communication.

www.feinc.net/cs-inv-p.htm
Crime Scene Investigation information by retired Sgt. Hayden B. Baldwin.

www.firearmsid.com
This site includes information on ammunition identification, gunshot residue, shotgun pattern testing, etc.

www.fitzcoinc.com
Site to order forensic collection and labeling supplies.

www.forensicentomology.com
This website contains forensic entomology information.

www.forensic-evidence.com
Website of information on forensic science, law, and public policy.
www.forensicpage.com/new04.htm
Website listing forensic journals.

www.georgialpa.org
The website of Georgia Legal Professionals for Animals.

www.geradts.com
Dr. Zeno's Forensic site, which contains forensic information about several disciplines.

www.gwu.edu/~forensic/listofli.htm
George Washington University forensic website links.

www.hsus2.org
This website contains The First Strike campaign materials and news stories on national cruelty cases.

www.indiana.edu/~diatom/diatom.html
Diatom home page for Indiana University.

www.k9sceneofcrime.co.uk
CSI Equipment.Com

www.lab.fws.gov
US Fish and Wildlife Service-National Fish and Wildlife Forensics Laboratory.

www.lynnpeavy.com
Lynn Peavy forensic supply company.

www-medlib.med.utah.edu/WebPath/FORHTML/FORIDX.html
Forensic Pathology website.

www/nabr.org/AnimalLaw/index.htm
Animal Law index.

www.ncjrs.gov/html/ojjdp
Newsletter from the Office of Juvenile Justice and Delinquency Prevention.

www.ncstl.org
National Clearinghouse for Science, Technology, and the Law, a program of the National Institute of Justice.

http://netvet.wustl.edu/law.htm
NetVet: Veterinary and animal government and law sites.

www.pet-abuse.com
This is a site that has started an animal abuse database. It also includes other helpful information and links.

www.questgen.biz
Animal DNA testing.

www.sirchie.com
Sirchie: a forensic supply company.

www.staggspublishing.com
Publishing company of forensic books.

http://texnat.tamu.edu/ranchref/predator/pred.htm
Site covering predation findings on wildlife and livestock.

www.thename.org
National Association of Medical Examiners. Source of the journal, *The American Journal of Forensic Medicine and Pathology*.

www.therionDNA.com
Laboratory that performs animal DNA testing.

www.tritechusa.com
Forensic supply company with veterinary and animal forensic kits.

www.tufts.edu/vet/cfa
Tufts University Center for Animals and Public Policy. This site features an animal law search feature and includes its own veterinary forensics site.

www.tufts.edu/vet/cfa/hoarding
The Hoarding of Animals Research Consortium. Contains the Tufts Animal Care and Condition Score.

www.veterinaryforensics.com
A veterinary forensics database.

www.vet.uga.edu/esp/IA/SRP/vfp/sitemap.html
The site of a University of Georgia senior student that focuses on wildlife forensics.

www.vgl.ucdavis.edu
Veterinary Genetics Laboratory of UC Davis. Features forensic animal DNA testing.

www.vifsm.org
The Virginia Institute of Science and Medicine. Provides on-location and on-line forensic education and training.

www.vu-wien.ac.at/i117/forensic/forensic.html
Institute of Pathology and Forensic Veterinary Medicine, Vienna, Austria.

Index

Abandonment, 75. *See also* Neglect
Abdomen
  blunt force trauma to, 98
  compression of, 158
Abrasion ring, 137
Abrasions
  artifacts and, 80
  dating of, 81
  in gunshot wound, 147*f*
  impact, 80
  overview of, 80
  patterned, 80
  scrape/brush, 80
Abuse. *See also* Emotional maltreatment; Neglect; Repetitive injuries
  by breed, 32
  types of, 75
Acceleration/deceleration injuries
diffuse axonal injury, 90–91
shaken baby syndrome, 91–92
subdural hematoma, 91
Accidental injury, 31
Acetaminophen, 190–91
Adipocere, 165, 247–48
Age, 32
Air-powered weapons, 149–50, 149*f*, 150*f*
Airway swelling/obstruction, 157–58
Alcohol, 197–98
Algor mortis, 245–46
American Animal Hospital Association, 5
American Board of Forensic Entomologists, 294–96
American Veterinary Medical Association, 5
Ammonia, 213
Ammunition, 133–34
Amphetamine, 193–94
Anemia, 207–8, 210
Angulation fractures, 84
Animal(s). *See also* Live animals
  behavior of, 34–35
  deceased, 126
  definition of, 4
  DNA testing for, 296–97
  as evidence, 7–8, 31–55
  seizure of, 6
Animal cruelty forensic kits, 305–6
Animal fighting
  cockfighting
    animal examination, 240
    disease testing, 240
    gamecocks, 239, 239*f*
    overview of, 239
  dog fighting
    animal examination, 237–39
    classifications, 236
    overview of, 235
    paraphernalia, 236–37
    pit bull, 235–36
    pit for, 26, 236
Animal hoarders
  crime scene findings, 212–13, 212*f*, 213*f*
  exam findings, 214–15, 214*f*
  overview of, 210–12
  warning signs, 211–12
Anorexia nervosa, 209
Anoxia, 155
Antemortem, 49
Anticoagulant rodenticides, 178–79
Antifreeze, 175
Antisocial personality disorder, 225
Anus, 230–31
Arrows, 105–6
Arterial spurt pattern, 25
Artifacts, 80
Asphyxia
  overview of, 155–56
  in sexual assault, 227
Associative evidence, 20
Attempted drowning, 164
Auto-loading pistols, 132

Autolysis, 246
Avian influenza, 240
Avulsion injury, 102–3

Backspatter, 136
Bacteria, 231. *See also* Zoonotic disease
Bait, 181
Ballistics, 135–36
BCS. *See* Body Condition Scoring
Behavior
  of animals, 34–35
  coping, 71
  of owner, 34
  during starvation, 205–6, 205*f*, 206*f*
Bench/non-jury trials, 4
Bestiality. *See* Sexual assault
Bioturbation, 27
Bite marks, 68–69
Blood
  clotting agents of, 240
  collection of, 50–51
  in CSI, 23–26, 24*f*
  DNA in, 67
Blood loss calculation, 42–43, 106
Blood spatter
  analysis, 25–26
  overview of, 23
Blood stain analysis, 23–24, 258
Blow fly, 251–53, 252*f*, 253*f*
Blunt force trauma
  to abdomen, 98
  overview of, 79
Bodies in bogs, 52
Bodily fluids
  collection of, 35–36
  at crime scene, 23
Body condition assessment form, 271
Body Condition Scoring (BCS), 40
Body, handling of, 52
Bond hearings, 4
Bone
  bullet wounds to, 135–36
  as DNA source, 67–68
  examination of
    in fire victims, 55
    overview of, 52
    pseudotrauma, 52–53
    scavengers and, 54–55
    sharp force injury, 53—54
    in trauma, 53
    water environments and, 55
Bone marrow fat analysis, 208–9, 297
Boredom, 73
Botany. *See* Forensic botany
Botany, forensic, 63–65, 259

Brady material, 9
Brain. *See also* Head trauma
  contusions, 88–89
  swelling, 90
Breed
  abuse and, 32
  poisoning by, 170*t*
Breeding stand, 237
Bromethalin, 179–80
Bruising
  dating of, 83
  overview of, 81–82
  patterned, 82–83, 83*f*
  postmortem findings of, 82
Bubble drops, 24
Buccal swabs, 67
Bullet wipe, 137
Burden of proof, 9–10
Burial features, 27–28
Burns
  chemical
    general findings in, 122–23
    overview of, 122
  classification of, 117–18, 117*t*
  degrees of, 118
  electrical
    general findings in, 123–24
    lightning electrocution, 124
    overview of, 123
    stun gun electrocution, 125
  eschar, 119*f*
  evidence pertaining to, 115–17
  histopathological findings in, 119
  interpretation of, 115, 116*f*
  smoke inhalation and, 125–29
  systemic effects of, 118–19
  thermal
    cigarette, 121
    microwave ovens, 120–21
    overview of, 119–20
    radiant heat, 120
    scalding, 121, 121*t*

Caffeine, 198
Caliber, 139
.22 caliber weapon, 143–44
Caliber nomenclature, 132
Callus formation, 85
Calories, 202, 203*t*
Cameras, 21, 36–37
Cannibalism, 205–6, 205*f*
Carbamate insecticides, 188–89
Carbon monoxide poisoning, 128–29
Cartridge cases, 151
Cast-off, 24*f*, 25

Cause of death, 4
Cavitation, 135
Centerfire rifle, 144–45
Certification of Medical Record, 286
Chain of custody
  evidence log for, 36, 265
  overview of, 36
  samples packaging form, 266
  samples receipt form, 267
Charging document, 8
Chemical burns
  general findings in, 122–23
  overview of, 122
Chest
  compression of, 158
  injury to, 97, 97*f*, 98*f*
Choking, 157
Cholecalciferol rodenticides, 181–82
Chop wounds, 109
Cigarette burns, 121
Circular fractures, 88
Clenbuterol, 238
Climate, 254–55
Clinical pathology, 41–42
Cocaine, 195–96
Cockfighting
  animal examination, 240
  disease testing, 240
  gamecocks, 239, 239*f*
  overview of, 239
Cold stress, 219
Collars, embedded, 220–21
Collecting tape, 62
Colon, 230–31
Coma, 94
Companionship, 75
Compliance, 8
Conditional evidence, 20
Conduct disorder, 225
Confessions, 11
Confidentiality, 5
Contact wounds, 141
Contamination, 60, 61
Contusions
  dating of, 83
  overview of, 81–82
  patterned, 82–83, 83*f*
  postmortem findings of, 82
Coping behaviors, 71
CPK. *See* Creatine phosphokinase
Creatine phosphokinase (CPK), 207
Credibility, 4
Crime scene
  immediate response to, 6
  photographs of, 21, 36–37
  teaching at, 3
  types of, 19
  veterinarian's at, 5
Crime scene investigation (CSI)
  animal as evidence in, 31–55
  blood, 23–26, 24*f*
  evidence in, 22–23, 22*f*
  grave detection and excavation, 26–29
  overview of, 19–20
  photography/videography in, 21
  of ritualistic crimes, 113
  in sexual assault, 226
  the veterinarian's role in, 20–21
  weather data and, 21
Criminal investigations, 19
Criterion of concordance, 167
Cruelty case samples packaging form, 36, 266
Cruelty case samples receipt form, 36, 267
Crush fracture, 84
CSI. *See* Crime scene investigation
"C.S.I." effect, 11, 17
Curriculum vitae (CV), 15
Cuts, 108
CV. *See* Curriculum vitae
Cyanide gas, 129

Daubert v. Merrell Dow Pharmaceuticals, Inc., 12
Dead game, 235
Deceased animal, 126
Deceleration/acceleration injuries
  diffuse axonal injury, 90–91
  shaken baby syndrome, 91–92
  subdural hematoma, 91
Decomposition
  necropsy and, 50
  overview of, 246–47
  sequence of, 247–48
Deep game, 235
Dehydration, 42, 204, 208
Demodicosis, 221
Deoxyribonucleic acid (DNA)
  animal examination and, 66
  collection from
    blood, 67
    buccal swabs, 67
    feces and urine, 68
    general, 66–67
    hair, 68
    muscle, organ and hide, 68
    teeth and bone, 67–68
  overview of, 65–66
  plant, 63, 64
  sample of, 41
Derringers, 132

Diabetes mellitus, 42
Diagnostic laboratories, 298–304
Diagnostic wounds, 49–50
Diatoms, 166–68, 297
DIC. *See* Disseminated intravascular coagulopathy
Diffuse axonal injury, 90–91
Digital cameras, 21, 37
Direct force fractures, 84
Discovery, 8–9
Dismemberment, 53–54
Disseminated intravascular coagulopathy (DIC), 218
Distant gunshot wounds, 142
Distress
- defined, 73
- examples of, 73

DNA. *See* Deoxyribonucleic acid
Documentation
- of evidence, 253–54
- of gunshot wounds, 152
- of live animals, 37–38
- of stab wounds, 103

Dog fighting
- animal examination, 237–39
- classifications, 236
- overview of, 235
- paraphernalia, 236–37
- pit bull, 235–36
- pit for, 26, 236

Domestic violence, 7
Dragging, 86
Drip pattern, 24
Drowning
- examinations in, 165–66
- overview of, 163–64
- submersion effects and, 164–65

Dry drowning, 164

Ears, 93, 93*f*
Education, 3
EG. *See* Ethylene glycol
Elected officials, 6
Electrical burns
- general findings in, 123–24
- lightning electrocution, 124
- overview of, 123
- stun gun electrocution, 125

Electrolyte, serum, 207
Embedded collars, 220–21
Emotional maltreatment. *See also* Neglect
- overview of, 74
- types of
  - emotional abuse, 75
  - emotional neglect, 74–75
  - physical abuse, 75
  - physical neglect, 74

Enclosed structures, 258
END. *See* Exotic Newcastle disease
Entomological sample log sheet, 293
Entomology. *See also* Forensic entomology
- body samples, 257–58
- climate/weather and, 254–55
- in enclosed structures, 258
- evidence collection, 255–57
- evidence documentation, 253–54
- of fires, 127
- overview of, 249–50, 249*t*, 251*f*
- time of death and, 249–58, 249*t*, 251*f*, 252*f*, 253*f*

Entomology specimen disposition/ID log, 292
Entrance wounds
- caliber determination, 139
- general characteristics of, 136–38
- intermediary targets, 138–39
- ricochet bullets, 139
- in skull, 139–40
- stippling, 140–41

Environment. *See also* Weather
- of animal hoarders, 212–13
- bioturbation and, 27
- CSI and, 21
- neglect and, 201–2
- poisoning and, 172
- water in, 55

Eosinopenia, 42
Epidural hematomas, 89
Eschar burn, 119*f*
Ethanol, 197
Ethylene glycol (EG)
- clinical signs, 176
- diagnostics, 176–77
- lesions, 177–78
- mechanism of action, 176
- sources of, 175

Evidence
- animal as, 7–8, 31–55
- associative, 20
- blood, 23–26, 24*f*
- botanical, 63–65
- chain of custody of, 36, 265
- CSI collection of, 35–36, 64–65, 255–57
- definition of, 36
- documentation of, 253–54
- federal rules for, 12
- integrity of, 9
- live animals as, 7–8
- MSBP and, 71

physical, 20
recognition and collection of, 22–23, 22*f*
tool mark, 27
trace, 59–62, 60*t*, 61*f*
weather and, 254–55
Evidence log, 36, 265
Examination
in animal fight, 237–40
of bone, 52–55
of DNA, 66
in drowning, 165–66
in excavation, 29
in gunshot wounds, 134–35
head trauma
ear, 93, 93*f*
nasal and oral, 93–94
neurological assessment, 94–95
ocular, 92
overview of, 92
physical, 38–40, 39*f*
PMI, 258–59
in sexual assault, 227–29, 229*f*
Examination report form, 38, 259, 268–76
Exam/necropsy report, 287–88
Excavation, 28–29
Exit wounds
caliber determination, 139
general characteristics of, 136–38
intermediary targets, 138–39
ricochet bullets, 139
in skull, 139–40
stippling, 140–41
Exotic Newcastle disease (END), 240
Expert witness
qualifying of, 15–17
testimony of, 11–14
External exam, 46–47
External wounds form
cat, 281
dog, 282
Eye, 92

Factual witness, 11–12
Falls, 85–86
Fat
bone marrow, 208–9, 297
lack of, 209–10
Fatal wounds, 109
Feces
at crime scene, 23
as DNA source, 68
sample of, 41
Federal laws, 4–5
Federal Rules of Evidence, 12
Feet, 39
Fight pit, 236
Final veterinary statement, 285
Firearms. *See also* Weapons
ammunition, 133–34
caliber nomenclature, 132
firing of, 134
handguns, 132
overview of, 131
rifles, 132
rifling, 132–33
shotgun, 132
Fires
bone analysis and, 55
deceased victims of, 126
entomology, 127
general exam and, 125
live victims of, 125–26
overview of, 125
First-degree burns, 118
Fixed tissue checklist, 283
Fleas, 45
Flow cytometry, 248
Flow pattern, 24
Foam cone, 165
Focal fracture, 84
Forensic botany
evidence collection in, 63–65
PMI and, 259
Forensic entomology. *See also* Entomology
body samples, 257–58
climate/weather and, 254–55
in enclosed structures, 258
evidence collection, 255–57
evidence documentation, 253–54
overview of, 249–50, 249*t*, 251*f*
PMI and, 249–58, 249*t*, 251*f*, 252*f*, 253*f*
Forensic entomology data form, 291
Forensic laboratories, 297
Forensic necropsy
gross necropsy
antemortem *vs.* postmortem injury, 49
decomposition, 50
external exam, 46–47
non-tissue collection, 50–51
technique, 47–49
therapeutic/diagnostic wounds, 49–50
vitreous, 51
overview of, 46
poisoning and, 172–73
Forensic palynology
evidence collection in, 64–65
overview of, 64
Forensic triad, 19

Fork stabbing, 105
Forth-degree burns, 118
Fractures
  circular, 88
  direct force, 84
  hangman's, 96
  indirect force, 84
  repetitive injuries and, 84–85
  rib, 41*f,* 97*f*
  ring, 88
  skull, 87–88, 91
  stellate, 88
Fur. *See also* Hair
  sample of, 41
  trace evidence on, 59–60

Gaffs, 239
Gamecocks, 239, 239*f*
Gameness, 235
Garroting, 160–61
Gastric emptying time, 249
Gauge, shotgun, 145
Gender, 32
Ghost drops, 24
Good Samaritan immunity, 4–5
Graves
  detection of
    bioturbation, 27
    burial features and, 27–28
    stratigraphy, 26–27
    tool mark evidence, 27
  excavation of, 28–29
  body examination and, 29
Graze wound, 138
Gross necropsy
  antemortem *vs.* postmortem injury, 49
  decomposition, 50
  external exam, 46–47
  non-tissue collection, 50–51
  technique, 47–49
  therapeutic/diagnostic wounds, 49–50
  vitreous, 51
GSR. *See* Gunshot residue
Gunshot range
  characteristics of, 141–42
  determination of
    .22 caliber weapon, 143–44
    air weapons, 149–50, 149*f,* 150*f*
    handguns, 142–43
    rifle, 144–45
    shotgun, 145–49, 147*f,* 148*f*
Gunshot residue (GSR)
  retrieval of, 150
  as trace evidence, 62
Gunshot wounds
  ballistics, 135–36
  cartridge case retrieval, 151
  documentation of, 152
  entrance/exit of, 136–41
  firearms, 131–34
  gunshot range and, 141–50, 147*f,* 148*f,* 149*f,* 150*f*
  overview of, 131
  projectile retrieval, 150–51
  trajectory of, 151–52
  victim examination in, 134–35
  weapon residue, 150

Hacking trauma, 109
Hair. *See also* Fur
  as DNA source, 68
  in starvation, 210
Hair/nails condition
  cat, 274
  dog, 275
  scale, 277
Handguns, 132, 142–43
Hanging, 161–63
Hangman's fracture, 96
HBC. *See* Hit-by car
Head trauma
  acceleration/deceleration injuries
    diffuse axonal injury, 90–91
    shaken baby syndrome, 91–92
    subdural hematoma, 91
  examination
    ear, 93, 93*f*
    nasal and oral, 93–94
    neurological assessment, 94–95
    ocular, 92
    overview of, 92
  impact injuries
    brain contusions, 88–89
    brain swelling, 90
    epidural hematomas, 89
    fractures, 87–88, 91
    subarachnoid hemorrhage, 89–90
    subdural hygromas, 90
Healing, 81
Hearsay, 34
Heartworms, 45
Heat stroke
  exam findings in, 216–17
  gross/microscopic findings in, 217–18
  overview of, 215–16
Heeling, 239
Helplessness, 73
Hemorrhage, 49
Hesitation marks. *See* Superficial incised wounds

Hide, 68
High rise syndrome, 86
High-velocity blood spatter (HVBS), 25
Hit-by car (HBC)
  history taking and, 33–34
  overview of, 85
Hoarders. *See* Animal hoarders
Hobbyist dog fighter, 236
Hog-dog rodeo, 235
Hookworms, 44
Hormones, 240
Housing, 22–23, 22*f*
Humanizing facts, 16
HVBS. *See* High-velocity blood spatter
Hyperextension, 96
Hyperthermia, 216, 217
Hypoglycemia, 207
Hypostasis, 242
Hypothermia
  exam findings, 219
  gross/microscopic findings, 219–20, 220*f*
  overview of, 218
Hypoxia, 155

Ibuprofen, 191–93
Ice pick wounds, 105
ICP. *See* Intracranial pressure
Identifiers, 68–69
Illness, falsifying of, 69
Immune system, 203–4, 208
Immunity, 4–5
Impact abrasions, 80
Impact injuries
  brain contusions, 88–89
  brain swelling, 90
  epidural hematomas, 89
  fractures, 87–88, 91
  subarachnoid hemorrhage, 89–90
  subdural hygromas, 90
Incised-stab wound, 107–8
Incised wounds
  appearance of, 108
  fatal, 109
  of neck, 109
  superficial, 108
Index of suspicion, 31, 69, 171
Indirect force fractures, 84
Inflammation, 42, 208
Inflicted submersion injury, 164
Initial report, 5
Injury. *See also* Head trauma; Non-accidental injury; Non-penetrating injuries; Penetrating injuries
  accidental, 31
  avulsion, 102–3
  chest, 97, 97*f*, 98*f*
  deceleration/acceleration, 90–92
  diffuse axonal, 90–91
  impact, 87–90, 91
  inflicted submersion, 164
  ligature, 99
  nasal, 93–94
  neck, 95
  ocular, 92
  oral, 93–94
  postmortem, 49
  repetitive, 31–32, 40, 84–85
  sharp force, 53–54
  spinal, 96–97
  swinging, 86
  thermal, 127–29
  untreated, 221–22
Insecticides
  carbamate, 188–89
  organophosphorus, 186–87
Insects. *See* Forensic entomology
Intermediate-range gunshot wounds, 142
Intracranial pressure (ICP), 95
Isolation, 75

Judicial hangings, 162
Juries, 14–15
Jurors, 14
Jury trial, 4

Kacey test, 177
KCW. *See* Knife-cut wounds
Ketogenesis, 42
Keyhole wound, 140
Kinetic energy, 135
Knife-cut wounds (KCW), 54
Knife-stab wounds (KSW), 54, 104–5
KSW. *See* Knife-stab wounds

Lacerations, 101–2, 102*f*
Langer's lines, 104
Law enforcement, 3
Laws, 4–5
Lead snowstorm, 145
Legal System
  animals as evidence and, 7–8, 31–55
  overview of, 5–7
  rules of discovery, 8–9
Leukocytosis, 42
Lichtenberg figures, 124
Lifters, 61–62
Ligature
  injuries, 99
  strangulation, 160–61
Lightning electrocution, 124

Linear acceleration, 90
Live animals
examination of
BCS, 40
blood loss calculation, 42–43, 106
clinical pathology, 41–42
documentation, 37–38
external, 38–40, 39*f*
parasites, 43–45
radiographs, 40–41, 41*f*
samples, 41
in fire, 125–26
overview of, 7–8
Live SOAP form, 268–69
Lividity, 82. *See also* Livor mortis
Livor mortis, 242–44, 243*f*
Local laws, 4–5
Locard, Edmond, 59
Locard's Exchange Principle, 19, 59
Low-velocity blood spatter (LVBS), 25–26
Lung
hypothermia of, 220*f*
lacerations of, 98*f*
LVBS. *See* Low-velocity blood spatter
Lymphopenia, 42

Macro crime scene, 19
Maltreatment, 74. *See also* Emotional maltreatment
Manual strangulation, 159–60
Marijuana, 194–95
Medical evaluation form, 259
Medium-velocity blood spatter (MVBS), 25
Metabolic rate, 202–3
Metaldehyde, 185–86
Methanol, 197
Micro crime scene, 19
Microwave oven burns, 120–21
Mikrosil, 54
Mitochondrial DNA (mtDNA), 66
Monocytosis, 42
Mortis
algor, 245–46
rigor, 244
MSBP. *See* Münchausen syndrome by proxy
mtDNA. *See* Mitochondrial DNA
Mummification, 247
Münchausen syndrome by proxy (MSBP)
evidence for, 71
outcomes of, 70
overview of, 69
symptoms, 70
Muscles
atrophy of, 209–10
as DNA source, 68
Mutilation, 110
MVBS. *See* Medium-velocity blood spatter
Myiasis, 221

Nandrolone, 238
Nasal injury, 93–94
Near contact wounds, 141–42
Neck
injury to, 95
wound interpretation of, 109
Necropsy. *See also* Forensic necropsy
forensic necropsy *v.*, 46
technique in, 47–49
Necropsy history form, 277
Necropsy report, 259
Necropsy worksheet, 278–80
Neglect. *See also* Abuse; Emotional maltreatment
demodicosis, 221
embedded collars, 220–21
environment and, 201–2
heat stroke, 215–18, 218*f*
hoarders, 210–15, 212*f*, 213*f*, 214*f*
hypothermia, 218–20, 220*f*
overview of, 74, 201
starvation
bone marrow fat analysis, 208–9, 297
cannibalism, 205–6, 205*f*
dehydration, 204
laboratory findings, 206–8
overview, 202
pica, 206, 206*f*
process of, 202–4, 202*t*
untreated injuries, 221–22
Neurological assessment, 94–95
Neutrophilia, 42
"No contact with animals" clause, 7
Non-accidental injury
animal history and, 33–34
hearsay and, 34
overview of, 31–32
patterns of
asphyxia and drowning, 155–68
in burns, 115–29, 116*f*, 117*t*, 119*f*, 121*t*
in gunshot wounds, 131–52, 147*f*, 148*f*, 149*f*, 150*f*
neglect, 201–22, 202*t*, 205*f*, 206*f*, 212*f*, 213*f*, 214*f*, 218*f*, 220*f*
in non-penetrating injuries, 79–99, 83*f*, 93*f*, 97*f*, 98*f*
in penetrating injuries, 101–13, 102*f*, 112*f*, 113*f*
poisoning, 169–99, 170*t*
practice setting and, 32–33
Non-penetrating injuries

abdominal, 98
abrasions, 80–81
blunt force trauma, 79, 98
bruising/contusions, 81–83, 83*f*
to chest, 97, 97*f*, 98*f*
falls, 85–86
fractures, 84–85
HBC, 85
head trauma, 86–95, 93*f*
ligature, 99
to neck, 95
to spine, 96–97
swinging/dragging, 86
Non-tissue samples, 50–51

Ocular injuries, 92
On call, 13
On-scene investigation, 5
Open records request, 5
OPs. *See* Organophosphorus insecticides
Oral injury, 93–94
Organophosphorus insecticides (OPs), 186–87
Organs
as DNA source, 68
starvation and, 204
Overpressuring, 75
Over-the-counter testing kits, 175
Owners, 34
Ownership, 8

Pain
overview of, 75–76
in physical exam, 39
signs of, 76*t*
Palo Mayombe, 111–13, 112*f*, 113*f*
Palynology, 64–65
Paraquat, 189–90
Parasites
fleas, 45
heartworms, 45
hookworms, 44
roundworms, 43
strongyloidiasis, 44–45
tapeworms, 44
whipworms, 43–44
Passive bloodstain patterns, 24
Patient records, 5
Patterned abrasions, 80
Patterned bruising, 82–83, 83*f*
Pattern evidence, 20
PCP. *See* Phencyclidine
Penetrating injuries
avulsion, 102–3
chop wounds, 109
incised wounds
appearance of, 108
fatal, 109
of neck, 109
superficial, 108
lacerations, 101–2, 102*f*
mutilation, 110
overview of, 101
ritualistic, 110–13, 112*f*, 113*f*
stab wounds
appearance of, 104–6
documentation, 103
evaluation of, 107
incised, 107–8
object removal in, 106
overview of, 103
weapons in, 106–7
therapeutic/diagnostic, 110
Perimeter blood stain, 24
Petechial hemorrhages, 156, 218*f*
Phencyclidine (PCP), 196–97
Photographs
of crime scene, 21, 36–37
of evidence, 35
for trial, 10
Photo logs, 21
Physical abuse, 75
Physical exam, 38–40, 39*f*
Physical needs, 74–75
Pica, 206, 206*f*
Pistols, 132
Pit bulls, 235–36
Plant DNA, 63, 64
PLR. *See* Pupillary light response
PMI. *See* Postmortem interval
Poisoning
agents
acetaminophen, 190–91
alcohol, 197–98
amphetamine, 193–94
anticoagulant rodenticides, 178–79
bromethalin, 179–80
caffeine, 198
carbamate insecticides, 188–89
cholecalciferol rodenticides, 181–82
cocaine, 195–96
ethylene glycol, 175–78
ibuprofen, 191–93
marijuana, 194–95
metaldehyde, 185–86
organophosphorus insecticides, 186–87
paraquat, 189–90
phencyclidine, 196–97
sodium monofluoroacetate, 184–85
strychnine, 182–83
zinc phosphide, 183–84

Poisoning *(continued)*
evidence and history, 171–72
overview of
demographics, 170, 170*t*
incidence, 169–70
index of suspicion and, 171
Polaroid cameras, 21, 36–37
Pollen samples, 64–65
Polydipsia, 207
Polyuria, 207
Postmortem
exam, 82
injury, 49
Postmortem interval (PMI), determination of, 242
crime scene examination and, 258–59
with forensic entomology, 249–58, 249*t*, 251*f*, 252*f*, 253*f*
Powder tattooing, 140–41
Practice setting, 32–33
Preliminary veterinary statement, 284
Primacy, 14–15
Proctitis, 230–31
Professional dog fighter, 236
Projected blood stains, 24
Projectiles, 150–51
Proof of intent, 4
Proptosis, 92
Prosecution offices, 6
Prosecutors, 3
Protein-calorie malnutrition, 202
Public awareness, 3–4
Pupa, 252–53, 253*f*
Pupillary light response (PLR), 94
Putrefaction, 246–47

Qualifying the expert, 15–17

Radiant heat burns, 120
Radiographs, 40–41, 41*f*
Rape stand, 237
Rectal prolapse, 231
Rectum, 230–31
Rejecting, 75
Re-offenders, 7
Repetitive injuries
fractures and, 84–85
overview of, 31–32
radiographs and, 40
Reporting requirements, 5
Reports
exam/necropsy, 287–88
final, 259–60
format for, 260–63
initial, 5
Revolvers, 132
Rib fracture, 41*f*, 97*f*
Ricochet bullets, 139
Rifles, 132, 144–45
Rifling, 132–33
Rigor mortis, 244
Ring fractures, 88
Ritualistic crimes
CSI for, 113
overview of, 110–11
Palo Mayombe, 111–13, 112*f*, 113*f*
Satanism, 111
Vampirism, 111
Rodenticides
anticoagulant, 178–79
cholecalciferol, 181–82
Roots, 52–53
Rotational acceleration, 90
Rotational fractures, 84
Roundworms, 43
Rule 702, 12
Rule 703, 12
Rule of primacy, 14–15
Rules of discovery, 8–9

Sabot slug, 146
Sadomasochism, 225
Saliva, 68
Salmonella pullorum, 240
Samples
collection of, 173–74
DNA, 41
entomologic, 257–58
feces, 41
fur, 41
live animal, 41
non-tissue, 50–51
pollen, 64–65
soil, 64–65
Satanism, 111
Saws, 53–54
Scalding burns, 121, 121*t*
Scavengers, 54–55
Scene markers, 258–59
Scissor stabbing, 105
Scrape/brush abrasions, 80
Screwdrivers, 105
Second-degree burns, 118
Seizure, animal, 6
Semen, 68, 232
Sentencing hearings, 4
Sexual assault
general findings in, 226–27
overview of, 225–26
sperm recovery, 232

suspicious findings
anus, rectum and colon, 230–31
vaginal, 230
victim examination, 227–29, 229*f*
zoonotic disease, 231–32
Shaken baby syndrome, 91–92
Shaken impact syndrome, 91
Sharp force injury, 53–54
Shotgun, 132, 145–49
Skin condition form
cat, 272
dog, 273
Skin tenting, 210
Skull. *See also* Head trauma
bullet wounds to, 139–40
fractures, 87–88, 91
Slug, 146, 147*f*
Smoke toxicity, 125–29
Smothering, 156–57
Sodium monofluoroacetate, 184–85
Soil
inhalation of, 29
samples of, 64–65
Soot patterns, 137
Spanish gamecocks, 239
Sperm, 232
Spinal injuries
head trauma and, 96
overview of, 96–97
Spores, 64
Spurs, 239
Stab wounds
appearance of, 104–6
documentation, 103
evaluation of, 107
incised, 107–8
object removal in, 106
overview of, 103
weapons in, 106–7
Starvation
bone marrow fat analysis, 208–9, 297
cannibalism, 205–6, 205*f*
dehydration, 204
hair in, 210
laboratory findings, 206–8
overview, 202
pica, 206, 206*f*
process of, 202–4, 202*t*
State's evidence, 7
Stellate fractures, 88
Steroids, 237, 238
Strangulation
general findings in, 158–59
ligature, 160–61
manual, 159–60
overview of, 158
yoking, 160
Stratigraphy, 26–27
Street fighter, 236
Stress
cold, 219
inflammation and, 208
laboratory findings and, 42
overview of, 71
physical manifestations of, 72
Striking a jury, 14
Strongyloidiasis, 44–45
Strontium, 168
Strychnine, 182–83, 240
Stun gun electrocution, 125
Subarachnoid hemorrhage, 89–90
Subdural hematomas, 91
Subdural hygromas, 90
Subpoena, 13
Suffering
boredom as, 73
definition of, 72
distress and, 73
emotional, 74–75
overview of, 72–73
physical, 75
Suffocation
airway swelling/obstruction, 157–58
chest/abdomen compression, 158
choking, 157
smothering, 156–57
vitiated atmosphere, 156
Superficial incised wounds, 108
Superficial perforating wounds, 138
Swabs, 35–36, 67
Swinging injuries, 86
Swipe pattern, 24

TACC. *See* Tufts Animal Condition and Care Scoring
Tache noire, 247
Tail, 227
Tape, collecting, 62
Tapeworms, 44
Tardieu spots, 243
Tattoos
as identifier, 68
powder, 140–41
Taunting, 75
TBSA. *See* Total body surface area
Teeth, 67–68
Teeth per inch (TPI), 54
Temporary Protective Orders (TPO), 7
Tension wedge fracture, 84
Terrorizing, 75

Therapeutic wounds, 49–50
Thermal burns
  cigarette, 121
  microwave ovens, 120–21
  overview of, 119–20
  radiant heat, 120
  scalding, 121, 121*t*
Thermal injury
  carbon monoxide poisoning, 128–29
  by cyanide, 129
  overview of, 127
  smoke toxicity, 127–28
Third-degree burns, 118
Throttling, 159–60
Time of death
  crime scene investigation and, 258–59
  determination of
    algor mortis, 245–46
    decomposition, 246–48
    flow cytometry, 248
    gastric emptying time, 249
    livor mortis, 242–44, 243*f*
    PMI and, 242
    rigor mortis, 244
    vitreous humor, 248–49
  entomology and, 249–58, 249*t*, 251*f*, 252*f*, 253*f*
  overview of, 241
Tool mark evidence, 27
Tools, for evidence collection, 35
Tooth mark artifacts, 55
Total body surface area (TBSA), 117–18
Toxicology testing
  chain of custody, 174
  in human labs, 174–75
  over-the-counter, 175
  sample collection/submission, 173–74
TPI. *See* Teeth per inch
TPO. *See* Temporary Protective Orders
Trace evidence
  on animal, 59–60
  collection and analysis of, 60–62, 61*f*
  overview of, 59
  types of, 60*t*
Traction fractures, 84
Trajectory, gunshot, 151–52
Transfer evidence, 20
Transferrin, 207
Transient evidence, 20
Trauma, 53
Trial
  bench/non-jury, 4
  jury, 4
  preparation for, 9–11
  visuals for, 10
Trier of fact, 13
Tufts Animal Condition and Care Scoring (TACC), 40, 289–90

United States v. Frye, 12–13
Untreated injuries, 221–22
Upside down suspension, 163
Urine
  at crime scene, 23
  as DNA source, 68
Urine specific gravity, 207
UV light, 61, 61*f*

Vaginal assault, 230. *See also* Sexual assault
Vaginal prolapse, 230
Vampirism, 111
Vertical compression fractures, 84
Veterinarian
  at crime scene, 5
  laws and, 4–5
  roles of, 3–4, 20–21
  statement forms for, 284–85
  trial preparation by, 9–11
  as witnesses, 4
Veterinary practice act, 5
Videography, 21, 36–37
Violent sex offenders, 225. *See also* Sexual assault
Visceral congestion, 155–56
Visuals, for trial, 10
Vitamin K, 240
Vitiated atmosphere, 156
Vitreous, 51
Vitreous humor, 248–49
Voir dire, 13, 14, 16
Vomit, 23

Wadding, 147, 148*f*, 150–51
Water environment, 55
Weapon cast-off blood spatter, 24*f*, 25
Weapons. *See also* Firearms; Gunshot wounds
  .22 caliber, 143–44
  air-powered, 149–50, 149*f*, 150*f*
  cast-off blood spatter from, 24*f*, 25
  for patterned bruising, 82–83, 86*f*
  residue from, 150
  in stab wounds, 106–7
Weather. *See also* Environment
  CSI and, 21
  entomological evidence and, 254–55
Webliography, 307–11
Weight change form, 268–69
Whipworms, 43–44

Wipe pattern, 24
Wischnewsky spots, 220
Witnesses
  calling of, 14–15
  expert, 11–14, 15–17
  factual, 11–12
  veterinarians as, 4

Yankee gamecocks, 239
Yoking, 160
Youth Subculture Satanists, 111

Zinc phosphide, 183–84
Zoonotic disease, 231–32